# Nutrition and the Origins of Disease

*Edited by*

CHARLES H. HALSTED
Division of Clinical Nutrition
Department of Internal Medicine
School of Medicine
University of California, Davis
Davis, California

ROBERT B. RUCKER
Department of Nutrition
College of Agricultural and Environmental Sciences
University of California, Davis
Davis, California

ACADEMIC PRESS, INC.
**Harcourt Brace Jovanovich, Publishers**
San Diego New York Berkeley Boston
London Sydney Tokyo Toronto

ACADEMIC PRESS, INC.
San Diego, California 92101

*United Kingdom Edition published by*
ACADEMIC PRESS LIMITED
24-28 Oval Road, London NW1 7DX

**Library of Congress Cataloging-in-Publication Data**

Nutrition and the origins of disease / edited by Charles H. Halsted,
Robert B. Rucker.
p. cm. — (Bristol-Myers nutrition symposia ; v. 7)
Papers presented at the Seventh Bristol-Myers Symposium on
Nutrition Research, held in San Francisco on Sept. 21-22, 1987.
Includes bibliographies and index.
ISBN 0-12-319640-X (alk. paper)
1. Nutritionally induced diseases—Congresses. 2. Nutrition
disorders—Congresses. 3. Nutrition—Congresses. I. Halsted,
Charles H., Date. II. Rucker, Robert B. III. Bristol-Myers
Symposium on Nutrition Research (7th : 1987 : San Francisco Calif.)
IV. Series.
[DNLM: 1. Disease—etiology—congresses. 2. Nutrition Disorders-
-complications—congresses. W3 BR323F v. 7 / QZ 105 N9754 1987]
RC622.N892 1988
616.3′9—dc19
DNLM/DLC′ 88-16789
for Library of Congress CIP

PRINTED IN THE UNITED STATES OF AMERICA
89 90 91 92 9 8 7 6 5 4 3 2 1

# Nutrition and the Origins of Disease

# Bristol-Myers Nutrition Symposia

*Series Editor*
JERRY L. MOORE
Nutritional Division
Mead Johnson & Company

1 R. W. Winters and H. L. Greene (Editors):
Nutritional Support of the Seriously Ill Patient, 1983

2 C. E. Butterworth, Jr., and Martha L. Hutchinson (Editors):
Nutritional Factors in the Induction and Maintenance of Malignancy, 1983

3 Morris Green and H. L. Greene (Editors):
The Role of the Gastrointestinal Tract in Nutrient Delivery, 1984

4 Samuel J. Fomon and William C. Heird (Editors):
Energy and Protein Needs during Infancy, 1986

5 Martha L. Hutchinson and Hamish N. Munro (Editors):
Nutrition and Aging, 1986

6 B. S. Lindbald (Editor):
Perinatal Nutrition, 1988

# Contents

## 3 Micronutrients, Chromatin Alterations, and Cancer

C. ELIZABETH CASTRO



## 4 Pathogenesis of Megaloblastic Anemias

VICTOR HERBERT



## 5 Regulation of Iron Exchange

CLEMENT A. FINCH

## 8 Vitamin D, Calcium, and Metabolic Bone Disease

HECTOR F. DELUCA



## 9 The Pathogenesis of Obesity

GEORGE A. BRAY



## 10 Essential Obesity and the Pathogenetic Role of a Low Metabolic Rate

CLIFTON BOGARDUS AND ERIC RAVUSSIN

# 18 Nitrogen Metabolism in the Intestine

NORMAN KRETCHMER AND RUTH HURWITZ



# 19 Role of Gastrointestinal Hormones in Adaptation

VAY LIANG W. GO



# 20 Nutrient Regulation of Intestinal Surface Membrane Hydrolases

GARY M. GRAY, ANN M. REISENAUER, AND RICHARD QUAN

## 21 Intestinal Adaptation to Parenteral Nutrition

ELLIOT WESER



## 22 Immunoregulation in the Mucosal Immune System and the Pathogenesis of Immunologic Diseases of the Gastrointestinal Tract

WARREN STROBER, MARJORIE E. KANOF, MARTIN ZEITZ, AND STEPHEN P. JAMES

# Contributors

Numbers in parentheses indicate the pages on which the authors' contributions begin.

*Thomas T. Aoki* (93), Division of Endocrinology, University of California, Davis, School of Medicine, Davis, California 95616

*William H. Beer* (285), Department of Medicine, Division of Gastroenterology and Nutrition, The University of Texas Health Science Center at San Antonio, and Audie L. Murphy Memorial Veterans' Hospital, San Antonio, Texas 78284

*Jonas Bergström* (185), Department of Renal Medicine, Karolinska Institute, and Huddinge University Hospital, S-141 86 Huddinge, Sweden

*Clifton Bogardus* (145), Clinical Diabetes and Nutrition Section, National Institute of Diabetes and Digestive and Kidney Diseases, National Institutes of Health, Phoenix, Arizona 85016

*George A. Bray* (129), Los Angeles County/USC Medical Center, and Division of Diabetes and Clinical Nutrition, Department of Medicine, University of Southern California, School of Medicine, Los Angeles, California 90033

*C. Elizabeth Castro* (31), Nutritional Sciences Division, University of California, Los Angeles, School of Public Health, Los Angeles, California 90024

*Russell W. Chesney*[1] (161), Department of Pediatrics, University of California, Davis, School of Medicine, Davis, California 95817

*Frank Chytil* (15), Departments of Biochemistry and Medicine, Vanderbilt University School of Medicine, Nashville, Tennessee 37232

[1]Present address: Department of Pediatrics, University of Tennessee, Memphis, The Health Science Center, Memphis, Tennessee 38103.

*William E. Connor* (69), Department of Medicine, Section of Clinical Nutrition and Lipid Metabolism, The Oregon Health Sciences University, Portland, Oregon 97201

*Robert J. Cousins* (1), Food Science and Human Nutrition Department, Center for Nutritional Sciences, University of Florida, Gainesville, Florida 32611

*Hector F. DeLuca* (109), Department of Biochemistry, College of Agricultural and Life Sciences, University of Wisconsin-Madison, Madison, Wisconsin 53706

*Jose Fernandez-Checa* (267), Liver Research Laboratory, Wadsworth Veterans Administration Hospital Center, Los Angeles, California 90073

*Clement A. Finch* (57), Division of Hematology, Department of Medicine, University of Washington School of Medicine and Hematology Research Laboratory, Providence Hospital, Seattle, Washington 98122

*Vay Liang W. Go*[2] (321), Division of Digestive Diseases and Nutrition, National Institute of Diabetes and Digestive and Kidney Diseases, Bethesda, Maryland, and Mayo Medical School, Rochester, Minnesota 55905

*Gary M. Gray* (333), Division of Gastroenterology and the Digestive Disease Center, Stanford University School of Medicine, Stanford, California 94305

*Charles H. Halsted* (249), Division of Clinical Nutrition and Clinical Nutrition Research Center, Department of Internal Medicine, University of California, Davis, School of Medicine, Davis, California 95616

*Victor Herbert* (47), Mount Sinai School of Medicine, New York, New York, and Bronx Veterans Administration Medical Center, Bronx, New York 10468

*Ruth Hurwitz* (309), Department of Nutritional Sciences, College of Natural Resources, University of California, Berkeley, Berkeley, California 94720

*Stephen P. James* (357), Mucosal Immunity Section, Laboratory of Clinical Investigation, National Institute of Allergy and Infectious Diseases, Bethesda, Maryland 20892

*Marjorie E. Kanof* (357), Mucosal Immunity Section, Laboratory of Clinical Investigation, National Institute of Allergy and Infectious Diseases, Bethesda, Maryland 20892

*Neil Kaplowitz* (267), Gastroenterology Section, University of California, Los Angeles, School of Medicine and Liver Research Laboratory, Wadsworth Veterans Administration Hospital Center, Los Angeles, California 90073

[2]Present address: Department of Medicine, University of California, Los Angeles, School of Medicine, Los Angeles, California 90024.

*Norman Kretchmer* (309), Department of Pediatrics, University of California, San Francisco, San Francisco, California, and Department of Nutritional Sciences, College of Natural Resources, University of California, Berkeley, Berkeley, California 94720

*Maria Anna Leo* (217), Mount Sinai School of Medicine, City University of New York, New York, and Section of Liver Disease and Nutrition, Alcohol Research and Treatment Center, Bronx Veterans Administration Medical Center, Bronx, New York 10468

*Charles S. Lieber* (217), Mount Sinai School of Medicine, City University of New York, New York, and Section of Liver Disease and Nutrition, Alcohol Research and Treatment Center, Bronx Veterans Administration Medical Center, Bronx, New York 10468

*Esteban Mezey* (203), Alcohol Research Center and Department of Medicine, The Johns Hopkins University School of Medicine, Baltimore, Maryland 21205

*Michael C. Okimura* (93), Division of Endocrinology, University of California, Davis, School of Medicine, Davis, California 95616

*Murad Ookhtens* (267), University of California, Los Angeles, School of Medicine and Liver Research Laboratory, Wadsworth Veterans Administration Hospital Center, Los Angeles, California 90073

*Richard Quan* (333), Department of Pediatric Gastroenterology–Nutrition, University of Texas Health Science Center at Dallas, Dallas, Texas 75235

*Eric Ravussin* (145), Clinical Diabetes and Nutrition Section, National Institute of Diabetes and Digestive and Kidney Diseases, National Institutes of Health, Phoenix, Arizona 85016

*Ann M. Reisenauer* (333), Division of Clinical Nutrition, University of California, Davis, School of Medicine, Davis, California 95616

*Steven Schenker* (285), Department of Medicine, Division of Gastroenterology and Nutrition, The University of Texas Health Science Center at San Antonio, and Audie L. Murphy Memorial Veterans' Hospital, San Antonio, Texas 78284

*Warren Strober* (357), Mucosal Immunity Section, Laboratory of Clinical Investigation, National Institute of Allergy and Infectious Diseases, Bethesda, Maryland 20892

*Robert M. Walter, Jr.* (93), Division of Endocrinology, University of California, Davis, School of Medicine, Davis, California 95616

*Elliot Weser* (343), Medicine Service, Audie L. Murphy Memorial Veterans' Hospital, University of Texas Health Science Center at San Antonio, San Antonio, Texas 78284

*Martin Zeitz* (357), Mucosal Immunity Section, Laboratory of Clinical Investigation, National Institute of Allergy and Infectious Diseases, Bethesda, Maryland 20892

# Editor's Foreword

While the pace of discovery of new essential nutrients has slowed, the understanding of the role of these nutrients in health and disease, apart from classical nutritional deficiency and toxicity syndromes, is beginning to accelerate.

To address these intriguing frontiers, the seventh annual Bristol-Myers Symposium, held in San Francisco on September 21–22, 1987, focused on "Nutrition and the Origins of Disease." Drs. Charles H. Halsted and Robert B. Rucker, of the University of California at Davis, assembled a distinguished panel of scientists to discuss several diseases and conditions in which nutrition may be a significant component or consideration.

The topics included the effects of alcohol intake on nutrient utilization; the pathogenesis of obesity; aminoacidurias and amino acid metabolism in renal diseases; the role of vitamins A and D, calcium, iron, zinc, and other micronutrients in the pathogenesis of disease; and new knowledge of gastrointestinal adaptation and immunoregulation in health and disease. These proceedings provide a valuable record of those presentations and discussions.

I congratulate the participants and the cochairpersons on the excellent results of their efforts. On behalf of Bristol-Myers and its Mead Johnson subsidiary, who sponsored the symposium and these proceedings, I express sincerest thanks for this important contribution to the advancement of nutrition research and knowledge.

*Jerry L. Moore*
*Series Editor*

# Foreword

Just over a century ago, the relationship between nutrition and illness might best have been summed up by the old English proverb, "Stuff a cold and starve a fever." Today, our understanding of that relationship has evolved to the point where scientific investigators are able to explore the role of diet in the regulation of gene expression.

The contents of this volume illustrate how far we have come in our understanding of the critical role of nutrition in the maintenance of good health as well as in the prevention and treatment of disease.

The papers within reflect the proceedings of the seventh annual Bristol-Myers Symposium on Nutrition Research, organized by the University of California at Davis and held September 21–22, 1987 in San Francisco.

Twenty-three distinguished clinical and research specialists representing a cross section of medical disciplines, participated in the symposium, which was co-chaired by Charles H. Halsted, M.D. and Robert B. Rucker, Ph.D.

The panelists presented new findings about the complex relationships between diet and the development of disease, covering such areas as molecular biology, metabolic and renal diseases, and alcoholic liver disease. For instance, we can now appreciate that nutritional factors such as vitamin A deficiency and/or excess, caused by alcohol and drug abuse, play an important role in the development of severe liver disease, which is among the top ten causes of death annually in the United States. Furthermore, the original research reported in this volume will enable readers to take a new look at the causes and treatment of such disorders as obesity and diabetes.

Identifying new pathways to the prevention and treatment of disease is a constant challenge to the research community. To help meet the challenge, Bristol-Myers Company has provided unrestricted medical research grants programs, sponsorship of scientific symposia, and awards to individuals for distinguished research achievement. Since 1977 the company has committed more than $20 million in no-strings-attached funding of nutrition, cancer, orthopaedics, pain, and neuroscience research.

Through the unrestricted nutrition research grant program, Bristol-Myers and its Mead Johnson nutritional division have awarded more than $4 million in unrestricted grants to leading nutrition research centers in the United States, Canada, Europe, South America, and Asia.

The 1988 recipient of the annual Bristol-Myers Award for Distinguished Achievement in Nutrition Research was Nevin S. Scrimshaw, Institute Professor Emeritus at the Massachusetts Institute of Technology. An independent peer-review committee selected Dr. Scrimshaw, honoring him for his pioneering work in linking malnutrition to infection and for developing the first successful vegetable weaning food for infants.

In their eighth year, the Bristol-Myers Symposia on Nutrition Research continue to further the goal of providing a forum through which researchers, clinicians, and academicians can exchange ideas and share knowledge.

The published proceedings of these symposia provide an even greater audience access to this information. We are pleased to be a part of this exchange.

*Richard L. Gelb*
*Chairman of the Board*
*Bristol-Myers Company*

# Preface

Less than 20 years ago, academic clinical nutrition was relegated to investigating the causes and pathophysiology of protein-calorie malnutrition and vitamin-deficiency diseases such as pellagra, beri-beri, and scurvy, all common in developing countries but infrequent in the United States. Modern clinical nutrition evolved rapidly from these basic advances in nutritional biochemistry. Discoveries in the 1930s, 1940s, and 1950s about requirements for essential nutrients and their biochemistry and physiology provided fresh insights into the pathophysiology of many diseases. Much of our knowledge about classifications and manifestations of nutritional anemias grew out of basic studies of iron, folic acid, and vitamin $B_{12}$ requirements and metabolism. After the pathophysiology of pellagra was identified as an abnormality of tryptophan and niacin metabolism, the disease was effectively eradicated in rural America. Although pellagra and scurvy appear occasionally, megaloblastic anemia of folate deficiency remains frequent among down-and-out alcoholics.

In the past two decades, scientific emphasis on defining energy and lipid metabolism has opened a new era of understanding of the nutritional bases of extremely common diseases such as obesity and atherosclerosis. We now recognize that many of the most common diseases, including those with highest mortality, are intrinsically related to diet. These include atherosclerosis and other forms of heart disease, many cancers, hypertension, diabetes, and alcoholic liver disease. Other common nutritional disorders, such as obesity, a disease of energy storage, and osteopenia, a disease of calcium and vitamin D imbalance, carry potentially life-threatening complications.

Indeed, together with chronic alcoholism, dietary factors are now clearly implicated in 8 of the 10 leading causes of death in the United States (Nutrition Policy Board, 1988). Thus, in a very short time, nutritional disorders have moved from relative obscurity to the forefront of clinical medicine. In this context, a modern definition of clinical nutrition is useful. We define it as a scientific and clinical discipline concerned with diseases that are caused by abnormalities in the intake, intestinal absorption, and metabolism of dietary substances and that can be treated by changes in the amount or composition of nutrients.

Even as clinical nutrition is becoming established as an essential medical discipline, basic advances in nutritional biochemistry continue to push back the frontiers of knowledge of the relationships between dietary factors and the basic mechanisms of disease. For example, we now know that the composition of fatty acids in the diet plays a major role in basic responses to tissue injury, including inflammation, vascular reactivity, and coagulability.

The new frontier of molecular biology also has immediate applications to nutrition science. We now have probes to investigate specific segments of a gene or to determine amounts of gene products, such as messenger RNA, that cause expression of given proteins and enzymes in response to nutrients. For example, certain essential trace minerals control the expression of specific genes that synthesize the proteins involved in transport or storage of these minerals. We now know zinc interacts with the gene promoter for metallothionein. Using molecular biology techniques, we have learned that metallothionein is probably a better measure of zinc status than serum zinc. In the present symposium, other examples of the use of molecular biology to solve nutritional problems focus on the role of vitamin A in regulating pulmonary secretions in the lung, the role of vitamin D in regulating key proteins associated with calcium absorption and ultimately with bone formation and metabolism, and the effect of malnutrition or nutrient deficiencies on maintenance of DNA structure, especially in neoplastic cells undergoing rapid turnover.

The present symposium brings together basic and clinical scientists from many specialties. The stage is set by three molecular biologists whose work illustrates the roles of elemental nutrients in cellular function that regulate health and are affected by disease. They are followed by a diverse group of state-of-the-art clinical presentations, ranging from metabolism to diseases of the blood, liver, intestine, and kidney.

Finally, we wish to express our deep appreciation to Bristol-Myers, whose unrestricted nutrition research grant program supported this symposium, and to Ann D. Wyant, who played a central role in copy-editing the manuscript.

*Charles H. Halsted*
*Robert B. Rucker*

## REFERENCE

Nutrition Policy Board (1988). Summary and recommendations. *In* "The Surgeon General's Report on Nutrition and Health." U.S. Department of Health and Human Services, Public Health Service; DHHS publication No. (PHS)88-50210.

# 1

# Molecular Biology and Micronutrient–Disease Relationships—Zinc as a Prototype

Robert J. Cousins

*Food Science and Human Nutrition Department*
*Center for Nutritional Sciences*
*University of Florida*
*Gainesville, Florida*



## I. INTRODUCTION

An understanding of the role of diet in regulating gene expression is emerging. Gene expression may be regulated indirectly via a complex array of hormones that regulate metabolic pathways for amino acids, carbohydrates, and lipids. Examples include regulation of the adipsin gene by food intake and of phosphoenolpyruvate carboxykinase by glucagon and glucocorticoids (Flier *et al.*, 1987; Lamers *et al.*, 1982). Other micronutrients regulate expression directly. Examples include transcriptional regulation of fibronectin- and calcium-binding protein genes by vitamins A and D, respectively (Kim and Wolf, 1987; Charles *et al.*, 1981). Furthermore, dietary iron has been shown to influence transferrin production (Idzerda *et al.*, 1986), and zinc has been shown to influence metallothionein production (McCormick *et al.*, 1981). Zinc interacts directly with the genome to increase synthesis of metallothionein, a protein involved in the subsequent metabolism and/or function of zinc; this unique system will be reviewed in terms of the molecular biology of micronutrient-related disease. Metabolic deficiencies of zinc have been reported for both plants and animals when the supply of this nutrient is limited (Hambidge *et al.*, 1986). In human subjects, zinc deficiency results in growth retardation, immune dysfunction, skin disease, and arrested sexual development. Acrodermatitis enteropathica, a congenital disease, is a zinc-malabsorption syndrome (Lombeck *et al.*, 1975). The skin lesions and impaired immunity associated with this disease can be reversed with supplemental physiologic doses of the metal (Moynahan, 1974). Although the metabolic basis of the disease is unknown, a change in intestinal compartmentalization that redirects zinc flux in the direction of net loss has been proposed as a biochemical mechanism (Cousins, 1976).

## II. ZINC METABOLISM

Zinc metabolism is well regulated via controlled intestinal absorption and tissue compartmentalization (Cousins, 1985). Absorption appears to be controlled by both brush-border membrane transport and intracellular compartmentalization. The latter controls release to the basolateral membrane. Recent evidence suggests that low dietary zinc levels stimulate brush-border transport. This, plus the small exchangeable intracellular zinc pool in the intestinal cells when the zinc supply is low, allows for rapid transfer from lumen to plasma (Hoadley *et al.*, 1987).

Plasma zinc concentration is maintained within narrow limits, usually 90–110 $\mu$g/dl in most species, even though only approximately 1 in 35 molecules of albumin, the major plasma carrier, contain bound zinc atoms (Cousins, 1985). This suggests that carefully regulated tissue uptake and excretion maintain plasma zinc levels. In zinc-depleted rats fed a zinc-rich meal, plasma zinc levels increased then returned to normal within hours (McCormick *et al.*, 1981). This subject has been reviewed in detail (Cousins, 1985). Why the plasma zinc concentration is so carefully controlled is unknown; however, it may relate to regulation of phagocytic activity of circulating cells involved in host defense (Chvapil *et al.*, 1982). Alternatively, because zinc within certain cellular pools exchanges rapidly with the extracellular environment and is markedly influenced by the external zinc concentration (Pattison and Cousins, 1986), accelerated uptake may activate intracellular functions. Plasma zinc levels fall in the presence of acute disease and stress (Falchuk, 1977).

## III. METALLOTHIONEIN

One well-studied aspect of zinc metabolism and function is its relationship to metallothionein. This low-molecular-weight (6.5 kDa) metalloprotein contains 25–35% cysteine residues and exists as two principal isoforms (Metallothioneins I and II). It binds up to 7 g atoms of zinc or 12 g atoms of copper as well as various other transition elements. Binding is within two clusters. Although the protein usually has a full complement of metal bound, the metal atoms rapidly exchange (in seconds and minutes) (Nettesheim *et al.*, 1985). The composition of metals bound determines the half-life of the protein. Copper metallothionein is poorly degraded in intracellular proteases, whereas zinc metallothionein is rapidly degraded. Apometallothionein is very rapidly degraded (Feldman *et al.*, 1978), and appreciable levels probably do not accumulate in cells. Numerous reviews on structural details of metallothionein have been published (Dunn *et al.*, 1987; Hamer, 1986).

Considerable recent attention has focused on metallothionein because of its interesting structural features and because of the possible link between its function and specific diseases. Fig. 1 shows the basis of regulation of metallothionein gene expression and its possible physiological functions. Studies have shown that metallothionein is inducible by a variety of agents; that it is transcriptionally regulated; and that its function may involve activation of copper and/or zinc apoenzymes, donation of metals by ligand exchange to specific cellular sites, or scavenging of free radicals (reviewed in Cousins, 1985; Dunn *et al.*, 1987).

### A. Dietary Regulation of Metallothionein

Feeding diets with low and elevated zinc levels have produced changes in zinc distribution in the cytosol fraction of liver and intestine (Richards and Cousins, 1976). Elevated dietary zinc resulted in substantially more zinc associated with metallothionein in both tissues. Studies have shown that $^{65}Zn$ is incorporated directly into newly synthesized metallothionein protein (McCormick *et al.*, 1981; Menard *et al.*, 1981). Protein synthesis inhibitors and cell-free translation systems were used to show that oral or intraperitoneal administration of sufficient amounts of zinc increased

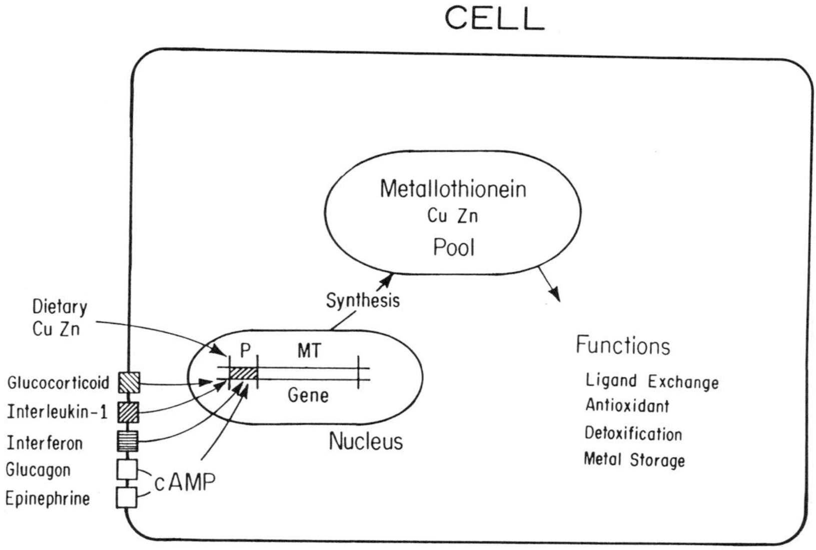


**Fig. 1.** Schematic of a hypothetical mammalian cell shows possible physiological inducers of metallothionein gene expression and potential functions of the protein. Functions may differ depending on cell type and physiological status.

the metallothionein mRNA pool available for translation (McCormick *et al.*, 1981; Menard *et al.*, 1981; Shapiro *et al.*, 1978). Acute increases in dietary zinc appear to influence metallothionein synthesis in both liver and small intestine. This seems logical because initial processing of a large amount of dietary zinc would be expected to involve hepatocytes and enterocytes. When zinc intake is very high, intestinal metallothionein may act as buffer that regulates its absorption (Menard *et al.*, 1981).

In contrast to acute changes in dietary zinc, constant levels of dietary zinc influence metallothionein gene expression principally in the kidney. When rats were fed diets containing 1, 6, or 36 mg copper/kg and 5, 30, or 180 mg zinc/kg, kidney metallothionein levels increased from 23 to 58 μg/g (Blalock *et al.*, 1988). Measurement of metallothionein mRNA levels by dot blot hybridization using a $^{32}$P-labeled oligonucleotide DNA probe demonstrated differences in control of the gene by copper and zinc. The surface response curve (Fig. 2) reveals a quadratic effect for zinc but a linear effect for copper on transcription of the gene. The highest mRNA levels (58 molecules per cell) were found when rats were fed 180 mg zinc/kg and 36 mg copper/kg. Brain and liver metallothionein mRNA levels were not influenced by these levels of dietary zinc and copper. However, when dietary copper was low and zinc was high, intestinal metallothionein mRNA levels increased. These findings suggest that, under ordinary

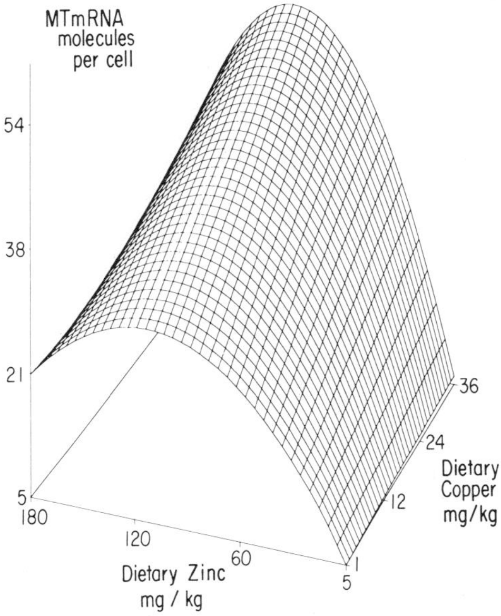


**Fig. 2.** Response surface shows the effect of dietary copper (Cu) and zinc (Zn) intake on metallothionein gene expression in rat kidney. Dietary Cu and Zn are in mg/kg diet. Gene expression is shown as molecules metallothionein mRNA per cell.

dietary conditions when zinc intake is fairly constant, kidney metallothionein gene expression increases directly in response to that concentration. However, optimal zinc intake for full expression may be about 120 mg/kg. Considerable amounts of zinc must be reabsorbed by the kidney epithelium because urinary zinc output is low, except in the presence of metabolic diseases that cause aminoaciduria or proteinuria. Metallothionein may regulate renal zinc processing, much like it is proposed to regulate intestinal zinc processing.

The sensitivity of metallothionein gene expression to the dietary zinc supply suggests that cellular factors closely monitor plasma or intracellular zinc levels and regulate transcription accordingly. Localized within the promoter region of the metallothionein gene are specific DNA sequences that impart metal regulation to the gene (Seguin and Hamer, 1987). These sequences of approximately 12 nucleotides are called "metal regulatory elements" (MRE). In theory, MRE sequences bind to transacting factors that activate transcription. We hypothesize that these factors are nuclear proteins that bind both the MRE and zinc (Cousins *et al.*, 1988).

To investigate this hypothesis, soluble extracts of isolated nuclei of liver and kidney cells were prepared, and the proteins were separated by gel electrophoresis and transferred to nitrocellulose sheets by Western blotting. The sheets were then incubated under neutral pH conditions with $^{65}$Zn and citrate to detect $^{65}$Zn-binding proteins. Equivalent sheets were incubated with $^{32}$P-labeled synthetic oligonucleotides with a MRE sequence ('5CCTTTGCGCCCG3'). Only one major $^{65}$Zn and $^{32}$P binding band was observed. This protein, tentatively called a "nuclear zinc regulatory protein" (NZRP), is about 35 kDa; attempts are now being made to purify it. We are also evaluating the effects of zinc binding to the NZRP. Preliminary evidence indicates that as intracellular metallothionein levels increase, zinc levels in kidney nuclei increase, suggesting that zinc binding to the NZRP could be greater when transcription rates are high. Confirmation of these observations could indicate that zinc binding by the NZRP serves as a positive effector.

## B. Hormonal Regulation of Metallothionein

Nearly a decade ago, our laboratory discovered that glucocorticoid hormones induce metallothionein synthesis in isolated hepatocytes and intact rats (Failla and Cousins, 1978; Etzel *et al.*, 1979). That response was associated with increased cellular uptake of zinc by hepatocyte cultures and a slight, but significant, reduction in plasma zinc levels in intact rats. It was later proposed that glucocorticoids, acting through metallothionein induction, were responsible in part for stress-related plasma zinc depressions associated with some forms of acute stress and disease (Cousins, 1985). Administration of glucocorticoids to human subjects produced changes in kinetics of $^{65}$Zn distribution similar to those shown in animal studies to be metallothionein-related (Henkin *et al.*, 1984), specifically, a substantial increase in zinc uptake by the liver with concomitant transfer from the plasma compartment.

Assuming that endocrine inputs associated with stress are multifaceted, we examined the effect of other hormones on metallothionein gene expression. We have observed that glucagon, epinephrine, and dibutyryl cAMP ($Bt_2$cAMP) all increased metallothionein levels in intact rats. These effects were tissue specific. In liver, metallothionein mRNA levels increased many fold after these agents were acutely administered (Cousins *et al.*, 1986). Of considerable significance was the inverse correlation between the serum zinc concentration and liver metallothionein. This indicates that cellular levels of the protein are in dynamic equilibrium with the plasma compartment. Because cellular zinc turnover is extremely rapid, with a half-life of 15 hr in hepatocytes (Pattison and Cousins, 1986), ligand exchange reactions within cells would be expected to alter zinc kinetics whenever disease produces significant changes in hormonal levels. The evidence suggests that cAMP may contribute significantly to physiological control of metallothionein gene expression. We have demonstrated through nuclear transcription rate measurements that $Bt_2cAMP$ administration *in vivo* activates transcription of this gene (Dunn and Cousins, 1987).

Metallothionein gene expression is also regulated by endotoxin and interleukin-1 (IL-1) (DiSilvestro and Cousins, 1984). Control via these mediators strongly suggests that a link may exist between synthesis of the protein and host-defense-related phenomena. Endotoxin and IL-1 induced metallothionein in zinc-deficient rats, suggesting induction does not depend on zinc status (DiSilvestro and Cousins, 1984). In recent experiments with purified, recombinantly produced human IL-1 alpha, this mediator acted as a potent inducer of liver metallothionein and as a weak inducer of kidney metallothionein; it was inactive in spleen and intestine (unpublished observations). In this study, liver metallothionein levels reached 359 μg/g, the highest we have observed by hormonal induction. Furthermore, the corresponding reduction in serum zinc concentration to only 28 μg/dl was the lowest produced by hormonal administration. Table I summarizes the approximate magnitude of tissue-specific dietary-, hormone-, and mediator-linked induction of metallothionein.

It has long been clear that metallothionein is an interactive ligand that participates in cellular activities and influences the metabolic fate of some transition metals. To evaluate the consequences of increased

**TABLE I**

**Tissue-Specific Regulation of Metallothionein Gene Expressiona**[a]

| Tissue | Inducer | Relative Potency |
|---|---|---|
| Intestine | Acute increase in dietary zinc | +++ |
| | Constant intake of high zinc and low copper diet | + |
| Liver | Acute increase in dietary zinc | +++ |
| | Glucocorticoid hormones | ++++ |
| | Endotoxin | ++++ |
| | Epinephrine | +++ |
| | Glucagon | +++ |
| | Dibutyryl cAMP | ++++ |
| | Interleukin-1 | +++++ |
| Kidney | Constant intake of high zinc diet | +++ |
| | Endotoxin | +++ |
| | Interleukin-1 | ++ |
| Bone marrow[b] | Dibutyryl cAMP | +++ |
| | Interleukin-1 | +++ |
| Thymus[b] | Interleukin-1 | +++ |

[a]The relative potency was derived from available hybridization data.
[b]These postulations were based on available kinetic data.

metallothionein gene expression, kinetic experiments with intravenously administered $^{65}Zn$ were conducted (Cousins and Leinart, 1988). Results showed that IL-1 alpha dramatically shifted the tissue distribution of $^{65}Zn$ (Fig. 3). When expressed as a percentage of dose taken up by tissues, IL-1 alpha stimulated uptake into liver, bone marrow, and thymus. Correspondingly less $^{65}Zn$ was taken up by bone, pancreas, small intestine, and skin. Muscle and kidney $^{65}Zn$ did not change. These data collectively indicate that IL-1 alpha, which has an important role in regulating host defense, can produce major changes in zinc distribution. The shift is clearly in the direction of highly proliferative tissues associated with host defense. We are now evaluating the extent to which metallothionein gene expression can be regulated in bone marrow cells and the thymus gland.

## C. Disease-Related Roles of Metallothionein

The functional significance of tissue-specific increases in metallothionein production is unclear. Currently available evidence suggests multiple functions for the protein. Metallothionein gene structure is highly conserved in both plant and animal phyla (Hamer, 1986). The ordered arrangement of the cysteine residues suggests a close structure–function relationship. Clearly, regulation of the gene by metals was the first of its control methods to evolve. Therefore, participation in metal exchange

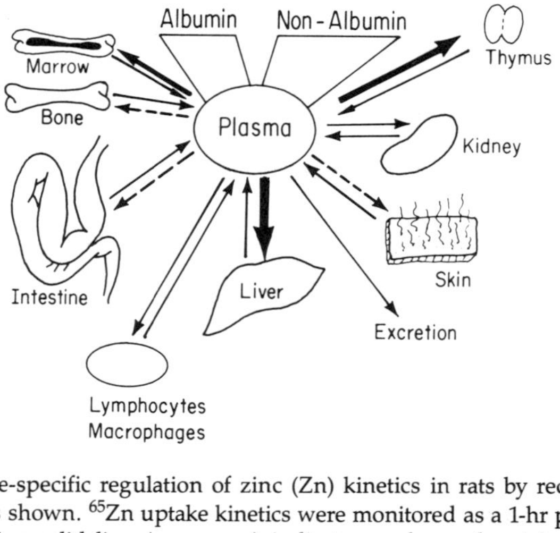


**Fig. 3.** Tissue-specific regulation of zinc (Zn) kinetics in rats by recombinant human interleukin-1 $\alpha$ is shown. $^{65}Zn$ uptake kinetics were monitored as a 1-hr pulse administered intravenously. Fine solid line (________) indicates unchanged uptake in response to a single dose of interleukin-1 alpha; heavy solid line (▬▬) indicates elevated uptake; and dotted line (__ __ __ __) indicates diminished uptake.

reactions and detoxification are probable functions. Intracellular accumulation of cadmium, mercury, copper, and other transition metals could be controlled and detoxified by metallothionein. Because the species of metal bound dictates the turnover rate and eventual excretory fate, a reduced turnover rate may act to detoxify (Cousins, 1985; Dunn *et al.*, 1987). Activation of apometalloenzymes by zinc–metallothionein has been demonstrated (Li *et al.*, 1980; Udom and Brady, 1980). Some mechanism for metal donation must exist for metal insertion into proteins during or after translation. A metal-rich protein like metallothionein, which readily exchanges zinc, would be an excellent metal-donor candidate. Because most metals bound to proteins exhibit a degree of ligand exchange with the aqueous environment, metallothionein may not be unique in this regard and may function as a metal donor *in vitro* only. Therefore, this function remains to be unequivocally established.

A broader view of metallothionein function is possible through discovery of regulation of the gene by hormones, host-defense mediators, and some environmental factors. The evidence that elevated metallothionein synthesis accounts for the acute fall in plasma zinc following administration of specific hormones including IL-1 alpha is convincing (Cousins *et al.*, 1986; DiSilvestro and Cousins, 1984). This suggests that selective metal uptake and redistribution of zinc accompany the plethora of effects reported for specific hormones. It has been suggested that the reduction in plasma zinc accounts for activation of phagocytic cells (Chvapil *et al.*, 1982). The kinetic evidence indicating zinc redistribution to sites that produce bursts of cell proliferation in response to disease supports this concept. The extensive involvement of zinc metalloenzymes in cell replication and protein synthesis (Cousins, 1986; Falchuk and Vallee, 1986) suggests these sites as appropriate targets for redistribution. Diversity of biological activities of IL-1, including thymocyte proliferation, release of neutrophils from bone marrow stores, and increased natural killer-cell activity, may place a critical demand on body zinc that requires these cells to induce metallothionein in order to selectively accumulate systemic zinc. This demand reduces zinc going to bone, skin, pancreas, and small intestine. Zinc may enhance activity in specialized cells. For example, natural killer activity in interferon-stimulated lymphocytes from AIDS patients is potentiated by zinc *in vitro* (Cunningham-Rundles, 1984). The critical, well-recognized role of zinc in immune response was initially demonstrated by Fraker and associates (1978).

Free-radical formation and associated tissue damage have been implicated in several disorders, including inflammatory diseases and cancer. Recent studies suggest that metallothionein functions as an intracellular antioxidant. *In vitro,* metallothionein shows pronounced activity against hydroxyl radicals compared to superoxide radicals

(Thornalley and Vasak, 1985). That is in contrast to superoxide dismutase, the intracellular protein that converts the superoxide ion to hydrogen peroxide. Activity of metallothionein against hydroxyl radicals occurs with concomitant loss of the metal and disulfide formation within the protein. Because radical formation increases in response to cellular injury, the induction of metallothionein to sequester hydroxyl radicals may have a teleological basis. Our experiments with cultured rat hepatocytes support these findings (Cousins and Coppen, 1987). As measured by both lipid peroxidation and electron spin resonance spectrometry, zinc supplementation appeared to suppress free-radical formation in these cell cultures. This cytoprotective effect of zinc, observed regardless of the agents used to induce radical formation, suggests a common zinc-related mechanism. Of considerable potential importance is that cytoprotection in the hepatocytes coincided with induction of metallothionein. Because IL-1 increases hydroxyl radical formation, its induction of metallothionein may be cytoprotective. The antioxidant role of this protein is being investigated.

### D. Human Metallothionein and Disease

Two decades have passed since metallothionein was isolated from a human tissue (Pulido *et al.*, 1966). Human metallothionein genes have now been isolated and cloned (Karin and Richards, 1982). In human adult liver, metallothionein primarily contains zinc (Buhler and Kagi, 1974). However, our knowledge of the function of metallothionein in human metabolism and disease must, by and large, be inferred from animal studies.

The circulating level of metallothionein in plasma is reported to be low in humans (Garvey, 1984) and experimental animals (Sato *et al.*, 1984). Until recently, little information has existed on tissue levels of metallothionein, except that they are highest in liver in the late prenatal and early neonatal period (Kagi and Nordberg, 1979; Ryden and Deutsch, 1978). Our laboratory has developed an ELISA method for human metallothionein, using IgG produced separately in sheep, against both human metallothioneins I and II. That assay is currently being evaluated. Table II compares liver metallothionein measurements using the cadmium-binding method (Eaton and Toal, 1982) to measurements using the ELISA method. Metallothionein levels are consistently high in neonates but variable in adults. That variation reflects a diagnosis of infectious disease. Patients who died from infectious disease had liver metallothionein concentrations 10–20 times above normal. The ELISA and cadmium-binding assays appear to give comparable values, supporting further use of the considerably more sensitive ELISA assay.

TABLE II

**Representative Examples of Metallothionein in Human Liver[a]**

| Subject | Age | Infectious disease | Metallothionein concentration[b] |
|---|---|---|---|
| Black female | 4 days | no | 1,777 |
| Black female | 19 years | no | 72 |
| White female | 61 years | no | 78 |
| White female | 34 years | yes | 1,484 |
| White female | 77 years | yes | 1,186 |
| White male | 22 years | no | 144 |
| | | | 160* |

[a]Data from unpublished observations.

[b]The cadmium-binding assay was used to measure metallothionein in all subjects; the enzyme-linked immunosorbant assay (ELISA) for human metallothionein was used to measure the second value (*) in the last subject. Values are stated in $\mu g/g$.

## IV. SUMMARY

The link between micronutrient status and human disease is strengthening. Zinc and some other micronutrients interact directly with the genome. This mode of transcriptional regulation points out the need to maintain an adequate dietary supply of micronutrients. As newer methods of molecular biology, cell biology, and high-level instrumentation support and complement traditional methods of analysis, many approaches now limited to experimental animal models can be extended to human studies of the effects of micronutrients on disease.

## ACKNOWLEDGMENTS

Research from the author's laboratory reported in this review is supported by NIH grants DK 31127 and DK 31651 and Boston Family Endowment Funds. The efforts of Drs. T. Lynn Blalock, Michael A. Dunn, Arthur Grider, and Annette S. Leinart in those experiments is gratefully acknowledged. The help of Dawn Mendoza for typing the manuscript and Walter Jones for drawing the figures is also appreciated.

## REFERENCES

Blalock, T. L., Dunn, M. A., and Cousins, R. J. (1988). Metallothionein gene expression in rats: Tissue specific regulation by dietary copper and zinc. *J. Nutr.* **118**, 222–228.

Buhler, R. H. O., and Kagi, J. H. R. (1974). Human hepatic metallothioneins. *FEBS Lett.* **39**, 229–234.

Charles, M. A., Martial, J., Zolock, D., Morrissey, R., and Baxter, J. D. (1981). Regulation of calcium-binding protein messenger RNA by 1,25-dihydroxycholecalciferol. *Calcif. Tissue Int.* **33**, 15–18.

Chvapil, M., Stankova, L.. Weldy, P., Bernhard, D., Campell, J., Carlson, E. C., Cox, T., Peacock, J., Bartos, Z , and Zukoski, C. (1982). The role of zinc in the function of some inflammatory cells: Clinical, biochemical and nutritional aspects of trace elements. *Curr. Top. Nutr. Dis.* **6**, 1–57.

Cousins, R. J. (1976). Zinc thionein and heritable diseases associated with aberrant zinc metabolism. *Lancet* **2**, 686–687.

Cousins, R. J. (1985). Absorption, transport and hepatic metabolism of copper and zinc: Special reference to metallothionein and ceruloplasmin. *Physiol. Rev.* **65**, 238–309.

Cousins, R. J. (1986). Molecular biology of zinc. *In* "Biotechnology for Solving Agricultural Problems. Beltsville Symposium on Agricultural Research." (D. C. Augustine, H. D. Danforth and M. R. Bakst, eds.), Vol. 10, pp. 207–219. Martinus Nijhoff Publishers, Boston.

Cousins, R. J., and Coppen, D. E. (1987). Regulation of liver zinc metabolism and metallothionein by cAMP, glucagon and glucocorticoids and suppression of free radicals by zinc. *In* "Metallothionein II" (J. H. R. Kagi and Y. Kojima, eds.). pp. 545–553. Birkhauser Verlag, Basel.

Cousins, R. J., and Leinart, A. S. (1988). Tissue-specific regulation of zinc metabolism and metallothionein genes by interleukin-1. *FASEB J.* **2**, in press.

Cousins, R. J., Dunn, M. A., Leinart, A. S., Yedinak, K. C., and DiSilvestro, R. A. (1986). Coordinate regulation of zinc metabolism and metallothionein gene expression in rats. *Amer. J. Physiol.* **251**, E688–E694.

Cousins, R. J., Dunn, M. A., Blalock, T. L., and Leinart, A. S. (1988). Coordinate regulation of zinc metabolism and metallothionein gene expression by cAMP, interleukin-1 and dietary copper and zinc. *In* "Trace Elements in Man and Animals" (L. S. Hurley, B. Lonnerdal, C. L. Keen, and R. B. Rucker. eds.), Vol. 6. Plenum Press, New York. (In press.)

Cunningham-Rundles, S. (1984). Nutritional factors in immune response. *In* "Malnutrition: Determinants and Consequences" (P. L. White and N. Selvey, eds.), pp. 233–244. Alan R. Liss, New York.

DiSilvestro, R. A., and Cousins. R. J. (1984). Mediation of endotoxin induced changes in zinc metabolism in rats. *Amer. J. Physiol.* **247**, E436–E441.

Dunn, M. A., and Cousins, R. J. (1987). Regulation of metallothionein gene transcription and kinetics of zinc metabolism by dibutyryl cAMP [Abstract]. *Fed. Proc.* **46**, 1643.

Dunn, M. A., Blalock, T. L., and Cousins, R. J. (1987). Metallothionein. *Proc. Soc. Exp. Biol. Med.* **185**, 107–119.

Eaton, D. L., and Toal, B. F. (1982). Evaluation of the Cd hemoglobin affinity assay for the rapid determination of metallothionein in biological tissues. *Toxicol. Appl. Pharmacol.* **66**, 134–142.

Etzel, K. R., Shapiro, S. G., and Cousins, R. J. (1979). Regulation of liver metallothionein and plasma zinc by the glucocorticoid dexamethasone. *Biochem. Biophys. Res. Commun.* **89**, 1120–1126.

Failla, M. L., and Cousins, R. J. (1978). Zinc accumulation and metabolism in primary cultures of rat liver cells: Regulation by glucocorticoids. *Biochim. Biophys. Acta* **543**, 293–304.

Falchuk, K. H. (1977). Effect of acute disease and ACTH on serum zinc proteins. *N. Engl. J. Med.* **296**, 1129–1134.

Falchuk, K. H., and Vallee, B. L. (1986). Zinc and chromatin structure, composition and function. *In* "Trace Element Metabolism in Man and Animals" (C. F. Mills, I. Bremner, and J. K. Chesters, eds.), Vol. 5, pp. 48–55. Commonwealth Agricultural Bureau, Slough, U.K.

Feldman, S. L., Failla, M. L.. and Cousins, R. J. (1978). Degradation of rat liver metallothioneins *in vitro*. *Biochim. Biophys. Acta* **544**, 638–646.

Flier, J. S., Cook, K. S., Usher, P., and Spiegelman, B. M. (1987). Severely impaired adipsin expression in genetic and acquired obesity. *Science* **237**, 405–408.

Fraker, P. J., DePasquale-Jardieu, P., Zwicki, C. M., and Luecke, R. W. (1978). Regeneration of T-cell helper function in zinc-deficient adult mice. *Proc. Nat. Acad. Sci. USA* **75**, 5660–5664.

Garvey, J. S. (1984). Metallothionein: Structure/antigenicity and detection/quantitation in normal physiological fluids. *Environ. Health Perspect.* **54**, 117–127.

Hambidge, K. M., Casey, C. E., and Krebs, N. F. (1986). Zinc. *In* "Trace Elements in Human and Animal Nutrition" (W. Mertz, ed.), 5th ed., pp. 1-109. Academic Press, New York.

Hamer, D. H. (1986). Metallothionein. *Ann. Rev. Biochem.* **55**, 913–951.

Henkin, R. I., Foster, D. M., Aamodt, R. L., and Berman, M. (1984). Zinc metabolism in adrenalcortical insufficiency: Effects of carbohydrate active steroids. *Metabolism* **33**, 491–501.

Hoadley, J. E., Leinart, A. S., and Cousins, R. J. (1987). Kinetic analysis of zinc uptake and serosal transfer by vascularly perfused rat intestine. *Amer. J. Physiol.* **252**, G825–G831.

Idzerda, R. L., Huebers, H., Finch, C. A., and McKnight, G. S. (1986). Rat transferrin gene expression: Tissue-specific regulation by iron deficiency. *Proc. Nat. Acad. Sci. USA* **83**, 3723–3727.

Kagi, J. H., and Nordberg, M. (1979). "Metallothionein." Birkhauser Verlag Basel.

Karin, M., and Richards, R. I. (1982). Human metallothionein genes: Molecular cloning and sequence analysis of the mRNA. *Nucl. Acid Res.* **10**, 3165–3173.

Kim, H. Y., and Wolf, G. (1987). Vitamin A deficiency alters genomic expression for fibronectin in liver and hepatocytes. *J. Biol. Chem.* **262**, 365–371.

Lamers, W. H., Hanson, R. W., and Meisner, H. M. (1982). cAMP stimulates transcription of the gene for cytosolic phosphoenolpyruvate carboxykinase in rat liver nuclei. *Proc. Nat. Acad. Sci. USA* **79**, 5137–5141.

Li, T. Y., Kramer, A. J., Shaw, C. F., III, and Petering, D. H. (1980). Ligand substitution reactions of metallothioneins with EDTA and apocarbonic-anhydrase. *Proc. Nat. Acad. Sci. USA* **77**, 6334–6338.

Lombeck, I., Schnippering, H. G., Ritzl, F., Feinendegen, L. E., and Bremer, H. J. (1975). Absorption of zinc in acrodermatitis enteropathica. *Lancet* **1**, 855.

McCormick, C. C., Menard, M. P., and Cousins, R. J. (1981). Induction of hepatic metallothionein by feeding zinc to rats of depleted zinc status. *Amer. J. Physiol.* **240**, E414–E421.

Menard, M. P., McCormick, C. C., and Cousins, R. J. (1981). Regulation of intestinal metallothionein biosynthesis in the rat by dietary zinc. *J. Nutr.* **111**, 1353–1361.

Moynahan, E. J. (1974). Acrodermatitis enteropathica: A lethal inherited human zinc deficiency disorder. *Lancet* **2**, 399–400.

Nettesheim, D. G., Engeseth, H. R., and Otvos, J. D. (1985). Products of metal exchange reactions of metallothionein. *Biochemistry* **24**, 6744–6751.

Pattison, S. E., and Cousins, R. J. (1986). Kinetics of zinc uptake and exchange by primary cultures of rat hepatocytes. *Amer. J. Physiol.* **250**, E677–E685.

Pulido, P., Kagi, J. H. R., and Vallee, B. L. (1966). Isolation and some properties of human metallothionein. *Biochemistry* **5**, 1768–1777.

Richards, M. P., and Cousins, R. J. (1976). Zinc binding protein: Relationship to short-term changes in zinc metabolism. *Proc. Soc. Exp. Biol. Med.* **153**, 52–56.

Ryden, L., and Deutsch, H. F. (1978). Preparation and properties of the major copper-binding component in human fetal liver. Its identification as metallothionein. *J. Biol. Chem.* **253**, 519–524.

Sato, M., Mehra, R. K., and Bremner, I. (1984). Measurement of plasma metallothionein-I in the assessment of the zinc status of zinc-deficient and stressed rats. *J. Nutr.* **114**, 1683–1689.

Seguin, C., and Hamer, D. H. (1987). Regulation *in vitro* of metallothionein gene binding factors. *Science* **235**, 1383–1387.

Shapiro, S. G., Squibb, K. S., Markowitz, L A., and Cousins, R. J. (1978). Cell-free synthesis of metallothionein directed by rat liver polyadenylated messenger RNA. *Biochem. J.* **175**, 833–840.

Thornalley, P. J., and Vasak, M. (1985). Possible role for metallothionein in protection against radiation-induced oxidative stress. Kinetics and mechanism of its reaction with superoxide and hydroxyl radicals. *Biochim. Biophys. Acta* **827**, 36–44.

Udom, A. O., and Brady, F. O. (1980). Reactivation *in vitro* of zinc-requiring apo-enzymes by rat liver zinc-thionein. *Biochem. J.* **187**, 329–335.

# 2

# Vitamin A, Gene Expression, and Pulmonary Problems in Neonates


Frank Chytil

*Departments of Biochemistry and Medicine*
*Vanderbilt University School of Medicine*
*Nashville, Tennessee*

# I. INTRODUCTION

Vitamin A (retinol) is an essential dietary component that must be supplied to animals in food of animal origin or in the form of its precursors—carotenes derived from plants (Fig. 1). Retinol is vital not only for vision but, along with an obligatory metabolite retinoic acid (Fig. 2), for cell differentiation. Recent work directed toward elucidating molecular mechanisms through which vitamin A participates in cell differentiation has been both intense and fascinating. Experimental evidence indicates that retinol availability is of prime importance during animal development, starting with spermiogenesis, egg fertilization, implantation, organogenesis, pregnancy maintenance, postnatal organ maturation, and immunity. The common demoninator in all of these processes is the participation of retinol or retinoic acid in cell differentiation.

This discussion focuses primarily on how vitamin A works at the molecular level. The role of retinol in the metabolism and development of the bronchopulmonary tree and in a relatively new syndrome of retinol deficiency and its consequences in premature human neonates will also be considered.

Retinol and retinoic acid are members of a family of naturally occurring compounds chemically derived from retinol and now called "retinoids" (Sporn *et al.*, 1976). In contrast, synthetic retinoids have been successfully used as potent therapeutic agents to treat hyperkeratic skin lesions (Peck, 1984). When possible, the terms "retinol" or "retinoic acid" will be used instead of "natural retinoids" to stress that these two compounds do not appear to have identical roles in cellular metabolism.

# II. CELLULAR EFFECTS OF RETINOL

## A. Lesions in Retinol Deficiency

Much information about the function of retinol can be derived from observing morphological alterations that occur in tissues of animals fed a retinol-deficient diet. Although clearly described long ago (Wolbach and

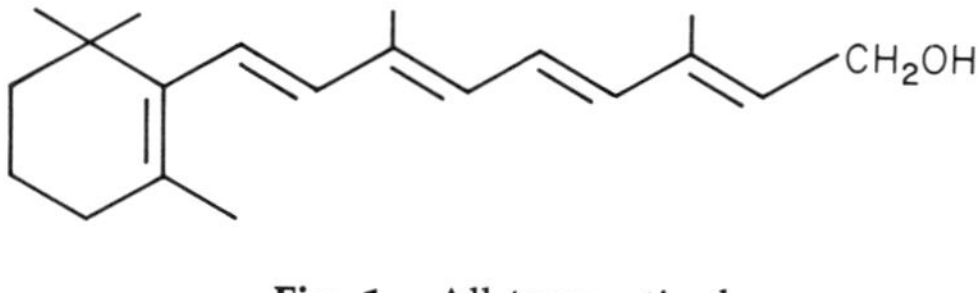


**Fig. 1.** All-*trans*-retinol.

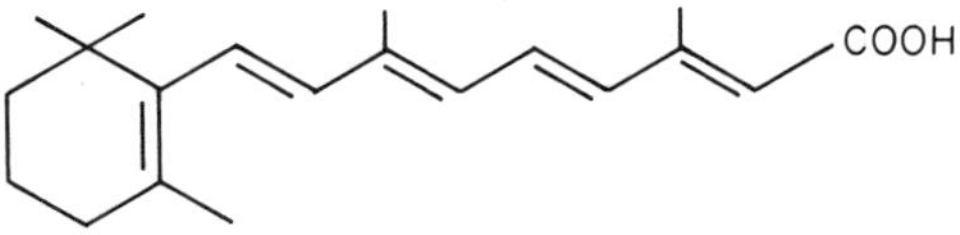


**Fig. 2.** All-*trans*-retinoic acid.

Howe, 1925), it is not yet common knowledge that retinol is required primarily to initiate and maintain differentiation of many if not all epithelia. These functions are not limited to epithelial cells; myeloid cells are also influenced by retinol or retinoic acid (Lotan, 1980; Strickland and Mahdavi, 1978; Murtaugh *et al.*, 1983).

The normal diet contains retinol or its precursor carotenoids but little retinyl aldehyde or retinoic acid. Thus, it is fair to assume that the biological effects of these retinoids may depend on the extent to which they are formed from retinol *in vivo*. Retinyl aldehyde is a known functional component of photoreceptors in the eye (Wald, 1968), but its role in cell differentiation remains to be delineated. Outside of the eye, retinyl aldehyde appears to be unstable and is quickly reduced to retinol or, to a limited extent, oxidized to retinoic acid. Although the molecular action of retinoic acid in this epithelia is unknown, it can, when added to a retinol-deficient diet, substitute for retinol in maintaining many epithelial tissues. However, retinoic acid cannot support visual function in the absence of retinol (Dowling and Wald, 1960). In addition, male animals fed a retinol-deficient diet containing retinoic acid show impaired spermiogenesis (Thompson *et al.*, 1964), even in the presence of normal circulating testosterone levels. This suggests a specific role of retinol distinct from retinoic acid (Appling and Chytil, 1981). With some oversimplification, the morphological alterations occurring in retinol deficiency can be divided into two categories. Some tissues, such as tracheal or urinary bladder epithelia, show metaplastic changes characterized by keratinization, whereas testicular seminiferous tubules show atrophy with no apparent expression of keratins. This striking difference in tissue reactivity to the lack of retinol must be taken into account when considering molecular mechanisms of retinol action. Moreover, this tissue specificity precludes a single molecular mechanism of action.

Also evident from experiments using retinol-deficient animals is the time dependency of observed sequelae. The sequences have been clearly described in rats (Wolbach and Howe, 1925) and in many other animal species including humans (Wolbach, 1937). Wolbach (1937) has described the time order of response to retinol deficiency, as judged by keratinizing metaplasia, in the rat. First affected are salivary glands, including submaxillary and all accessory glands of the tongue, buccal cavity, and pharynx. Then comes the respiratory tract, including nares, maxillary sinuses, Jacobson's organ, trachea, and bronchi. Genitourinary tract follows, including the renal pelves, ureters, bladder, epididymis, prostate, seminal vesicles, coagulating glands, uterus, oviducts, and accessory sex glands of the vulva. The last group of tissues morphologically influenced by the lack of retinol are the eyes and parocular glands—including corneal conjunctiva and the Hardenian, intraorbital, and extraorbital lacrimal glands—and the meibomian glands. The sequence of lesions appears to be similar in other species, including human infants suffering from retinol deficiency (Wolbach, 1937).

These apparently primary alterations are followed by secondary changes such as weight loss (resulting from fat loss and muscle atrophy), anemia, cessation of bone growth, degenerative lesions of skeletal muscle, and lymphoid hypoplasia of the spleen (Wolbach and Howe, 1925). Although these morphological observations indicate that the primary function of retinol is in differentiation it is unclear whether retinol serves as growth-promoting agent in cell replication.

These data indicate that retinol plays a role in many tissues, with few species differences in its action. Consequently, the rat is an adequate experimental model for elucidating the mechanisms of retinol action.

### B. Recovery from Retinol Deficiency

The sequelae attributable to retinol deficiency disappear time dependently when dietary retinol is restored (Wolbach and Howe, 1933). In the rat, changes in metaplastic respiratory epithelia, starting with the trachea, begin as early as the fifth day after a retinol-sufficient diet is restored. In organs like the testes, complete regeneration of function requires several months. It is not known why the initiation of observed sequelae and subsequent recovery are time dependent.

## III. MOLECULAR MECHANISMS OF VITAMIN A ACTION

Any viable hypothesis of molecular mechanisms of action of retinol and/or retinoic acid should attempt to explain not only how cell differentiation is initiated and maintained, but also why tissue specificity and reversibility of action occur. It is also important to elucidate the relationship between retinol and retinoic acid during these processes and during animal development.

### A. Older Hypotheses

The evolution of hypotheses and experimental designs to explain the molecular activities of retinol and retinoic acid has paralleled progress in biochemistry, physiology, and molecular biology. Early studies suggested that the primary activities of natural retinoids were mediated via interactions with cell membranes (Roels, 1967). More recently, it was proposed that phosphorylated retinol, conjugated with mannose, acts as a coenzyme in the transfer of glycosidic residues to specific glycoproteins (DeLuca, 1977). This theory is deficient in several respects. First, *in vivo* studies have failed to provide convincing evidence of the transfer reaction or of the requisite intermediate compounds (Creek *et al.*, 1986). Second, retinoic acid is a very potent biological compound, but its terminal carboxylic acid group is not amenable to phosphorylation, and the existence of its putative hydroxyl derivative that could eventually be phosphorylated has not been demonstrated. Most importantly, even if the putative retinol-mediated glycosidic transfers do occur, such reactions are unlikely to represent the principal target for cell differentiation.

## B. Effects of Retinol and/or Retinoic Acid on Gene Expression

The only viable hypothesis is that retinol and/or retinoid acid act on the cell nucleus and affect cell differentiation by influencing gene expression. It is not coincidental that the first cellular retinol-binding protein (CRBP) was discovered using this working hypothesis before any specific genomic effects were known (Bashor *et al.*, 1973). Evidence supporting the genomic expression mechanism has since accumulated rapidly. In addition to numerous global changes in mRNA synthesis (Omori and Chytil, 1982), expression of more than 40 gene products (proteins) is known to be influenced by retinol or retinoic acid (Chytil, 1986). More genes have since been reported to be influenced by retinoids. Thus, available evidence leaves little doubt that retinol and/or retinoic acid affect genomic expression and somehow mediate cell differentiation.

The exact molecular mechanisms by which natural or synthetic retinoids affect cell differentiation remain to be elucidated, but recent research indicates that both retinol and retinoic acid affect genomic expression by interacting with the cell nucleus (Chytil and Sherman, 1987). Whether this interaction is direct or indirect has not been unequivocally settled. Cell-culture and whole-animal studies have shown that both retinol and retinoic acid affect genomic expression by simultaneously activating and repressing specific genes. These multiple effects, which have been shown for genes for cytoskeleton proteins, enzymes, and membrane receptors (Chytil, 1986), parallel extensive changes in nuclear chromatin structure described in retinol-deficient animals (Porter *et al.*, 1986).

Retinol and retinoic acid affect genomic expression time dependently, with some genes influenced in an hour or less (Omori and Chytil, 1982; Murtaugh *et al.*, 1983) and others after a considerably longer time (Fuchs and Green, 1981). If one gene is influenced first, interaction with this "early" gene may trigger a mechanism that later affects other genes time dependently. Alternatively, retinol or retinoic acid may interact simultaneously with regulatory sequences of many genes. Furthermore, retinol may serve only as a precursor of retinoic acid, which, in turn, could be the active metabolite responsible for changes in the genome.

## C. Modes of Interaction of Retinol or Retinoic Acid with the Genome

Several modes of interaction of retinol or retinoic acid with the genome have been proposed.

### 1. *Mode of Interaction in Nonepithelial Cells*

Retinol may enter the target cell from the bloodstream and interact directly with nuclear chromosomal material whose composition and expression is tissue specific (Chytil and Spelsberg, 1971; Derman *et al.*, 1981) (Fig. 3). Free retinol or retinoic acid entering the nucleus from the blood or formed *in situ* could interact with a nuclear informative molecule with high affinity and specificity for particular regulatory regions. This molecule, probably complexed with a DNA-binding protein, could then alter transcription of nearby gene(s) by exposing the DNA sequences, thus altering the affinity of RNA polymerase for the affected promoter site. These activities could be followed by transcriptional enhancement (activation) or diminution (repression), each occurring in response to retinol or retinoic acid (Fuchs and Green, 1981; Omori and Chytil, 1982). Such mechanisms may operate in nonepithelial cell-culture systems such as human promyelocytic leukemia cells HL 60 (Breitman *et al.*, 1980), histolytic lymphoma cells (Chomienne *et al.*, 1986), or peritoneal macrophages (Murtaugh *et al.*, 1983), in which retinoic acid has induced

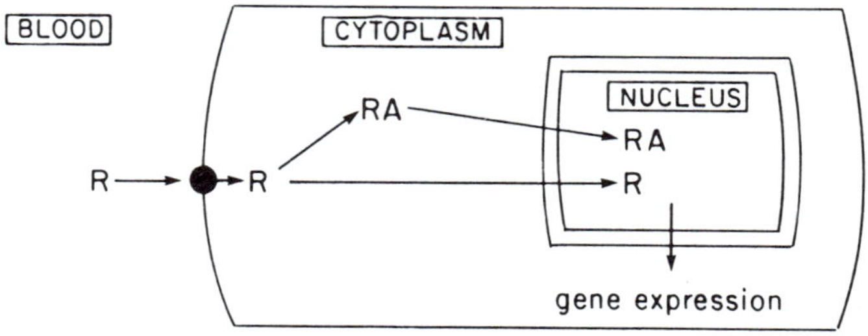


**Fig. 3.** Molecular effects of retinol (R) and/or retinoic acid (RA) on gene expression may be mediated by interaction of *free* R or RA with the cell nucleus.

differentiation and specific gene expression. Similar direct intercellular transfer of a small molecule without participation of a cytosolic binding component was proposed for triiodothyronine (Oppenheimer, 1983; Samuels, 1983).

### 2. *Mode of Interaction in Epithelial Cells*

Retinol or retinoic acid may interact differently with the genome in epithelial cells, which, in contrast to myeloid cells, contain cellular retinol-binding protein (CRBP) and cellular retinoic acid-binding protein (CRABP) (Fig. 4). CRBP and CRABP, both of which have been extensively characterized, may facilitate interaction of their respective ligands with the genome, thereby altering its expression (Chytil and Ong, 1984). This contention is supported by observations that the affinity of certain retinoids for CRBP and CRABP correlates well with their ability to influence various biological systems (Chytil and Ong, 1984). F9 embryonal carcinoma cells also contain CRABP and differentiate in response to retinoic acid (Strickland and Mahdavi, 1978; Jetten, 1986; Sherman, 1986). In isolated mutant cell lines that have lost responsiveness to retinoic acid, CRABP is also missing. However, in retinoic acid-sensitive revertants, CRABP is once again detectable (Sherman, 1986).

In another set of *in vitro* experiments, nuclei and chromatin were found to accept retinol from its complex with CRBP (Takase *et al.*, 1979; Liau *et al.*, 1981; Barkai and Sherman, 1987) and retinoic acid from its complex with CRABP in a specific, saturable, and temperature-dependent fashion (Takase *et al.*, 1986; Barkai and Sherman, 1987). Retinol and retinoic acid recognize physically distinct sites within chromatin. CRBP and CRABP apparently shuttle their ligands to these sites because they do not remain bound (Liau *et al.*, 1981; Takase *et al.*, 1986). More recently, it was reported

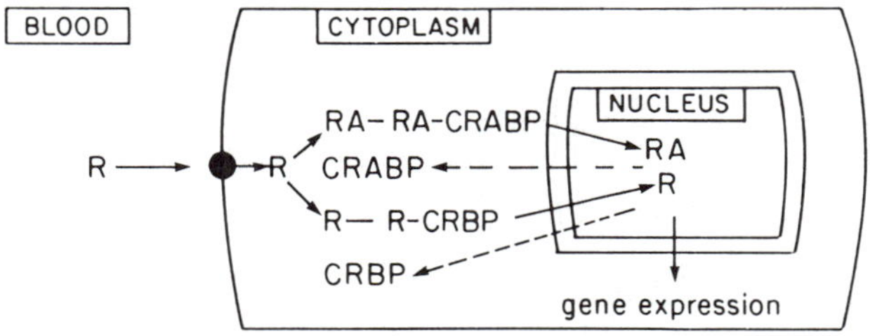


**Fig. 4.** Molecular effects of retinol (R) and/or retinoic acid (RA) on gene expression may be mediated by interaction of the complexes of R with cellular retinol-binding protein (CRBP) or RA with cellular retinoic acid-binding protein (CRABP) with cell nucleus.

that only CRBP—and not other retinol-binding proteins—can compete effectively for retinol-specific binding sites within chromatin (Crow *et al.*, 1987). No direct evidence has shown that the interaction of retinol or retinoic acid with the nucleus requires the presence of CRBP or CRABP or leads to altered genomic expression, but available data strongly suggest that these binding proteins are involved in retinoid-induced cell differentiation.

Finally, the recent observation of very rapid induction of CRBP mRNA in the lungs four hours after administration of retinyl acetate to retinol-deficient rats suggests that CRBP is important in recovery from the effects of deficiency in this organ (Sherman *et al.*, 1987). The speed with which this affects expression of a specific gene in the whole animal suggests a direct effect of retinol on the genome.

### 3. *Other Modes of Interaction*

Another possibility is that the primary interaction of retinol takes place on the plasma membrane or on some intracellular cytoplasmic entity (Fig. 5). Through such an interaction with retinol or retinoic acid formed inside the cell, a "second messenger" may be formed. This messenger could enter the nucleus, later affecting gene expression. Further work is needed to identify this proposed second messenger.

# IV. VITAMIN A AND DEVELOPMENT

## A. Role of Retinol in Gene Expression during Pregnancy and Perinatal Development

The supply of retinol to the fetus from the mother is essential for normal fetal development and maintenance of the pregnancy (Moore, 1967). It is reasonable to assume that retinol and/or retinoic acid play an essential

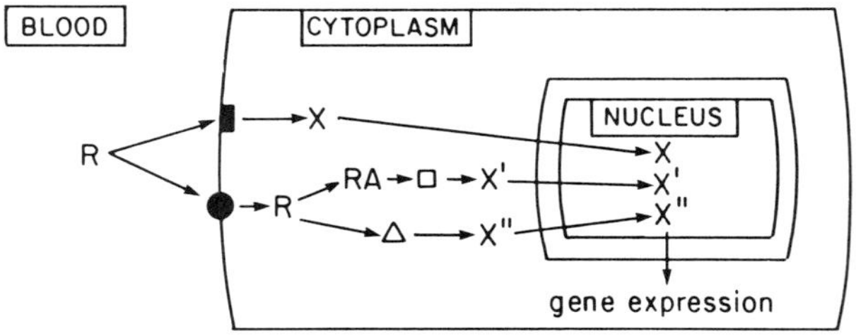


**Fig. 5.** Molecular effects of retinol (R) and/or retinoic acid (RA) on gene expression may be mediated by a "second messenger" (X, X', X"), which, in turn, interacts with cell nucleus.

role in gene expression and in the appearance or disappearance of various gene products accompanying these processes. During the perinatal period, changes in certain enzymes, and cytological alterations in many cells are also observed (Knox, 1972). This suggests that the biological information stored in DNA has a regulated pattern of expression and that the developmental process involves time-dependent activation and repression of nuclear genes. Although the molecular activities underlying these processes are unclear, alterations in nuclear chromatin composition may be linked to fetal and perinatal development in animals (Chytil *et al.*, 1974).

Little evidence is available to explain how retinol is transferred from the mother to the fetus. Studies of the growth and accumulation of vitamin A in rat fetuses have delineated three distinct phases during the 21-day gestation period (Takahashi *et al.*, 1977). The first phase (days 7 to 9) is characterized by accumulation of a high concentration of retinol in the conceptus, suggesting a need for retinol in organogenesis. Indeed, the most recent report implicates retinoic acid in organogenesis (Thaller and Eichele, 1987). The second phase (days 11 to 14) involves parallel accumulation of retinol transferred from maternal circulation. The third phase (days 16 to 20) marks the start of retinol storage in the fetal liver. After birth, retinol stores in the liver are limited (Takahashi *et al.*, 1977). Only after weaning (day 21 postnatally) does retinol accumulate substantially in the liver (Kylberg *et al.*, 1981). Thus, retinol and/or retinoic acid appear to be necessary for gene expression throughout fetal development. Because the fetus only stores small amounts of retinol in the liver, the mother must provide an adequate supply throughout the pregnancy.

## B. Vitamin A and Gene Expression in the Developing Lungs

Several lines of evidence indicate that retinol is involved in differentiation and perinatal development of the bronchopulmonary tree. Experimental animals with retinol deficiency develop focal squamous keratinizing metaplasia of the trachea and bronchopulmonary tree (Wolbach and Howe, 1925). These respiratory lesions precede the well-known consequences of retinol deficiency in visual processes that eventually result in xerophthalmia (Bloch, 1921; Bloch, 1924). In retinol-deficient human infants, keratinized metaplasia of the trachea and bronchi are very early sequelae (Blackfan and Wolbach, 1933). Moreover, it has long been recognized that defects in differentiation and regeneration of the epithelium of the respiratory mucosa explain the frequency, severity, and persistence of pneumonias in the presence of vitamin A deficiency. Atelectasis and high susceptibility to infection appear long before the epithelium is replaced by stratified keratinized structures (Blackfan and Wolbach, 1933).

Differentiation of the lungs to form the alveolar system, a timely process leading to maturity in humans, occurs mainly during the third trimester of pregnancy (Stahlman, 1984). In contrast, perinatal lung development in the rat, which involves differentiation of alveoli from primitive saccules, occurs during the first three weeks postnatally (Burri *et al.*, 1974). Because of this delay in lung maturation, rats have been used to study the time-dependent expression of intracellular vitamin A-binding proteins during perinatal development. The presence of CRBP and CRABP has been detected in humans (Bashor *et al.*, 1973) and in fetal and adult rats (Ong and Chytil, 1975). Striking changes in CRBP and CRABP levels were observed (Ong and Chytil, 1976) (Fig. 6). CRABP levels rose soon after birth, peaked on day 10 postnatally, and were not detectable by the method then used on day 21 postnatally. These changes coincided with rat lung differentiation, when rat pulmonary morphology changed from primitive saccules to fully differentiated alveoli (Burri *et al.*, 1974; Powell and Whitney, 1980) (Fig. 6). The experiments also showed that, during perinatal lung development, pulmonary cells may require and use retinol differently than retinoic acid. These results lead to a working hypothesis that retinol is involved in lung maturation (Chytil, 1985).

## V. VITAMIN A STATUS AND PULMONARY PROBLEMS IN PREMATURE INFANTS

### A. Vitamin A Status of Premature Infants

Premature delivery deprives the human infant of the maternal supply of retinol, which often leads to impaired pulmonary differentiation, chronic respiratory distress, and chronic lung disease and bronchopulmonary dysplasia (BPD) (Stahlman, 1984).

Although the etiology of pulmonary distress syndrome is multifactorial, some features of its acute period are reminiscent of the sequelae observed in vitamin A-deficient animals. These include widespread alveolar atelectasis and, more importantly, patchy loss of ciliated cells with keratinizing metaplasia and necrosis of the bronchiolar mucosa (Northway *et al.*, 1967; Stahlman, 1984). The focally occurring keratinizing metaplasia suggests activation of keratin genes and has led to the suspicion that vitamin A metabolism may be compromised in these infants.

Several studies have examined vitamin A status in premature infants. In studies comparing premature and term neonates, serum retinol and retinol-binding protein (RBP) levels were significantly lower in the premature babies (Shenai *et al.*, 1985a). The very low liver retinol concentrations found in premature infants provided more evidence that their vitamin A status is jeopardized (Olson *et al.*, 1984; Shah and Rajalakshmi, 1984; Hustead *et al.*, 1984; Shenai *et al.*, 1985a).

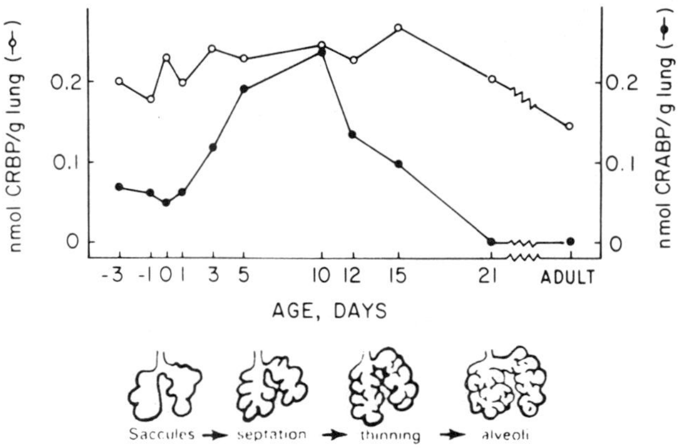


**Fig. 6.** Upper panel: Levels of cellular retinol-binding protein (CRBP) and cellular retinoic acid-binding protein (CRABP) during perinatal rat lung development are plotted. (Redrawn from Ong and Chytil, 1976. Reprinted with permission.) Lower panel: Morphology during perinatal development of rat lung alveoli is shown. (From Powell and Whitney, 1980. Reprinted with permission.)

Vitamin A status has been prospectively assessed and compared in two groups of preterm neonates—a group with clinical and radiographic evidence of BPD and a control group with no significant lung disease (Shenai *et al.*, 1985b). BPD infants required prolonged mechanical ventilation and supplemental oxygen therapy and had a higher incidence of cardiorespiratory complications than controls. Their mean plasma retinol concentrations were significantly lower than controls at four sampling times in the first postnatal month. Plasma vitamin A concentrations in BPD infants declined substantially from initial values, and a high percentage of these infants had severe deficiencies, with plasma concentrations less than 10 μg/dl. Delayed establishment of gastrointestinal feeding and a lower vitamin A intake in BPD infants than in controls may explain these suboptimal plasma vitamin A concentrations, which continued for extended periods. It was speculated that necrotizing bronchiolitis and squamous metaplasia of conduction airways associated with vitamin A deficiency may influence orderly lung repair in mechanically ventilated neonates and may contribute to the pathophysiology of BPD (Shenai *et al.*, 1985b).

## B. Effect of Retinyl Palmitate Administration on Perinatal Lung Development of Premature Infants

The above findings suggested that premature neonates with poor vitamin A status might benefit from retinol supplementation. A randomized, double-blind controlled trial was conducted to determine whether early postnatal vitamin A supplementation would reduce morbidity associated with BPD in very low birthweight neonates (Shenai *et al.*, 1987). The trial involved 40 neonates with birthweights ranging from 700 to 1,300 g and gestational ages ranging from 26 to 30 weeks; all were oxygen-dependent and required mechanical ventilation for at least 72 hours after birth. Both groups had comparable gestational maturity, clinical characteristics, initial lung disease, and vitamin A status at entry into the trial. The two groups received either 2,000 IU retinyl palmitate or 0.9% saline on postnatal day 4 and on alternate days thereafter, for a total of 14 intramuscular injections over 28 days.

Infants receiving retinyl palmitate achieved significantly higher mean plasma concentrations of vitamin A and RBP and experienced a lower incidence of BPD than controls. Moreover, the need for supplemental oxygen, mechanical ventilation, and intensive care was reduced in vitamin A-supplemented infants, as were airway infection and retinopathy of prematurity. These results demonstrated that vitamin A supplementation at the dosage tested not only improved vitamin A status of very low birthweight neonates but also decreased morbidity associated with BPD (Shenai *et al.*, 1987). This study also suggested that vitamin A deficiency contributes to the etiology of chronic lung disease in newborns.

## VI. CONCLUSIONS

Evidence indicates that retinol and its obligatory metabolite, retinoic acid, affect gene expression in epithelial and nonepithelial cells. Although the molecular mechanisms remain to be elucidated, both retinol and retinoic acid rapidly affect the animal genome, resulting in repression and activation of many specific genes.

Moreover, retinol and retinoic acid are essential to organogenesis and perinatal maturation of lungs and other organs. The essential role of retinol in orderly lung development is supported by observations that premature human neonates are retinol deficient and that morbidity resulting from prematurity can be lowered by postnatal supplementation with retinyl palmitate as a source of retinol.

## ACKNOWLEDGMENTS

This work was supported by grants from the U.S. Public Health Service HD-09195, HL-14214, and from General Foods Corporation. The author is indebted to L. Chytil, M. Hunt, and T. Hamilton for their assistance in animal experimental studies as well as in writing this manuscript and to Drs. M. T. Stahlman and J. P. Shenai for collaboration and discussions during the work on premature infants.

## REFERENCES

Appling, D. R., and Chytil, F. (1981). Evidence for a role of retinoic acid (vitamin A acid) in the maintenance of testosterone production in male rats. *Endocrinology* **108**, 2120–2123.

Barkai, U., and Sherman, M. I. (1987). Analysis of the interactions between retinoid-binding proteins and embryonal carcinoma cells. *J. Cell Biol.* **104**, 671–678.

Bashor, M. M., Toft, D. O., and Chytil, F. (1973). *In vitro* binding of retinol to rat tissue components. *Proc. Nat. Acad. Sci. USA* **70**, 3483–3487.

Blackfan, K. D., and Wolbach, S. B. (1933). Vitamin A deficiency in infants. *J. Pediatr.* **3**, 679–706.

Bloch, C. E. (1921). Clinical investigations of xerophthalmia and dystrophy in infants and young children (Xerophthalmia et Dystrophia Alipogenetica). *J. Hygiene* **19**, 283–307.

Bloch, C. E. (1924). Blindness and other diseases in children arising from deficient nutrition/lack of fat-soluble A factor. *Amer. J. Dis. Child.* **27**, 139–148.

Breitman, T. R., Selonick, S. E., and Collings, S. J. (1980). Induction of differentiation of the human promyelocytic leukemia cell line (HL-60) by retinoic acid. *Proc. Nat. Acad. Sci. USA* **77**, 2936–2940.

Burri, P. H., Dbaly, J., and Weibel, E. R. (1974). The postnatal growth of the rat lung. *Anat. Rec.* **178**, 711–730.

Chomienne, C., Balitrand, N., Degos, L., and Abita, J. P. (1986). L-β-D-arabino-furanosyl cytosine and all-*trans* retinoic acid in combination accelerates and increases monocyte differentiation of myeloid leukemic cells. *Leukemia Res.* **10**, 631–636.

Chytil, F. (1985). Function of vitamin A in the respiratory tract. *Acta Vitaminol. Enzymol.* **7** (Suppl.), 27–31.

Chytil, F. (1986). Retinoic acid: Biochemistry and metabolism. *J. Amer. Acad. Dermatol.* **15**, 741–747.

Chytil, F., and Ong, D. E. (1984). Cellular retinoid-binding proteins. *In* "The Retinoids" (M. B. Sporn and A. B. Roberts, eds.), Vol. 2, pp. 89–123. Academic Press, Orlando.

Chytil, F., and Sherman, D. R. (1987). How do retinoids work? *Dermatologia* **175** (Suppl. 1), 8–12.

Chytil, F., and Spelsberg, T. C. (1971). Tissue differences in antigenic properties of non-histone protein-DNA complexes. *Nature New Biol.* **233**, 215–218.

Chytil, F., Glasser, S. R., and Spelsberg, T. C. (1974). Alterations in liver chromatin during perinatal development of the rat. *Dev. Biol.* **37**, 295–305.

Creek, K. E., Rimoldi, D., Clifford, A. J., Silverman-Jones, C. S., and DeLuca, L. M. (1986). Mannosylation of endogenous and exogenous phosphatidic acid by liver microsomal membranes. *J. Biol. Chem.* **261**, 3490–3500.

Crow, J. A., Ong, D. E., and Chytil, F. (1987). Specificity of cellular retinol-binding protein in the transfer of retinol to nuclei and chromatin. *Arch. Biochem. Biophys.* **254**, 372–375.

DeLuca, L. M. (1977). The direct involvement of vitamin A in glycosyl transfer reactions of mammalian membranes. *Vitam. Hormon.* **35**, 1–57.

Derman, E., Krauter, K., Walling, L., Weinberger, C., Ray, M., and Darnell, J. E., Jr. (1981). Transcriptional control in the production of liver-specific mRNAs. *Cell* **23**, 731–739.

Dowling, J. E., and Wald, C. (1960). The role of vitamin A acid. *Vitam. Hormon.* **18**, 515–541.

Fuchs, E., and Green, H. (1981). Regulation of terminal differentiation of cultured human keratinocytes by vitamin A. *Cell* **25**, 617–625.

Hustead, G. A., Gutcher, G. R., Anderson, S. A., and Zachman, R. D. (1984). Relationship of vitamin A (retinol) status to lung disease in the preterm infant. *J. Pediatr.* **105**, 610–615.
Jetten, A. M. (1986). Induction of differentiation of embryonal carcinoma cells by retinoids. *In* "Retinoids and Cell Differentiation" (M. I. Sherman, ed.), pp. 106–159. CRC Press, Inc., Boca Raton, Florida.
Knox, W. E. (1972). "Enzyme Patterns in Fetal, Adult, and Neoplastic Rat Tissues." Karger, Basel.
Kylberg, H. K., Ong, D. E., and Chytil, F. (1981). Cellular retinol binding protein during postnatal development of the rat small intestine. *Biol. Neonate* **39**, 100–104.
Liau, G., Ong, D. E., and Chytil, F. (1981). Interaction of the retinol cellular retinol-binding protein complex with isolated nuclei and nuclear compounds. *J. Cell Biol.* **91**, 63–68.
Lotan, R. (1980). Effects of vitamin A and its analogues (retinoids) on normal and neoplastic cells. *Biochim. Biophys. Acta* **605**, 33–91.
Moore, T. (1967). Effect of vitamin A deficiency in animals. *In* "The Vitamins" (W. H. Sebrell and R. S. Harris, eds.), pp. 245–266. Academic Press, New York.
Murtaugh, M. P., Mehta, K., Johnson, J., Myers, M., Juliano, R. J., and Davies, P. J. A. (1983). Induction of tissue transglutaminase in mouse peritoneal macrophages. *J. Biol. Chem.* **258**, 11074–11081.
Northway, W. H., Rosan, R. O., and Porter, D. (1967). Pulmonary disease following respiratory therapy of hyaline membrane disease. *N. Engl. J. Med.* **276**, 357–368.
Olson, J. A., Gunning, D. B., and Tilton, R. A. (1984). Liver concentrations of vitamin A and carotenoids, as a function of age and other parameters, of American children who died of various causes. *Amer. J. Clin. Nutr.* **39**, 903–910.
Omori, M., and Chytil, F. (1982). Mechanism of vitamin A action: gene expression in retinol-deficient rats. *J. Biol. Chem.* **257**, 14370–14374.
Ong, D. E., and Chytil, F. (1975). Retinoic acid binding protein in rat tissue. *J. Biol. Chem.* **250**, 6113–6117.
Ong, D. E., and Chytil, F. (1976). Changes in levels of cellular retinol-binding and retinoic acid-binding proteins of liver and lung during perinatal development. *Proc. Nat. Acad. Sci. USA* **73**, 3976–3978.
Oppenheimer, J. H. (1983). The nuclear receptor-triiodothyronine complex: relationship to thyroid hormone distribution, metabolism, and biological action. *In* "Molecular Basis of Thyroid Hormone Action" (J. H. Oppenheimer and H. H. Samuels, eds.), pp. 1–34. Academic Press, New York.
Peck, G. L. (1984). Synthetic retinoids in dermatology. *In* "The Retinoids" (M. B. Sporn and A. B. Roberts, eds.), Vol. 2, pp. 391–411. Academic Press, New York.
Porter, S. B., Ong, D. E., and Chytil, F. (1986). Vitamin A status affects chromatin structure. *Internat. J. Vit. Nutr. Res.* **56**, 11–20.
Powell, J. T., and Whitney, P. L. (1980). Postnatal development of rat lung. *Biochem. J.* **188**, 1–8.
Roels, O. A. (1967). Biochemical systems. *In* "The Vitamins" (W. H. Sebrell and R. S. Harris, eds.), Vol. 1, pp. 167–245. Academic Press, New York.
Samuels, H. H. (1983). Identification and characterization of thyroid receptors and action using cell culture techniques. *In* "Molecular Basis of Thyroid Hormone Action" (J. H. Oppenheimer and H. H. Samuels, eds.), pp. 35–65. Academic Press, New York.
Shah, R. S., and Rajalakshmi, R. (1984). Vitamin A status of the newborn in relation to gestation age, body weight, and maternal nutritional status. *Amer. J. Clin. Nutr.* **40**, 794–800.
Shenai, J. P., Chytil, F., and Stahlman, M. T. (1985a). Liver vitamin A reserves of very low birth weight neonates. *Pediatr. Res.* **19**, 892–893.
Shenai, J. P., Chytil, F., and Stahlman, M. T. (1985b). Vitamin A status of neonates with bronchopulmonary dysplasia. *Pediatr. Res.* **19**, 185–188.

Shenai, J. P., Kennedy, K. A., Chytil, F., and Stahlman, M. T. (1987). A clinical trial of vitamin A supplementation in infants susceptible to bronchopulmonary dysplasia. *J. Pediatr.* **111**, 269–277.

Sherman, D. R., Lloyd, R. S., and Chytil, F. (1987). Rat cellular retinol-binding protein gene: cDNA sequence and rapid retinol-dependent accumulation of mRNA. *Proc. Nat. Acad. Sci. USA* **84**, 3209–3213.

Sherman, M. I. (1986). How do retinoids promote differentiation? *In* "Retinoids and Cell Differentiation" (M. I. Sherman, ed.), pp. 161–186. CRC Press, Inc., Boca Raton, Florida.

Sporn, M. B., Dunlop, N. M., Newton, D. L., and Smith, J. M. (1976). Prevention of chemical carcinogenesis by vitamin A and its synthetic analogs (retinoids). *Fed. Proc.* **35**, 1332–1338.

Stahlman, M. T. (1984). Chronic lung disease following hyaline membrane disease. *In* "Neonatal Medicine" (L. Stern and P. Vert, eds.), pp. 454–473. Masson Publ. USA, New York.

Strickland, S., and Mahdavi, V. (1978). The induction of differentiation in teratocarcinoma stem cells by retinoic acid. *Cell* **15**, 393–403.

Takahashi, Y. I., Smith, J. E., and Goodman, D. S. (1977). Vitamin A and retinol binding protein metabolism during fetal development in the rat. *Amer. J. Physiol.* **233**, E263–E272.

Takase, S., Ong, D. E., and Chytil, F. (1979). Cellular retinol-binding protein allows specific interaction of retinol with the nucleus *in vitro*. *Proc. Nat. Acad. Sci. USA* **76**, 2204–2208.

Takase, S., Ong, D. E., and Chytil, F. (1986). Transfer of retinoic acid from its complex with cellular retinoic acid-binding protein to the nucleus. *Arch. Biochem. Biophys.* **247**, 328–334.

Thaller, C., and Eichele, G. (1987). Identification and spatial distribution of retinoids in the developing chick limb bud. *Nature* **327**, 625–629.

Thompson, J. N., Howell, J. M., and Pitt, G. A. (1964). Vitamin A and reproduction in rats. *Proc. R. Soc. Biol.* **159**, 510–535.

Wald, G. (1968). Molecular basis of visual excitation. *Science* **162**, 230–239.

Wolbach, S. B. (1937). The pathologic changes resulting from vitamin deficiency. *J. Am. Med. Assn.* **108**, 7–17.

Wolbach, S. B., and Howe, P. R. (1925). Tissue changes following deprivation of fat-soluble vitamin A. *J. Exp. Med.* **42**, 753–777.

Wolbach, S. B., and Howe, P. R. (1933). Epithelial repair in recovery from vitamin A deficiency. *J. Exp. Med.* **57**, 511–526.

# 3

# Micronutrients, Chromatin Alterations, and Cancer

C. Elizabeth Castro

*Nutritional Sciences Division*
*University of California, Los Angeles*
*School of Public Health*
*Los Angeles, California*



## I. CHROMATIN AND GENE EXPRESSION

The eukaryotic genetic apparatus is extremely dynamic. Alterations may occur by mutations resulting from substitutions, deletions, frameshifts, gene amplification, translocations, sister chromatid exchanges, viral integration, and DNA repair processes. The precise relationship between chromatin or chromosomal alterations and tumorigenesis is far from understood. However, the structural configuration of chromatin is a key factor in its alteration and in the regulation of gene expression. Alteration of chromatin may confer a primary, or *coarse*, level of gene regulation preceding the processes of *fine* regulation (Weintraub, 1985). Specific and/or global changes in chromatin structure probably preface the regulation of gene expression.

The condensation of approximately 50 cm of DNA in a eukaryotic nucleus of 10 $\mu$m diameter is achieved by an elaborate hierarchy of organization (Berlin *et al.*, 1982; Igo-Kemenes *et al.*, 1982; McGhee *et al.*, 1980). Extensive, in-depth reviews describe chromatin arrangement in the nucleus (Nelson *et al.*, 1986; Castro, 1987a; Castro, 1987b). This discussion centers on the impact of selected micronutrients on chromatin structure.

Early studies of dietary effects on chromatin first examined the role of starvation or feeding patterns on the chromatin template. Barbiroli and associates (1973a) demonstrated that liver cells respond to food intake with an increased rate of RNA synthesis that could be ascribed to increased availability of the chromatin template (Barbiroli *et al.*, 1973b; Barbiroli *et al.*, 1975) and to increased activity of preexisting RNA polymerase molecules (Barbiroli *et al.*, 1975). It was further demonstrated that refeeding after a 16-hour fast induced changes in the ultraviolet absorption spectra of liver chromatin (Barbiroli *et al.*, 1976).

It was later shown that changes in the macronutrient components of diets fed to rats altered the higher order organization of liver chromatin. Sensitivity to micrococcal nuclease (EC3.1.31.1) is one measure of alteration of chromatin structure. Micrococcal nuclease preferentially cleaves transcriptionally active chromatin (Bloom and Anderson, 1978). Diets with varied proportions of fat, protein, or carbohydrate altered the sensitivity of rat liver chromatin to nuclease in a diet-dependent manner (Castro and Sevall, 1980). A carbohydrate-rich, fat-free diet increased the sensitivity of chromatin to digestion by nuclease, indicating a more diffuse state of chromatin. In contrast, protein-free diets containing low or adequate carbohydrate decreased sensitivity, indicating increased condensation of chromatin. This phenomenon was reproducible regardless of age (Fig. 1). Chromatin from rats fed a protein-free, low-carbohydrate diet was digested to mononucleosome (the fundamental packaging unit of eukaryotic chromatin) at a reduced rate compared with that of chromatin from control rats (Castro, 1983).

The enhanced condensation of chromatin associated with low-protein diets is particularly interesting with respect to human health. In developing countries, such diets are common for children after weaning. However, the nutrients responsible for specific chromatin alterations remain to be identified. It is known, for example, that the level of dietary protein also affects the availability of trace minerals like zinc (Zn). Rats retained less less of a dose of $^{65}$Zn when fed a low-protein diet than when fed a high-protein diet (Van Campen and House, 1974; Chan *et al.*, 1979). Further,

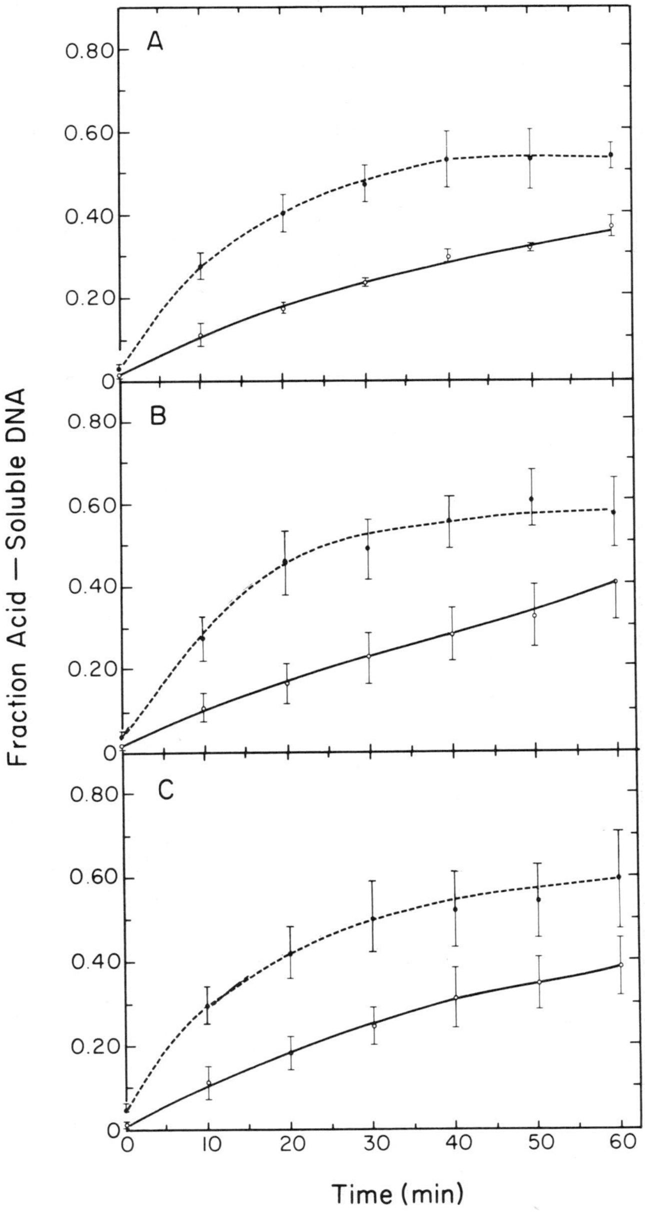


**Fig. 1.** Liver nuclei were isolated from AXC rats fed a basal diet (● - - - ●) or a protein-free, low-carbohydrate diet (○-----○). Panel A shows two-month-old rats, panel B shows 12-month-old rats, and panel C shows 24-month-old rats. (Data from unpublished observations.)

this phenomenon is complicated by the composition of the protein sources. Snedeker and Greger (1983) showed that zinc absorption is greater when rats are fed a high-protein diet (45% lactalbumin) or a low-protein diet (15% lactalbumin) supplemented with histidine, proline, and cysteine than when they are fed a low-protein diet supplemented with only proline or proline and histidine.

Therefore, we tested the possibility that the increased nuclease sensitivity, and hence the altered higher order organization of chromatin associated with feeding protein-free diets to rats, is related to secondary deficiencies of zinc and magnesium (Mg), trace minerals that are critical for maintaining chromatin structure and function.

## II. ZINC DEFICIENCY AND CHROMATIN STRUCTURE

### A. Nuclease Sensitivity

Zinc deficiency can be established in young rats by feeding a low-zinc diet (0.9 ppm) for 28 days (Castro *et al.*, 1986a). One group of control rats was fed *ad libitum* a 40 ppm zinc-supplemented diet, while a second control group was fed the zinc-supplemented diet in the same amount as that consumed by the zinc-deficient group. This second control group constituted a pair-fed cohort, which was necessary because zinc deficiency causes low food intake and hence decreased weight gain. When liver nuclei were isolated from zinc-deficient rats and digested with micrococcal nuclease, only 35% of total chromatin was rendered acid-soluble by the enzyme, compared with 54% of that from pair-fed and 45% of that from *ad libitum*-fed controls (Castro *et al.*, 1986b). The amount of acid-soluble DNA after micrococcal nuclease digestion in nuclei of zinc-deficient rats was quantitatively similar to that from rats fed a protein-free, low-carbohydrate diet (Castro and Sevall, 1980).

Decreased nuclease sensitivity associated with zinc deficiency has also been demonstrated in a lower eukaryote, *Euglena gracilis* (Stankiewicz *et al.*, 1983). Micrococcal nuclease digested *E. gracilis* chromatin grown in zinc-containing medium 10 to 30 times faster than chromatin grown in zinc-depleted medium. Zinc deficiency in *E. gracilis* was related to repression of genome function and transcription (Falchuk *et al.*, 1975) and to virtual extinction of histone proteins (Mazus *et al.*, 1984).

With regard to potential mechanisms, zinc ions have been shown to condense chicken erythrocyte chromatin from a 10 nm fiber into a 30 nm solenoid (Sen and Crothers, 1986a). Zinc ligands, such as zinc chloride–diethylenetriamine or zinc chloride–tris(2-aminoethyl)amine, were efficient inducers *in vitro* of Z-form DNA (Fazakerley, 1984; Zacharias *et al.*, 1982;

Russell *et al.*, 1983). Such ligands can bind to alternating purine-pyrimidine sequences [poly (dG-dC)] and shift a right-handed B form of DNA to a left-handed Z form (Fazakerley, 1984). Recently, zinc was shown to promote sequence-directed DNA bending of a 200 base pair (bp) segment from *Crithidia fasciculata* kinetoplast minicircles (Laundon and Griffith, 1987). When this segment of DNA was flanked by 207 bp by plasmid DNA on one side and 460 bp on the other side, the fraction with the most extreme bend measured by electron microscopy was increased from 2% to 50% by increasing the concentration of zinc or of cobalt, barium, or manganese. The prominent effect of zinc in promoting bending may be relevant to the exciting discovery that several DNA-binding proteins contain zinc bound to regions that strongly interact with the DNA molecule.

## B. DNA-Binding Proteins

Zinc may play a role in gene expression by maintaining the stability and function of DNA-binding proteins. Transcription factor IIIA (TFIIIA) from *Xenopus laevis* was the first eukaryotic transcription factor to be sequenced (Miller *et al.*, 1985; Wu and Wu, 1987). It facilitates RNA polymerase III transcription of 5S RNA *in vitro.* 5S is synthesized by immature *Xenopus* oocytes prior to synthesis of other rRNAs. The 5S RNA complexes with TFIIIA and activates the transcription of the 5S gene by binding to an internal control region (Sakonju *et al.*, 1980). Proteolytic digestion of TFIIIA yields intermediate products spaced at 3K intervals. Based upon this characteristic pattern and on the presence of 7 to 11 zinc atoms per molecule, Miller and associates (1985) proposed that TFIIIA contains repetitive zinc-binding domains. The linear pattern of these repetitive folding domains, each centered on a zinc ion, allows TFIIIA to bind an internal control region of the 5S gene and stay bound during the passage of an RNA polymerase molecule. The DNA sequence bound by TFIIIA contains a corresponding repeat with a periodicity of 5 bp (Rhodes and Klug, 1986).

The repetitive structural motif of TFIIIA occurs in other nucleic-acid binding proteins. A zinc-binding sequence is inherent in the single-stranded DNA-binding protein, gene32 protein (g32P), required for replication, recombination, and translational control in the phage T4 life cycle (Coleman *et al.*, 1987). Berg (1986) has identified sequences that are putative metal-binding domains in five classes of proteins involved in nucleic-acid binding or gene regulation. These proteins, including liver alcohol dehydrogenase, aspartate carbamoyltransferase, metallothionein, rubredoxin, superoxide dismutase, and others, contain short Cys or His sequences that provide two ligands to single metal ions. Histone H3 also has a similar conserved sequence, Cys-Ala-Ile-His (Saavedra, 1986).

Because each nucleosome has two molecules of H3, the apposition of the two H3 sequences yields a potential structure capable of coordinating a metal ion. Saavedra (1986) postulated that the two copies of H3, interacting through the coordination of a metal ion, suggest that other interactions that effect gene expression may occur within the nucleosome.

Another zinc-containing nucleic-acid-binding protein is poly(A) polymerase, an enzyme essential for eukaryotic mRNA processing. As a constituent of this enzyme, zinc may exert a role in tumorigenesis (Wu and Wu, 1987). Rose and associates (1978) have measured two to three times the amount of zinc in poly(A) polymerase from Morris hepatoma as in the corresponding liver enzyme.

Histone H1 is another nucleoprotein essential for maintaining higher order chromatin structure. The most diverse of all the histones, it consists of at least five closely related molecular subtypes (Bustin and Cole, 1968) that differ in amino-acid sequence (Cole, 1984), molecular size, and postsynthetic modifications (Lennox *et al.*, 1982; Langan, 1982). Rodent liver contains at least six different types of H1, with H1.1, H1.2, and H1° the most abundant (Lennox, 1984; Roche *et al.*, 1985). The H1 subvariant profiles vary during developmental growth, partial pancreatectomy, liver regeneration, or tumorigenicity (Larue *et al.*, 1983; Lennox and Cohen, 1983; Ohba *et al.*, 1984; Varricchio *et al.*, 1977; Tan *et al.*, 1982).

We examined whether nutritional zinc deficiency would alter the histone H1 pattern in rat liver. Histone H1 was isolated from the liver of zinc-deficient, control, and pair-fed-control rats by the method of Goodwin and associates (1977). The H1 class of histones was separated by polyacrylamide gel electrophoresis in the presence of sodium dodecyl sulfate (Fig. 2) (Castro *et al.*, 1986a). Densitometric scanning (Fig. 3) indicated that the relative ratio of the subvariants was altered in zinc deficiency. The proportion of H1° to total H1 was 5.6% from *ad libitum*-fed and 7.8% from pair-fed rat liver, in general agreement with the 7% measured in normal adult rat liver (Roche *et al.*, 1985). By contrast, the proportion of H1° to total H1 from zinc-deficient rat liver was 3.8%. This reduced relative ratio of H1° may be responsible for the altered chromatin structure reflected in increased resistance to micrococcal nuclease.

The potential relevance of decreased histone H1° associated with zinc deficiency may lie in promoting varied chromatin structures that may be important in regulating gene expression and cell differentiation (Lennox, 1984; Jin and Cole, 1986). It has been demonstrated that H1° segregates nonrandomly on chromatin, is depleted in template-inactive chromatin, and is enriched in template-active chromatin (Delabar, 1985). Variable H1 subtypes may be a coarse control mechanism that precludes the necessity for fine control in genomic regions that are infrequently or never expressed (Newrock *et al.*, 1978; Weintraub, 1985). Rudimentary control of gene

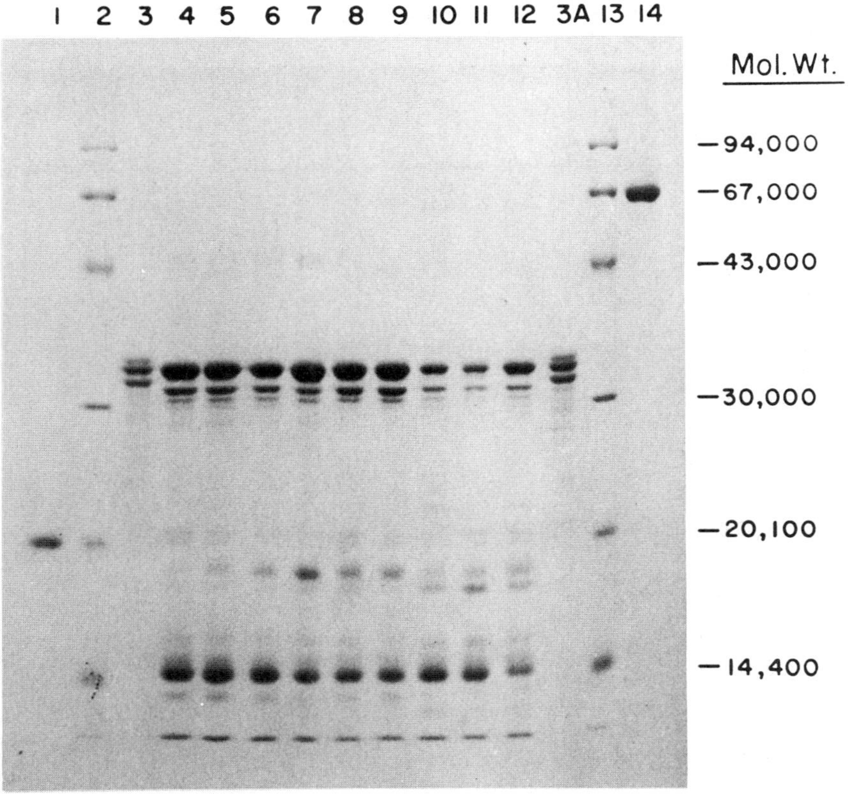


**Fig. 2.** Histone H1 was isolated from liver of zinc-deficient, pair-fed control, or control rats. Lane 1 is 5 μg soybean trypsin inhibitor; lanes 2 and 13 are 5 μg molecular weight standards; lanes 3 and 3A are 3 μg bovine histone H1; lanes 4–6 are 5 μg protein from *ad libitum*-fed control rats; lanes 7–9 are 5 μg protein from pair-fed control rats; lanes 10–12 are 5 μg protein from zinc-deficient rats; lane 14 is 2 μg bovine serum albumin. (From Castro *et al.*, 1986a. Reprinted with permission.)

expression afforded by H1 subvariants may coexist with precise control mechanisms necessary for specific gene regulation.

## C. Zinc Deficiency and Cancer

Zinc is essential for many mechanisms involved in regulating DNA replication and transcription. In teratogenesis, the primary effects of zinc deficiency are probably exerted in nucleic-acid and protein synthesis (Hurley, 1981). In tumorigenesis, zinc deficiency may affect both DNA replication and RNA polymerization, as well as regulation of gene

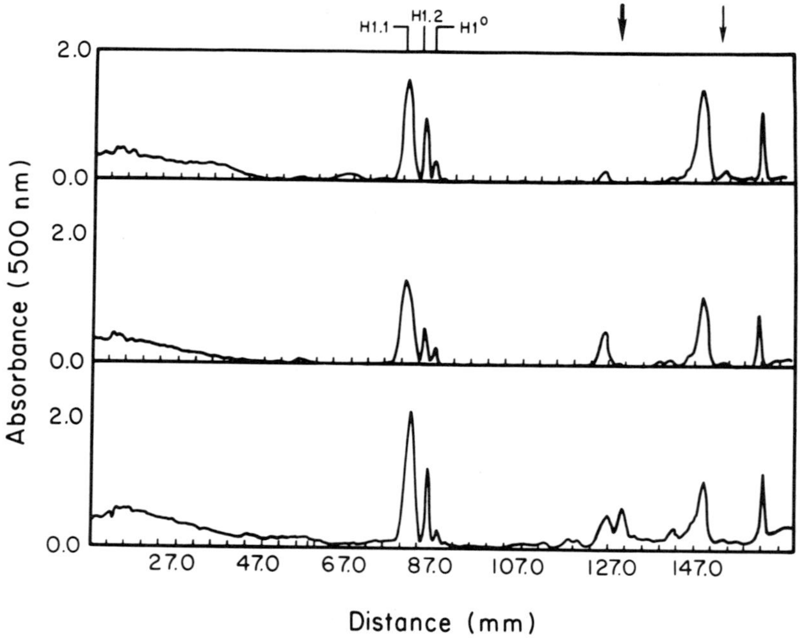


**Fig. 3.** Densitometric scan of a portion of the gel in Fig. 2 shows absorbance of histone H1 proteins from *ad libitum*-fed rat (top panel), pair-fed rat (center panel), and zinc-deficient rat (bottom panel). The relative amount of the H1° subvariant to the total of H1.1 + H1.2 + H1° is reduced in zinc deficiency to 50% of the comparable ratio from rats pair-fed a zinc-supplemented diet ($p = 0.05$). (Data from unpublished observations.)

expression, as exemplified by the role of zinc in DNA-binding transcription factors or in proteins essential for chromatin structure. Furthermore, the roles of zinc in transcription and nucleic-acid synthesis as well as in maintaining chromatin organization dictate that the micronutrient exhibit major influence over gene expression in many cell types, including cells involved in immune function (Fraker *et al.*, 1986).

Not unexpectedly, zinc has a variable role in tumorigenesis. Zinc deficiency inhibited the growth of solid tumors in certain rodent models (McQuitty *et al.*, 1970). When the Walker 256/M1 tumor was transplanted into zinc-deficient rats, the ratio of tumor-to-carcass weight was significantly less than in control rats (Mills *et al.*, 1981). When rats were implanted with R323OAC mammary adenocarcinoma and consequently made zinc deficient, tumor growth was inhibited approximately 35% (Mills *et al.*, 1984a).

In contrast, zinc deficiency enhanced methylbenzylnitrosamine-induced esophageal carcinogenesis in rats (Schrager *et al.*, 1986). Here the enhancement is probably related to hyperplasia in the stratified squamous epithelium of the esophagus induced by zinc deficiency (Hurley, 1981). In another case in which Balb/c mice were inoculated with an allogeneic tumor from DBA/2 mice, zinc deficiency enhanced tumorigenesis. However, the mechanism was related to a reduction in T-cell-mediated cytotoxicity (Frost *et al.*, 1981). Zinc deficiency clearly affects tumorigenic processes in a multitude of ways, depending on the state of cellular proliferation of host and tumor and on other variables.

## III. MAGNESIUM DEFICIENCY AND CHROMATIN STRUCTURE

A major feature of chromatin condensation is one of charge neutralization. Chromatin packaging is promoted by the addition of cations to the negatively charged chromatin fiber (Lewis and Laemmli, 1982; Sen and Crothers, 1986a). Maintenance of the 30-nm solenoidal structure of chromatin depends on the presence of a monovalent cation concentration of at least 50 m*M* (Thoma *et al.*, 1979) or a divalent cation concentration of at least 0.2 m*M* (Sen and Crothers, 1986a; Ausio *et al.*, 1984).

The magnesium ion is a very efficient promoter of chromatin folding. Higher order structure was induced by 0.3 m*M* of magnesium compared with 75 m*M* for sodium chloride (Ausio *et al.*, 1984). In fact, other multivalent cations, including spermine and spermidine, will compact chromatin. The concentration of multivalent ion required for optimal compaction decreases as cationic charge increases (Sen and Crothers, 1986a).

### A. Nuclease Sensitivity

We have investigated the effect of a nutritional deficiency of magnesium on compaction of the chromatin fiber *in vivo*. We established magnesium deficiency in rats by feeding a diet containing approximately 30 ppm of magnesium for 16 or 45 days (Teklad Test Diets, Madison, WI). A control diet containing 650 ppm of magnesium was fed *ad libitum* to a second group. Liver nuclei were isolated and incubated with 1 U micrococcal nuclease/0.4 $\mu$g nuclear DNA for 0 to 60 minutes.

Table I shows that the maximum percentage of nuclease-solubilized chromatin from liver of magnesium-deficient rats after 16 days of magnesium deficiency was 38.7 $\pm$ 4.4%. This value was similar to the amount of acid-soluble DNA generated from rats fed a protein-free diet or a zinc-deficient diet. When rats were fed a magnesium control diet, 49.4 $\pm$ 4.6% of the chromatin was solubilized (unpublished observation). These results demonstrate that a magnesium-deficient diet alters the higher order compaction of liver chromatin.

TABLE I

**Percentage of Acid-Soluble Liver DNA from Rats Fed Magnesium-Deficient or Control Diets**[a]

| | | Percent Acid-Soluble DNA | | |
|---|---|---|---|---|
| Minutes | Micrococcal Nuclease | Control | Mg Deficient 16 days | Mg Deficient 45 days |
| 0 | + | 4.51 ± 1.29 (*n* = 12) | 3.97 ± 1.17 (*n* = 9) | 4.90 ± 1.00 (*n* = 3) |
| 10 | + | 33.08 ± 4.59 (*n* = 12) | 27.76 ± 5.45 (*n* = 8) | 23.02 ± 1.64 (*n* = 3) |
| 20 | + | 42.32 ± 4.28 (*n* = 12) | 36.38 ± 4.67 (*n* = 9) | 33.69 ± 4.62 (*n* = 3) |
| 40 | + | 48.35 ± 2.85 (*n* = 12) | 38.65 ± 4.41 (*n* = 9) | 42.46 ± 0.97 (*n* = 3) |
| 60 | + | 49.35 ± 4.61 (*n* = 12) | 38.35 ± 7.57 (*n* = 8) | 46.35 ± 1.17 (*n* = 3) |
| 0 | — | 0.94 ± 0.57 (*n* = 10) | 1.06 ± 0.52 (*n* = 9) | 0.88 ± 0.26 (*n* = 3) |
| 60 | — | 1.28 ± 0.68 (*n* = 8) | 1.80 ± 0.71 (*n* = 9) | 1.23 ± 0.03 (*n* = 2) |

[a]Data from unpublished observations.

Surprisingly, after 45 days of magnesium deficiency, 46.4 ± 1.2% of the DNA was solubilized by micrococcal nuclease. This percentage was similar to control values. At least two explanations seemed plausible. After the extended period of magnesium deficiency, the animals' adaptation to reduced food intake and body weight may have produced a response similar to that produced by starvation. However, the similar body weights for all three groups at the end of the feeding period did not support this conclusion. Alternatively, the extended deficiency may have resulted in mobilization of magnesium from bone because bone is a source of easily available magnesium in rats, although availability decreases with age (Ferment and Touitou, 1985). If this mobilization occurred, it would mean that the effects of magnesium deficiency on higher order chromatin structure are reversible.

## B. Histone H1

Higher order chromatin compaction depends on histone H1 as well as on cation concentration. H1 binds to DNA as the fiber enters and exits the nucleosome (Boulikas *et al.*, 1980). We isolated histone H1 from liver of control rats and of rats made magnesium-deficient for 16 days or 45 days and separated the proteins on polyacrylamide gels (Fig. 4). The histone H1 family exhibited an $M_r$ of 30,000 to 34,000. Two additional electrophoretic species in the H1 class were seen more clearly in densitometric scan of representative lanes (Fig. 5). The electrophoretic pattern seen after 45 days was consistent with nuclease digestion experiments in which the percentage of acid-soluble DNA after 45 days approached that of control liver (Table I).

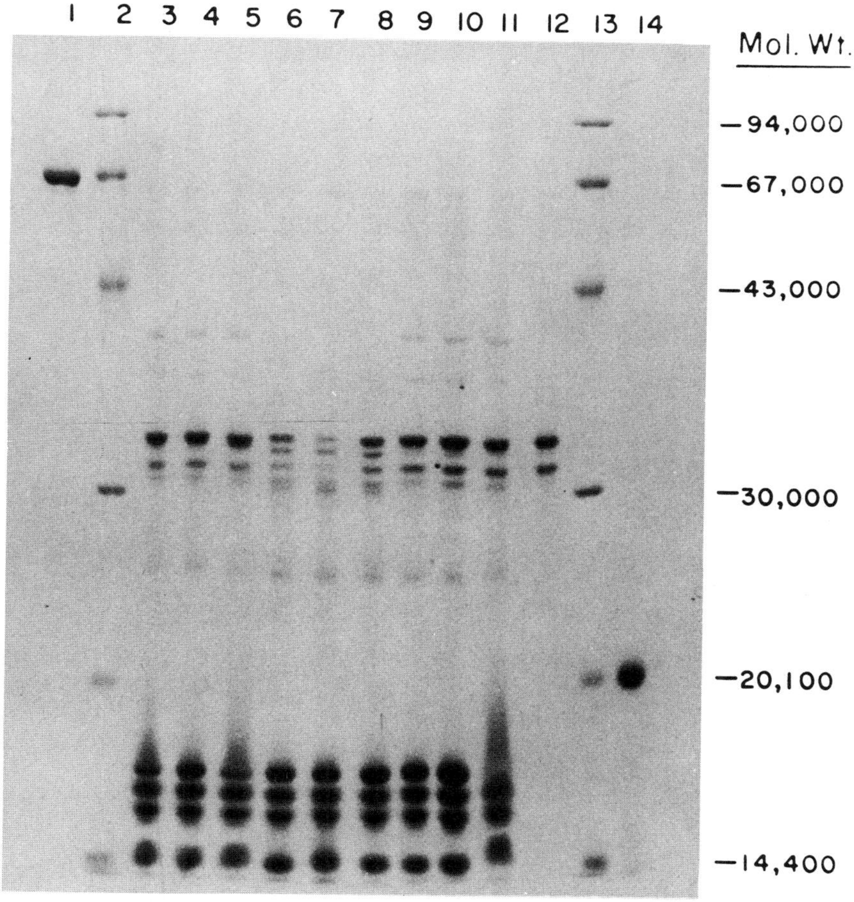


**Fig. 4.** Histone H1 proteins were isolated from magnesium-deficient or control rats. Lanes 1–2 and 12–14 contain molecular weight standards. (For orientation of the H1 family of proteins, bovine H1 is in lane 12.) Lanes 3–5 are 10 μg nuclear proteins from three control rats; lanes 6–8 are 10 μg proteins from rats fed magnesium-deficient diet for 16 days; lanes 9–11 are 10 μg protein from rats fed magnesium-deficient diet for 45 days. (Data from unpublished observations.)

## C. Relevance to Cancer

Although the biological significance of molecular changes induced by magnesium deficiency are unclear, they may relate to the prominent role of magnesium in growth processes. The rates of DNA, RNA, and protein biosynthesis were inhibited in magnesium-deficient cells (Ebel and Gunther, 1980). Our results provide evidence that inhibition is associated with altered chromatin compaction and changes in histone H1, a nucleoprotein essential for chromatin condensation.

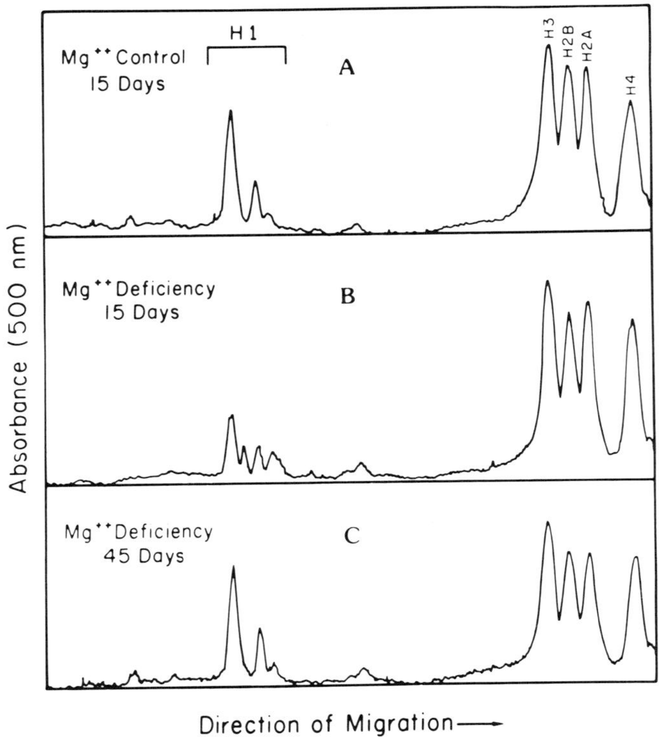


**Fig. 5.** Densitometric scan shows absorbance of H1 proteins isolated from control rats (panel A), rats made magnesium ($Mg^{2+}$)-deficient for 16 days (panel B), and rats made magnesium-deficient for 45 days (panel C). (Data from unpublished observations.)

An understanding of the molecular changes caused by magnesium deficiency is important to understanding tumorigenesis. Growth of transplanted Yoshida hepatoma and Walker's sarcoma was inhibited by magnesium deficiency (Young and Parsons, 1977). Similarly, the growth of an established mammary adenocarcinoma (R3230AC) was inhibited 46% after rats were made magnesium deficient (Mills *et al.*, 1984b). In addition, the degree of condensation of chromatin conferred by magnesium may influence the DNA-binding capacity of various drugs (Sen and Crothers, 1986b). Such drugs may have pharmacological function or DNA-damaging potential (Castro, 1987a; Castro, 1987b).

## IV. SUMMARY

The higher order compaction of chromatin is an integral feature of gene expression and regulation. Deficiencies of several nutrients, including protein, zinc, and magnesium, alter the higher order configuration of chromatin determined by nuclease sensitivity and are associated with alterations in histone H1 proteins. An understanding of the molecular basis by which micronutrients alter chromatin is essential because this may offer an opportunity to intervene in the processes of tumorigenesis.

## ACKNOWLEDGMENTS

The author thanks Jacqueline Armstrong and Maria Ramirez-Ortega for technical assistance.

## REFERENCES

Ausio, J., Borochov, N., Seger, D., and Eisenberg, H. (1984). Interaction of chromatin with NaCl and $MgCl_2$. Solubility and binding studies, transition to and characterization of the higher-order structure. *J. Mol. Biol.* **177**, 373–398.

Barbiroli, B., Moruzzi, M. S., Monti, M. G., and Tadolini, B. (1973a). Diurnal rhythmicity of mammalian DNA-dependent RNA polymerase activities I and II: Dependence on food intake. *Biochem. Biophys. Res. Commun.* **54**, 62–68.

Barbiroli, B., Monti, M. G., Tadolini, B., and Moruzzi, M. S. (1973b). Regulation of RNA synthesis in the liver of rats maintained under controlled feeding schedules. *FEBS Lett.* **37**, 159–161.

Barbiroli, B., Tadolini, B., Moruzzi, M. S., and Monti, M. G. (1975). Modification of the template capacity of liver chromatin for form-B ribonucleic acid polymerase by food intake in rats under controlled feeding schedules. *Biochem. J.* **146**, 687–696.

Barbiroli, B., Monti, M. G., Moruzzi, M. S., Tadolini, B., and Mezzetti, G. (1976). Food-induced changes in UV-absorption spectra of isolated chromatin from liver of rats under controlled feeding schedules. *Experientia* **32**, 442–443.

Berg, J. M. (1986). Potential metal-binding domains in nucleic acid binding proteins. *Science* **232**, 485–487.

Berlin, J., Castro, C. E., Bailey, F., and Sevall, J. S. (1982). Adaptation of rat parenchymal hepatocyte to nutritional variation: Quantitation by stereology. *Nutr. Res.* **2**, 51–63.

Bloom, K. S., and Anderson, J. N. (1978). Fractionation of hen oviduct chromatin into transcriptionally active and inactive regions after selective micrococcal nuclease digestion. *Cell* **15**, 141–150.

Boulikas, T., Wiseman, J. M., and Garrard, W. T. (1980). Points of contact between histone H1 and the histone octamer. *Proc. Nat. Acad. Sci. USA* **77**, 127–131.

Bustin, M., and Cole, R. D. (1968). The applicability of extraction by trichloroacetic acid to the preparation of very lysine-rich histones from the mammary gland. *Arch. Biochem. Biophys.* **127**, 457–462.

Castro, C. E. (1983). Nucleosomal repeat length in rat liver nuclei is decreased by a high carbohydrate, fat-free diet. *J. Nutr.* **113**, 557–565.

Castro, C. E. (1987a). Nutrient effects on DNA and chromatin structure. *Ann. Rev. Nutr.* **7**, 407–421.

Castro, C. E. (1987b). Nutritional influences on chromatin: Toxicological implications. *In* "Nutritional Toxicology" (J. Hathcock, ed.), pp. 129–155. Academic Press, San Diego.

Castro, C. E., and Sevall, J. S. (1980). Alteration of higher order structure of rat liver chromatin by dietary composition. *J. Nutr.* **110**, 105–116.

Castro, C. E., Alvares, O. F., and Sevall, J. S. (1986a). Zinc deficiency decreases histone H1° in rat liver. *Nutr. Rep. Internat.* **34**, 67–74.

Castro, C. E., Armstrong-Major, J., and Ramirez, M. E. (1986b). Diet-mediated alteration of chromatin structure. *Fed. Proc.* **45**, 2394–2398.

Chan, W., Calhoun, N. R., Howard, M. P., and Smith, J. C., Jr. (1979). $^{65}$Zinc retention, plasma and bone zinc concentration: Affected by level of dietary protein in rats [Abstract]. *Fed. Proc.* **38**, 606.

Cole, R. D. (1984). A minireview of microheterogeneity in H1 histone and its possible significance. *Anal. Biochem.* **136**, 24–30.

Coleman, J. E., Giedroc, D. P., Keating, K. M., and Williams, K. R. (1987). Role of zinc in the structure and function of ssDNA binding proteins [Abstract]. *Fed. Proc.* **46**, 2238.

Delabar, J. M. (1985). Nonrandom location of H1-H1° histones on chromatin of mouse liver and brain. *J. Biol. Chem.* **260**, 12622–12628.

Ebel, H., and Gunther, T. (1980). Magnesium metabolism: A review. *J. Clin. Chem. Clin. Biochem.* **18**, 257–270.

Falchuk, K. H., Fawcett, D. W., and Valley, B. L. (1975). Role of zinc in cell division of *Euglena gracilis*. *J. Cell Sci.* **17**, 57–78.

Fazakerley, G. V. (1984). Zinc Z-DNA. *Nucl. Acid Res.* **12**, 3643–3648.

Ferment, O., and Touitou, Y. (1985). Magnesium: Metabolism and hormonal regulation in different species. *Comp. Biochem. Physiol.* **82A**, 753–758.

Fraker, P. J., Jardieu, P., and Wirth, J. (1986). The immunopathobiological consequences of zinc deficiency. *In* "Nutritional Diseases: Research Directions in Comparative Pathobiology" (D. G. Scarpelli and G. Migaki, eds.), pp. 197–213. Alan R. Liss, Inc., New York.

Frost, P., Rabbani, P., Smith, J., and Prasad, A. (1981). Cell mediated cytotoxicity and tumor growth in zinc deficient mice. *Proc. Soc. Exp. Biol. Med.* **167**, 333–341.

Goodwin, G. H., Rabbani, A., Nicolas, R. H., and Johns, E. W. (1977). The isolation of the high mobility group nonhistone chromosomal protein HMG 14. *FEBS Lett.* **80**, 413–416.

Hurley, L. S. (1981). Teratogenic aspects of manganese, zinc, and copper nutrition. *Physiol. Rev.* **61**, 249–295.

Igo-Kemenes, T., Horz, W., and Zachau, H. G. (1982). Chromatin. *Ann. Rev. Biochem.* **51**, 89–121.

Jin, Y., and Cole, R. D. (1986). H1 histone exchange is limited to particular regions of chromatin that differ in aggregation properties. *J. Biol. Chem.* **261**, 3420–3427.

Langan, T. A. (1982). Characterization of highly phosphorylated subcomponents of rat thymus H1 histone. *J. Biol. Chem.* **257**, 14835–14846.

Larue, H., Bissonnette, E., and Belanger, L. (1983). Histone H1° expression during developmental growth of rat liver. *Can. J. Biochem. Cell Biol.* **61**, 1197–1200.

Laundon, C. H., and Griffith, J. D. (1987). Cationic metals promote sequence-directed DNA bending. *Biochemistry* **26**, 3759–3762.

Lennox, R. W. (1984). Differences in evolutionary stability among mammalian H1 subtypes. Implications for the roles of H1 subtypes in chromatin. *J. Biol. Chem.* **259**, 669–672.

Lennox, R. W., and Cohen, L. H. (1983). The histone H1 complements of dividing and non-dividing cells of the mouse. *J. Biol. Chem.* **258**, 262–268.

Lennox, R. W., Oshima, R. G., and Cohen, L. H. (1982). The H1 histones and their interphase phosphorylated states in differentiated and undifferentiated cell lines derived from murine teratocarcinomas. *J. Biol. Chem.* **257**, 5183–5189.

Lewis, C. D., and Laemmli, U. K. (1982). Higher order metaphase chromosome structure: Evidence for metalloprotein interactions. *Cell* **29**, 171–181.

Mazus, B., Falchuk, K. H., and Vallee, B. L. (1984). Histone formation, gene expression, and zinc deficiency in *Euglena gracilis*. *Biochemistry* **23**, 42–47.

McGhee, J. D., Rav, D. C., Charney, E., and Felsenfeld, G. (1980). Orientation of the nucleosome within the higher order structure of chromatin. *Cell* **22**, 87–96.

McQuitty, J. T., DeWys, W. D., Monaco, L., Strain, W. H., and Rob, C. G. (1970). Inhibition of tumor growth by dietary zinc deficiency. *Cancer Res.* **30**, 1387–1390.

Miller, J., McLachlan, A. D., and Klug, A. (1985). Repetitive zinc-binding domains in the protein transcription factor IIIA from *Xenopus* oocytes. *EMBO J.* **4**, 1609–1614.

Mills, B. J., Broghamer, W. L., Higgins, P. J., and Lindeman, R. D. (1981). A specific dietary requirement for the growth of the Walker 256/M1 tumor in the rat. *Amer. J. Clin. Nutr.* **34**, 1661–1669.

Mills, B. J., Broghamer, W. L., Higgins, P. J., and Lindeman, R. D. (1984a). Inhibition of tumor growth by zinc depletion of rats. *J. Nutr.* **114**, 746–752.

Mills, B. J., Broghamer, W. L., Higgins, P. J., and Lindeman, R. D. (1984b). Inhibition of tumor growth by magnesium depletion of rats. *J. Nutr.* **114**, 739–745.

Nelson, W. G., Pienta, K. J., Barrack, E. R., and Coffey, D. S. (1986). The role of the nuclear matrix in the organization and function of DNA. *Ann. Rev. Biophys. Chem.* **15**, 457–475.

Newrock, K. M., Alfageme, C. R., Nardi, R. V., and Cohen, L. H. (1978). Histone changes during chromatin remodeling in embryogenesis. *Cold Spring Harbor Symp. Quant. Biol.* **42**, 421–431.

Ohba, Y. Higurashi, M., and Hayashi, Y. (1984). Phosphorylation of H1 subtypes in regenerating rat liver. *J. Biol. Chem.* **259**, 2942–2948.

Rhodes, D., and Klug, A. (1986). An underlying repeat in some transcriptional control sequences corresponding to half a double helical turn of DNA. *Cell* **46**, 123–132.

Roche, J., Girardet, J.-L., Gorka, C., and Lawrence, J.-J. (1985). The involvement of histone H1° in chromatin structure. *Nucl. Acid Res.* **13**, 2843–2853.

Rose, K. M., Allen, M. S., Crawford, I. L., and Jacob, S. T. (1978). Functional role of zinc in poly(A) synthesis catalysed by nuclear poly(A) polymerase. *Eur. J. Biochem.* **88**, 20–36.

Russell, W. C., Precious, B., Martin, S. R., and Bayley, P. M. (1983). Differential promotion and suppression of Z leads to B transitions in poly [d(G-C)] by histone subclasses, polyamino acids and polyamines. *EMBO J.* **2**, 1647–1653.

Saavedra, R. A. (1986). Histones and metal-binding domains (Letter). *Science* **234**, 1589.

Sakonju, S., Bogenhagen, D. F., and Brown, D. D. (1980). A control region in the center of the 5S RNA gene directs specific initiation of transcription: I. The 5′ border of the region. *Cell* **19**, 13–25.

Schrager, T. F., Busby, W. F., Jr., Goldman, M. E., and Newberne, P. M. (1986). Enhancement of methylbenzylnitrosamine-induced esophageal carcinogenesis in zinc-deficient rats: Effects on incorporation of [$^3$H]thymidine into DNA of esophageal epithelium and liver. *Carcinogenesis* **7**, 1121–1126.

Sen, D., and Crothers, D. M. (1986a). Condensation of chromatin: Role of multivalent cations. *Biochemistry* **25**, 1495–1503.

Sen, D., and Crothers, D. M. (1986b). Influence of DNA-binding drugs on chromatin condensation. *Biochemistry* **25**, 1503–1509.

Snedeker, S. M., and Greger, J. L. (1983). Metabolism of zinc, copper and iron as affected by dietary protein, cysteine and histidine. *J. Nutr.* **113**, 644–652.

Stankiewicz, A. J., Falchuk, K. H., and Vallee, B. L. (1983). Composition and structure of zinc-deficient *Euglena gracilis* chromatin. *Biochemistry* **22**, 5150–5156.

Tan, K. B., Borun, T. W., Charpentier, R., Cristofalo, V. J., and Croce, C. M. (1982). Normal and neoplastic human cells have different histone H1 compositions. *J. Biol. Chem.* **257**, 5337–5338.

Thoma, F., Koller, T., and Klug, A. (1979). Involvement of histone H1 in the organization of the nucleosome and of the salt-dependent superstructures of chromatin. *J. Cell Biol.* **83**, 403–427.

Van Campen, D., and House, W. A. (1974). Effect of a low protein diet on retention of an oral dose of $^{65}$Zn and on tissue concentrations of zinc, iron, and copper in rats. *J. Nutr.* **104**, 84–90.

Varricchio, F., Mabogunje, O., Kim, D., Fortner, J. G., and Fitzgerald, P. J. (1977). Pancreas acinar cell regeneration and histone (H1 and H1°) modifications after partial pancreatectomy or after a protein-free ethionine regimen. *Cancer Res.* **37**, 3964–3969.

Weintraub, H. (1985). Assembly and propagation of repressed and derepressed chromosomal states. *Cell* **42**, 705–711.

Wu, F. Y.-H., and Wu, C.-W. (1987). Zinc in DNA replication and transcription. *Ann. Rev. Nutr.* **7**, 251–272.

Young, G. A., and Parsons, F. M. (1977). The effects of dietary deficiencies of magnesium and potassium on the growth of transplanted tumors and host tissues in the rat. *Eur. J. Cancer* **13**, 103–113.

Zacharias, W., Larson, J. E., Klysik, J., Stirdivant, S. M., and Wells, R. D. (1982). Conditions which cause the right-handed to left-handed DNA conformational transitions. Evidence for several types of left-handed DNA structures in solution. *J. Biol. Chem.* **257**, 2775–2782.

# 4

# Pathogenesis of Megaloblastic Anemias

Victor Herbert

*Mount Sinai School of Medicine*
*New York, New York*
*Bronx Veterans Administration Medical Center*
*Bronx, New York*



## I. INTRODUCTION

Megaloblastic anemia or ''giant germ cell anemia'' is the morphological expression of slowed DNA synthesis resulting from any cause (Herbert, 1985; Herbert and Colman, 1988). For example, drugs like 6-mercaptopurine (6-MP) and 5-fluorouracil (5-FU) which slow DNA synthesis will produce megaloblastosis with enlargement of immature red blood cells in the bone marrow. In more than 95% of cases, however, megaloblastic anemia is caused by deficiencies of vitamin $B_{12}$ (cobalamin) or folic acid (folate). As is the case in all vitamin deficiencies, vitamin $B_{12}$ or folate deficiency may be caused by inadequate ingestion, malabsorption, poor utilization, increased requirement, increased excretion, increased rate of destruction, or a combination of these factors.

## II. DIAGNOSIS OF MEGALOBLASTIC ANEMIA

### A. Vitamin $B_{12}$ Deficiency

In the United States, vitamin $B_{12}$ deficiency most often results from inadequate absorption (Herbert, 1987b; Herbert and Colman, 1988). The most frequent cause of vitamin $B_{12}$ malabsorption is age-dependent loss of gastric secretions of acid, enzymes, and, later, intrinsic factor, which produces a form of megaloblastic anemia called "pernicious anemia." The diagnostic triad for pernicious anemia includes: megaloblastosis, vitamin $B_{12}$ malabsorption caused by inadequate gastric secretions, and a serum "true vitamin $B_{12}$" level below 112 pg/ml. A serum vitamin $B_{12}$ level of 112 pg/ml normally includes about 100 pg/ml of vitamin $B_{12}$ on the storage proteins holohaptocorrin—also known as "holohap," holotranscobalamins (I+III), [TC (I+III)] and holocobalophilin—and about 12 pg/ml of vitamin $B_{12}$ on the delivery protein holotranscobalamin II—also known as "holo-TC II" or "TC II." The prefix "holo" describes the protein with vitamin $B_{12}$ attached, the prefix "apo" describes the protein without vitamin $B_{12}$, and no prefix may mean either or both, depending on the context.

### B. Inability to Absorb Vitamin $B_{12}$ from Food

Free vitamin $B_{12}$ is not found in food. Its absorption from animal protein requires gastric acid and enzymes, which split vitamin $B_{12}$ from food peptides, and intrinsic factor, a glycoprotein secreted by gastric parietal cells, which binds free vitamin $B_{12}$ for intestinal transit to the ileum. Here vitamin $B_{12}$ is released, undergoes intestinal transport, and is bound to transcobalamins for transport to other tissues. Disruption at any step of this process results in vitamin $B_{12}$ malabsorption.

The age-related gastric atrophy that leads to pernicious anemia begins with gradual losses of gastric acid and enzymes, which usually precede the loss of gastric intrinsic factor by months or years. Losses of gastric acid and enzymes decrease the availability of free vitamin $B_{12}$, which is reflected in low serum holo-TC II levels (Herzlich and Herbert, 1988), negative vitamin $B_{12}$ balance, and gradual tissue depletion of vitamin $B_{12}$.

The classic demonstration of vitamin $B_{12}$ malabsorption is the crystalline $B_{12}$ Schilling test. This test involves two stages—feeding free radioactive vitamin $B_{12}$ alone to measure its absorption, and feeding free radioactive vitamin $B_{12}$ with gastric intrinsic factor to correct subnormal vitamin $B_{12}$ absorption. The first stage of the Schilling test remains normal in the early phases of pernicious anemia because even 10% of the normal secretion of intrinsic factor is adequate for absorption of 1 $\mu$g of free vitamin $B_{12}$. Thus, the standard Schilling test is only diagnostic for advanced loss of intrinsic factor.

The inability to absorb bound vitamin $B_{12}$ in food can be diagnosed using a food Schilling test, such as the "omelet Schilling test" devised by Doscherholmen and associates (1976) or a food Schilling test involving any other protein (chicken meat, chicken serum, etc.) to which radioactive vitamin $B_{12}$ is bound. In the omelet Schilling test, free radioactive vitamin $B_{12}$ is added to a raw egg. The radioactive vitamin $B_{12}$ binds to the protein in the egg, which is made into an omelet and fed to the patient. Our studies of aging veterans suggest that most elderly patients with a low serum vitamin $B_{12}$ level but a normal crystalline Schilling test would prove to be unable to absorb vitamin $B_{12}$ from food if given a food Schilling test (Herbert 1987d).

## C. Folate Deficiency

Folate deficiency would rarely occur if everyone had fruit juice or one fresh uncooked fruit or vegetable each day. Folate is ubiquitous in uncooked food but is oxidatively destroyed by prolonged cooking (Herbert, 1987a; Herbert 1987e; Herbert, 1987f). Lightly stir-fried vegetables, as in Chinese wok cooking, retain most of their folate, whereas vegetables cooked for a long time in boiling water do not (Herbert, 1987f).

Clinical conditions such as chronic alcohol consumption may lead to folate deficiency. Alcoholics may become folate deficient via a combination of causes—inadequate nutrition, reduced absorption, and altered hepatobiliary metabolism of folate (Halsted, 1988; Herbert and Colman, 1980). In addition, our group has recently demonstrated that products of alcohol metabolism cause direct destruction of folate (Shaw *et al.*, 1987).

Folate deficiency can produce mental symptoms such as "megaloblastic madness," paranoia, irritability, and forgetfulness, all of which disappear dramatically after one or two days of folate therapy.

## D. Laboratory Tests of Nutrient Status

We have proposed models delineating the sequence of abnormalities in laboratory tests at each stage in the development of vitamin $B_{12}$ or folate deficiency or excess (Herbert, 1987d; Herbert, 1987e; Herbert, 1988; Herbert and Colman, 1988) (Figs. 1 and 2). Because serial changes from

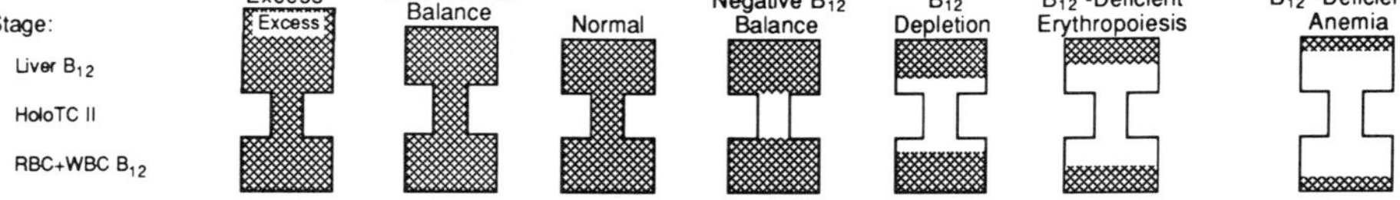


| Stage: | Excess | Positive $B_{12}$ Balance | Normal | Negative $B_{12}$ Balance | $B_{12}$ Depletion | $B_{12}$-Deficient Erythropoiesis | $B_{12}$-Deficiency Anemia |
|---|---|---|---|---|---|---|---|
| HoloTC II (pg/ml) | >50 | >40 | >30 | <20 | <20 | <12 | <12 |
| TC II % sat. | >5% | >5% | >5% | <5% | <2% | <1% | <1% |
| Halohap (pg/ml) | >500 | >300 | >150 | >150 | <150 | <100 | <100 |
| dU Suppression | Normal | Normal | Normal | Normal | Normal | Abnormal | Abnormal |
| Hypersegmentation | No | No | No | No | No | Yes | Yes |
| TBBC % sat. | >50% | >40 | >15% | >15% | >15% | <15% | <10% |
| Hap % sat. | >50% | >40 | >20% | >20% | >20% | <20% | <10% |
| RBC Folate (ng/ml) | >160 | >160 | >160 | >160 | >160 | <140 | <100 |
| Erythrocytes | Normal | Normal | Normal | Normal | Normal | Normal | Macroovalocytic |
| MCV | Normal | Normal | Normal | Normal | Normal | Normal | Elevated |
| Hemoglobin | Normal | Normal | Normal | Normal | Normal | Normal | Low |
| TC II | Normal | Normal | Normal | Normal | Normal | Elevated | Elevated |
| Methylmalonate ↑ | No | No | No | No | No | ? | Yes |
| Myelin Damage | No* | No | No | No | No | ? | Frequent |

**Fig. 1.** This model delineates the biochemical and hematological sequence of changes in laboratory tests as negative vitamin $B_{12}$ balance progresses. The shaded boxes on the first three lines show the relative quantities of vitamin $B_{12}$ in each compartment in normal subjects, and the increasingly unshaded areas show its proportional disappearance during successive stages of development of vitamin $B_{12}$ deficiency. Unshaded boxes enclose laboratory abnormalities that characterize the onset of the stage indicated in the column heading. Laboratory measurements include: liver vitamin $B_{12}$; pg/ml of holotranscobalamin II—transcobalamin II bound to vitamin $B_{12}$ (Holo TC II); white- and red-blood-cell vitamin $B_{12}$ (WBC + RBC $B_{12}$); Percentage of total transcobalamin II bound to vitamin $B_{12}$ (TC II % sat); pg/ml of holohaptocorrin—transcobalamin (I + III) bound to vitamin $B_{12}$ (Holohap); dU suppression, a measure of vitamin $B_{12}$ deficiency in bone marrow or lymphocytes; hypersegmentation, a measure of the increase in lobes in granulocytic white-cell nuclei; total vitamin $B_{12}$ binding capacity of plasma (TBBC % sat); percentage of total TC (I + III) bound to vitamin $B_{12}$ (Hap % sat); ng/ml of red-blood-cell folate (RBC Folate); erythrocytes; mean corpuscular volume (MCV); hemoglobin; TC II; elevation of methylmalonate in serum and urine; and myelin damage. (Copyright 1987, Victor Herbert. Reprinted with permission.)

individual norms precede deviations from the laboratory norm, recognition of individual changes allows for earlier diagnosis (Herbert *et al.*, 1986).

Our vitamin $B_{12}$ model postulates that the earliest abnormality in developing vitamin $B_{12}$ deficiency is loss of the vitamin from its transport protein TC II (Herzlich and Herbert, 1988). Our evidence suggests that as vitamin $B_{12}$ absorption shuts off, absorbed vitamin $B_{12}$ is no longer available to attach to TC II. As a result, vitamin $B_{12}$ is no longer transported to cells, and tissue vitamin $B_{12}$ stores decrease compensatorily. The desaturation of TC II is much more rapid than the desaturation of

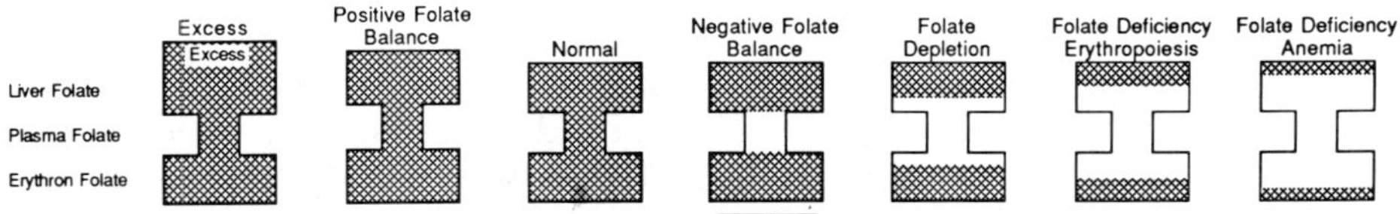


| | Excess | Positive Folate Balance | Normal | Negative Folate Balance | Folate Depletion | Folate Deficiency Erythropoiesis | Folate Deficiency Anemia |
|---|---|---|---|---|---|---|---|
| Serum Folate (ng/ml) | >10 | >10 | >5 | <3 | <3 | <3 | <3 |
| RBC Folate (ng/ml) | >400 | >300 | >200 | >200 | <160 | <120 | <100 |
| Diagnostic dU Suppression | Normal | Normal | Normal | Normal | Normal | Abnormal | Abnormal |
| Lobe Average | <3.5 | <3.5 | <3.5 | <3.5 | <3.5 | >3.5 | >3.5 |
| Liver Folate (μg/g) | >5 | >400 | >3 | >3 | <1.6 | <1.2 | <1 |
| Erythrocytes | Normal | Normal | Normal | Normal | Normal | Normal | Macroovalocytic |
| MCV | Normal | Normal | Normal | Normal | Normal | Normal | Elevated |
| Hemoglobin (g/dL) | >12 | >12 | >12 | >12 | >12 | >12 | <12 |
| Plasma Clearance of Intravenous Folate | Normal | Normal | Normal | Normal | Normal | Increased | Increased |

**Fig. 2.** This model delineates the biochemical and hematological sequence of changes in laboratory tests as negative vitamin folate balance progresses. The shaded boxes on the first three lines show the relative quantities of folate in each compartment in normal subjects, and the increasingly unshaded areas show its proportional disappearance during successive stages of folate deficiency development. Unshaded boxes enclose laboratory abnormalities that characterize the onset of the stage indicated in the column heading. Laboratory measurements include: liver folate; plasma folate; erythron folate; ng/ml of serum folate; red-blood-cell folate (RBC folate); diagnostic dU suppression, a measure of folate deficiency in bone marrow or lymphocytes; lobe average, a measure of hypersegmentation—the increase in lobes in granulocytic white-cell nuclei; mcg/g of liver folate; erythrocytes; mean corpuscular volume (MCV); g/dL of hemoglobin; and plasma clearance of intravenous folate. In our laboratory, 100 normal adults were found to have an arithmetic mean serum folate of 8.125 ± 5.06 ng/ml and a geometric mean serum folate of 6.92, giving a range of 1.89–21.8 ± 2 SD. The same subjects were found to have an arithmetic mean RBC folate of 359.5 ± 158.2 ng/ml and a geometric mean RBC folate of 329.7, giving a range of 129.8–773.3 ± 2 SD. (Copyright 1987, Victor Herbert. Reprinted with permission.)

TC (I+III) because the turnover of vitamin $B_{12}$ on TC II is much more rapid than on TC (I+III). Vitamin $B_{12}$ bound to TC II is analogous to iron bound to transferrin—it is in equilibrium with metabolically active vitamin $B_{12}$ in bone marrow hematopoietic cells via the hematopoietic cell TC II receptors, just as iron bound to transferrin is in equilibrium with transferrin receptors, some of which may circulate (Kohgo *et al.*, 1987). Vitamin $B_{12}$ bound to TC (I+III) appears to be in equilibrium with storage vitamin $B_{12}$, much as iron bound to ferritin is in equilibrium with storage iron. After a period of negative vitamin $B_{12}$ balance, the amount of vitamin $B_{12}$ bound to TC (I+III) falls, just as after a period of negative iron balance, the amount of iron bound to ferritin falls.

## E. Megaloblastosis Hidden by Iron Deficiency or Hemoglobinopathy

Iron deficiency is present in more than half of patients with folate deficiency (Herbert, 1987c; Herbert, 1987d) and in a third of patients with vitamin $B_{12}$ deficiency (Herbert, 1982). When the iron deficiency or hemoglobinopathy is more severe than the vitamin deficiency, red cell morphology may reveal defective hemoglobin synthesis but not the macroovalocytic red cells of slowed DNA synthesis. Red cell morphology will reveal both the small red cells of iron deficiency and the large red cells of folate or vitamin $B_{12}$ deficiency only when the concurrent vitamin and mineral deficiencies are relatively equal in severity. The presence of both is diagnostic for dimorphic anemia. Either or both of the following two evaluatory procedures will reveal the slowed DNA synthesis of megaloblastosis otherwise hidden by iron deficiency or hemoglobinopathy.

### 1. *Hypersegmentation*

An early indication of slowed DNA synthesis is hypersegmentation of nuclei of the granulocytes, manifested by a lobe average greater than 3.5 or by other measures of the number of lobes (Herbert, 1987d). If hypersegmentation is present, it may be possible to diagnose coincident folate or vitamin $B_{12}$ deficiency in patients with conditions involving defective hemoglobin synthesis, such as iron deficiency or hemoglobinopathy. However, two red herrings, congenital hypersegmentation and the hypersegmentation of chronic renal disease, must be ruled out. As with many laboratory tests, hypersegmentation for the individual precedes hypersegmentation for the laboratory (Herbert *et al.*, 1986). The clearest proof that there was hypersegmentation is a fall in the lobe average within two weeks after therapy with the missing vitamin. Normal segmentation for the individual has returned if a lobe average within the laboratory normal range—but above the laboratory median—falls below the laboratory median after therapy.

### 2. *Diagnostic dU Suppression Test*

The diagnostic deoxyuridine (dU) suppression test, another indicator of slowed DNA synthesis, is useful in patients whose folate or vitamin $B_{12}$ deficiency is hidden by concurrent iron deficiency or hemoglobinopathy and in patients with liver disease or myeloproliferative disorders whose serum vitamin $B_{12}$ is elevated despite $B_{12}$ deficiency (Herbert, 1987d). This test measures specific deficiency of either vitamin in bone marrow or lymphocytes by the in vitro suppression of incorporation of $[^3H]$thymidine into DNA when nonradioactive dU plus the deficient vitamin are added (Herbert, 1983).

In folate deficiency, the dU suppression test is abnormal first in bone marrow and then in lymphocytes when folate content falls below 250 ng folate/$10^9$ cells (Colman and Herbert, 1980a). However, in folate or $B_{12}$ deficiency with concomitant iron deficiency the dU suppression test is abnormal first in lymphocytes and later in bone marrow. A dU suppression test carried out on bone marrow cells becomes normal within six hours after the patient is treated with the missing vitamin. However, lymphocytes take up vitamins only when they are triggered to make DNA. Therefore, a dU suppression test carried out on peripheral blood lymphocytes remains abnormal for up to two months after treatment, thus allowing for diagnosis of a past deficiency of vitamin $B_{12}$ or folate—unless the patient has an intercurrent viral infection that triggers lymphocytes to make DNA.

Other useful tests for detecting vitamin $B_{12}$ deficiency include measurements of methylmalonate elevation in serum or urine (Herbert, 1985).

### F. Nervous System Damage

The myelin damage found in combined systems disease occurs only with vitamin $B_{12}$ deficiency but never with folate deficiency (Jacob and Herbert, 1980; Colman and Herbert, 1980b). This vitamin $B_{12}$ deficiency causes defective myelin synthesis, with secondary deterioration of the axon and eventual irreversible deterioration of the nerve head. Myelin damage present for less than one year can be gradually corrected to normal with vitamin $B_{12}$ therapy. Damage present for one to two years may also be corrected if the nerve head has not been destroyed, but damage present for more than two years cannot be corrected, since the head is gone.

The possible significance of relatively high levels of vitamin $B_{12}$ analogs in predicting nerve damage in vitamin $B_{12}$ deficiency is being studied (Carmel *et al.*, 1987; Herbert, 1987d). Our group is also testing the hypothesis that slowed nerve conduction may predict subsequent neurological damage just as hypersegmentation predicts subsequent anemia.

## III. SUMMARY

Megaloblastic anemia is the morphological expression of slowed DNA synthesis. Its most common cause is vitamin $B_{12}$ or folic acid deficiency. Vitamin $B_{12}$ deficiency most frequently results from age-dependent gastric atrophy, which leads to inadequate absorption and pernicious anemia. The diagnostic triad for pernicious anemia includes: megaloblastosis, a serum "true vitamin $B_{12}$" level below 112 pg/ml, and inadequate secretions of gastric acid, enzymes, and intrinsic factor. Free vitamin $B_{12}$ is not found in food, and inadequate gastric secretions prevent food $B_{12}$ release and absorption. Because losses of gastric acid and enzymes usually precede losses of intrinsic factor, the crystalline Schilling test is useful only in diagnosing late intrinsic factor loss. A food Schilling test can measure inability to absorb food vitamin $B_{12}$, allowing for diagnosis of vitamin $B_{12}$ deficiency even when substantial intrinsic factor is still present. Folate deficiency can be prevented by consuming fruit juice or one uncooked fruit or vegetable each day. Clinical conditions like chronic alcoholism can produce deficiency, which is rapidly reversed by folic acid therapy.

We have proposed models delineating the sequence of abnormalities in laboratory tests at each stage in the development of vitamin $B_{12}$ or folate deficiency or excess. Our vitamin $B_{12}$ model postulates that the earliest abnormality is loss of the vitamin from the vitamin $B_{12}$ transport protein TC II. Diagnostic tests include those for hypersegmentation and dU suppression, both of which are early indicators of slowed DNA synthesis. These tests allow for diagnosis of coincident folate or vitamin $B_{12}$ deficiency in patients with iron deficiency, hemoglobinopathy, myeloproliferative disorders, or liver disease. Because serial changes from individual norms precede deviations from the laboratory norm, recognition of individual changes allows for earlier diagnosis. Vitamin $B_{12}$ deficiency also affects the nervous system by causing myelin damage. Vitamin $B_{12}$ therapy can gradually correct this damage if the nerve head has not been destroyed. Current studies are exploring the hypotheses that relatively high levels of vitamin $B_{12}$ analogs may predict nerve damage and that slowed nerve conduction may predict subsequent neurological damage.

## ACKNOWLEDGMENTS

This work was supported by the Research Service of the U.S. Veterans Administration and USPHS Grant No. DK37509 and by donations to the Committee to Strengthen Nutrition, Mount Sinai Medical Center, New York, New York.

## REFERENCES

Carmel, R., Karnaze, D. S., and Werner, J. M. (1987). ''Analogue'' values in cobalamin deficiency: Neurologic dysfunction is associated with higher levels than is anemia [Abstract]. *Blood* **70** (Suppl. 1), 45a.

Colman, N., and Herbert. V. (1980a). Abnormal lymphocyte deoxyuridine suppression test: A reliable indicator of decreased lymphocyte folate levels. *Amer. J. Hematol.* **8**, 169–176.

Colman, N., and Herbert, V. (1980b). Folate metabolism in brain. *In* ''Biochemistry of Brain'' (S. Kumar, ed.), pp 103–125. Pergamon Press, New York.

Doscherholmen, A., McMahon, J. H. and Ripley. D. (1976). Inhibitory effects of eggs on vitamin $B_{12}$ absorption: Description of a simple ovalbumin $^{57}$Co-vitamin $B_{12}$ absorption test. *Brit. J. Haemat.* **33**, 261–272.

Halsted, C. H. (1989). Alcoholism and folate homeostasis. *In* "Nutrition and the Origins of Disease" (C. H. Halsted and R. B. Rucker, eds.), pp. 249–266. Academic Press, San Diego.

Herbert, V. (1982). Megaloblastic anemia with two nutrient deficiencies: Two cases. *Medical Grand Rounds* **1**, 320–336.

Herbert, V. (1983). The inhibition of some cancers and the promotion of others by folic acid, vitamin $B_{12}$, and their antagonists. *In* "Nutritional Factors in the Induction and Maintenance of Malignancy" (C. E. Butterworth and M. L. Hutchinson, eds.), pp. 273–287. Academic Press, New York.

Herbert, V. (1985). The megaloblastic anemias. *Lab. Invest.* **52**, 3–19.

Herbert, V. (1987a). Recommended dietary intakes (RDI) of folate in humans. *Amer. J. Clin. Nutr.* **45**, 661–670.

Herbert, V. (1987b). Recommended dietary intakes (RDI) of $B_{12}$ in humans. *Amer. J. Clin. Nutr.* **45**, 671–678.

Herbert, V. (1987c). Recommended dietary intakes (RDI) of iron in humans. *Amer. J. Clin. Nutr.* **45**, 679–686.

Herbert, V. (1987d). The 1986 Herman award lecture: Nutrition science as a continually unfolding story: The folate and vitamin $B_{12}$ paradigm. *Amer. J. Clin. Nutr.* **46**, 387–402.

Herbert, V. (1987e). Making sense of laboratory tests of folate status: Folate requirements to sustain normality. *Amer. J. Hematol.* **26**, 199–207.

Herbert, V. (1987f). Recommended dietary intake (RDI) of folate in humans: Reply to letter by Baggott. *Amer. J. Clin. Nutr.* **46**, 1057.

Herbert, V. (1988). Staging nutrient status from too little to too much by appropriate laboratory tests. *In* "Nutritional Status Assessment of the Individual" (G. E. Livingston, J. E. Vanderveen, and J. M. Iacono, eds.). Food and Nutrition Press, Westport, CT.

Herbert, V., and Colman, N. (1980). Hematologic complications of alcoholism: Overview. *Amer. J. Hematol.* **17**, 164–176.

Herbert, V., and Colman, N. (1988). Folic acid and vitamin $B_{12}$. *In* "Modern Nutrition in Health and Disease" (M. E. Shils and V. R. Young, eds.), pp 388–416. Lea and Febiger, Philadelphia.

Herbert, V., Memoli, D., McAleer. E., and Colman, N. (1986). What is normal? Variation from the individual's norm for granulocyte "lobe average" and holotranscobalamin II (holo-TC II) diagnoses vitamin $B_{12}$ deficiency before variation from the laboratory norm [Abstract]. *Clin. Res.* **34**, 718A.

Herzlich, B., and Herbert, V. (1988). Depletion of serum holotranscobalamin II: An early sign of negative $B_{12}$ balance. *Lab. Invest.* **58**, 332–337.

Jacob, E., and Herbert, V. (1980). Vitamin $B_{12}$ and the nervous system. *In* "Biochemistry of the Brain" (S. Kumar, ed.), pp. 127–142. Pergamon Press, New York.

Kohgo, T., Niitsu, Y., Kondo, H. Tsushima, N., Sasaki, K., Hirayama, M., Numata, T., Nishisato, T., and Urushizaki, I. (1987). Serum transferrin receptors as a new index of erythropoiesis. *Blood* **70**, 1955–1958.

Shaw, S., Jayatilleke, E., Herbert, V., and Colman, N. (1987). Cleavage of 5-methyltetrahydrofolate (5MTHF) during ethanol metabolism: Role of acetaldehyde-xanthine oxidase-generated superoxide [Abstract]. *Clin. Res.* **35**(3), 644A.

# 5

# Regulation of Iron Exchange

Clement A. Finch

*Division of Hematology*
*Department of Medicine*
*University of Washington School of Medicine*
*Seattle, Washington*



## I. INTRODUCTION

Human iron metabolism is built on a scaffold of three proteins: transferrin, which moves iron through extracellular fluids; specific membrane receptors for transferrin, which determine the amount of iron taken up by individual tissues; and ferritin, which stores intracellular iron. This discussion concerns the behavior of these compounds and the nature of various disorders of iron metabolism that occur in humans.

## II. INTERNAL IRON EXCHANGE

Exchange of iron between tissues is accomplished by a plasma protein with a molecular weight of about 80,000 and two iron-binding sites (Huebers and Finch, 1987). There are actually several human transferrins that differ in their glycan sidechains. Plasma transferrin is found in the body's extracellular fluids and in the intestinal lumen; other transferrins are found in sanctuary areas in the testes and central nervous system. Iron loads randomly, one atom at a time, on the iron-binding sites of transferrin from donor cells—reticuloendothelial (RE) cells, hepatocytes, and intestinal mucosal cells. Thus, the proportions of iron as apotransferrin, monoferric transferrin, and diferric transferrin are predictable on the basis of transferrin saturation (Huebers *et al.*, 1984).

Transferrin molecules attach on specific membrane receptors, and the iron–transferrin complex is internalized in a vacuole from which all iron is released (Dautry-Varsat *et al.*, 1983). Then the apotransferrin–receptor complex is returned to the cell membrane, where transferrin is released to the plasma (Klausner *et al.*, 1983).

The interaction of the transferrin molecule with receptors differs according to its iron status. Receptors have a very low affinity for apotransferrin and bind it only when iron-bearing molecules are insufficient to saturate receptor binding sites. Receptors have a 3.5-fold greater affinity for diferric transferrin than for monoferric transferrin (Huebers *et al.*, 1985). Therefore, diferric transferrin delivers iron more effectively and constitutes the major source of iron for tissues. As the amount of diferric transferrin increases, plasma iron uptake by body tissues increases (Cazzola *et al.*, 1985). The tissue distribution of iron depends on the number of receptors in a given tissue. Because the erythroid marrow dominates iron uptake, most of the body's transferrin receptors are located in that tissue. The total number of body transferrin receptors parallels the degree of erythroid proliferation and increases when plasma iron supply is inadequate.

Ferrokinetic studies carried out with radioactive iron have contributed to our knowledge of iron exchange (Fig. 1) and also to our understanding of erythropoiesis (Bothwell *et al.*, 1979; Cavill and Ricketts, 1980). The erythron and the RE cells hold some 75% of body iron and together constitute the major circuit for iron in the body. Every day about 20 mg of iron is taken up by the erythroid marrow, incorporated into circulating red cells, and eventually processed by RE cells. Wastage of iron also occurs during erythropoiesis. Some plasma iron moves extravascularly and returns through lymphatics. The hepatocytes exchange iron with plasma transferrin and also process the iron of any hemoglobin resulting from intravascular hemolysis. These are the major pathways of iron within the body.

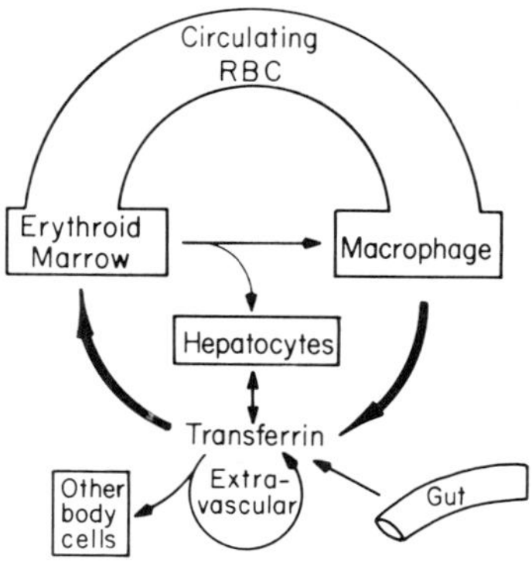


**Fig. 1.** The format of internal iron metabolism is depicted above. Body iron is primarily concerned with the hemoglobin synthesis in developing red cells and with their circulation and subsequent destruction in reticuloendotheliel (RE) cells by phagocytosis or in the hepatocyte after hemolysis. Transferrin completes the cycle by moving iron from the RE cell or hepatocyte through the plasma and back to the erythroid marrow. Other pathways of limited quantitative importance include extravascular flux and uptake by other body tissues. A small amount of iron goes from plasma transferrin to mucosal cells and is lost through exfoliation (not shown). (From Finch and Huebers, 1982. Reprinted with permission.)

By measuring plasma iron turnover, it is possible to estimate the number of functioning erythroid marrow receptors, which is equivalent to the number of developing red cells (Cazzola *et al.*, 1987). This is done by eliminating the extravascular flux of iron, which is proportionate to the plasma iron (Cook *et al.*, 1970). Then the tissue iron uptake is converted to iron-bearing transferrin uptake by correcting for the relative amounts of mono) and diferric transferrin iron in circulation (Cazzola *et al.*, 1985). Finally, the amount of nontransferrin uptake is subtracted. This simplified procedure, which requires only a few hours, involves the determination of plasma iron, total iron-binding capacity, the rate of radioiron disappearance, and the hematocrit (Cazzola *et al.*, 1985).

Recent measurements of plasma transferrin–transferrin receptor complexes suggest that the number of receptor complexes in plasma may reflect the number in body tissues (Kohgo *et al.*, 1986; Kohgo, 1986). If iron deficiency is excluded, the number of receptor complexes would appear to be the equivalent of the erythron transferrin uptake as an index of erythropoiesis.

The determination of plasma iron and total iron-binding capacity together characterize iron supply. Although plasma iron supply undergoes diurnal fluctuation, it is not affected by the size of iron stores within a wide range. Plasma iron is reduced by a critical deficiency in body iron, by the inflammatory block, and by a marked depletion of transferrin. It is increased when receptors are reduced below one-third of basal, as in aplastic anemia; when increased absorption occurs, as in idiopathic hemochromatosis; and when ineffective erythropoiesis or hepatic damage occurs. The last finding suggests that the liver is involved in regulation. At some point, massive iron stores may overwhelm the regulation of plasma iron.

## III. EXTERNAL IRON EXCHANGE

Special mechanisms for iron procurement and conservation satisfy the body's requirements for iron. Excretion, occurring principally from the gut (blood, desquamated mucosal cells, bile), is extremely limited and amounts to only about 1 mg/day in humans (Green *et al.*, 1968). Because iron loss varies from 0.5 to 2.0 mg according to iron status, some regulation of iron loss does occur. Of greater importance is the regulation of dietary iron absorption, which changes to maintain iron balance, but only over a range from < 1 mg to 3–4 mg (Bothwell *et al.*, 1979).

The absorptive process is influenced by gastrointestinal secretions and motility and by mucosal activity in the upper small intestine. The stomach facilitates iron absorption by secreting acid to solubilize dietary iron and by slowly releasing iron to the upper intestine. The reduced absorption of iron in achlorhydric subjects illustrates the relative importance of acid (Cook *et al.*, 1964); however, iron deficiency does not occur unless other factors are also involved. On the other hand, operations that destroy the hopper function of the stomach produce iron deficiency anemia in a large proportion of patients (Magnusson *et al.*, 1979).

### A. Dietary Iron Absorption

It was previously estimated that about 10% of food iron was absorbed, and determinations of dietary adequacy were based on matching this estimate to individual requirements. The critical periods of iron absorption are during the high-growth stage in infancy, during menstruation and pregnancy in the female, and to a lesser degree during the growth spurt of adolescence. The increased prevalence of iron deficiency during these periods attests to the additional requirements of as little as 1 to 2 mg/day.

The iron content of food is usually 5 to 6 mg/1,000 kcal unless fortified to higher levels (Wretlind, 1968). Paradoxically, higher levels were found in some developing countries in association with a high prevalence of iron-deficiency anemia. The prevalence of hookworm, which is accompanied by increased blood loss, was not the sole cause of this anemia. Further exploration showed that the amount of dietary iron did not correlate with the amount absorbed and that, in some instances, the high iron content resulted from contaminating iron that was insoluble and unabsorbable (Bothwell *et al.*, 1979).

Precise measurements using radioiron-labeled foods showed impressive differences in the absorption of iron from one food versus another (Layrisse *et al.*, 1969; Bjorn-Rasmussen *et al.*, 1974; Cook *et al.*, 1972; Hallberg and Bjorn-Rasmussen, 1972). In these studies, available iron in food fell into two categories—hemoglobin, or heme, iron and ionized, or nonheme, iron. The iron in heme compounds was the most available and was independent of other dietary substances. On the other hand, ionized iron availability was influenced by the presence of certain enhancing substances, such as ascorbate and meat, and by the presence of blocking substances, particularly tannic acid and phosphate compounds. Although heme and ionized iron absorption were both affected by the individual's iron status, heme iron was less affected than nonheme iron. Iron-depleted subjects on an otherwise excellent diet may absorb as much as 3 mg/day of excess iron. This excess absorption was shown in superdonors (Monsen *et al.*, 1983) and in patients bled for treatment of polycythemia vera (Haskins *et al.*, 1952). On the other hand, subjects consuming a diet low in meat and ascorbate may be unable to increase absorption above basal or may have low iron absorption despite the presence of iron deficiency (Monsen *et al.*, 1978).

## B. Intestinal Regulation of Iron Absorption

The intestinal mucosa also regulate iron absorption. Three pathways of food iron absorption exist in the upper small intestine: one for ionized iron, one for hemoglobin iron, and one for transferrin-bound iron. Absorption by all three pathways adjusts to changes in body iron to reestablish a normal iron balance.

Despite many attempts to understand the molecular details of the absorptive process, these mechanisms have been an enigma for the past 40 years. It was first proposed that ferritin within the mucosal cell might regulate absorption through its capacity to bind iron (Crosby, 1963). Thus, the more ferritin in the mucosal cell, the lower the absorption. Although the inverse relationship between mucosal ferritin and iron absorption was documented, subsequent studies could not account for direct binding of iron by ferritin (Brittin and Raval, 1971). It seems more likely that ferritin serves as a storage compound for excess iron in mucosal cells as it does in other body cells. Although we do not know exactly how iron is taken up and passed through the mucosal cell, changes in the capacity of this uptake–throughput process appear to be of primary importance. In the absorptive pathways for hemoglobin and transferrin, mucosal receptors for these compounds appear to increase in iron deficiency.

An attractive hypothesis originally suggested by Conrad and Crosby (1963) is that mucosal iron content may determine the capacity of the absorptive process. The iron content of the cell is influenced by luminal iron input and by loading of transferrin iron from the plasma. However, it is difficult to ignore the possibility that an internal messenger other than transferrin iron also informs the mucosa of internal needs.

### C. Evaluation of Overall Iron Balance

Overall iron balance reflects the success or failure of the absorptive process, and iron balance is best evaluated by determining the individual's iron stores. Iron is stored in most body cells as ferritin and, in its denatured state, as hemosiderin. The largest iron deposits are located in RE cells and hepatocytes. The most convenient way for the clinician to evaluate iron stores is to measure plasma ferritin, which monitors the aggregate of both (Finch *et al.*, 1986). Plasma ferritin appears to be a secretory product of body cells and quantitatively reflects the amount being synthesized; this synthesis is usually proportionate to the cell's ferritin content. The appropriateness of the plasma ferritin level depends on an individual's age and sex because these parameters normally affect iron stores. Changes in plasma ferritin—its depression in iron deficiency and elevation in iron overload—are useful in detecting changes in iron balance. This is particularly so in iron deficiency because depletion may be detected and therapy may be instituted before essential body iron is altered. However, plasma ferritin can be affected by conditions unrelated to iron stores, including disturbances in metabolic rate, tissue damage, neoplastic disease, and ascorbate deficiency.

## IV. CLINICAL DISORDERS OF IRON METABOLISM

### A. Iron Deficiency

In certain situations, iron supply to the erythroid marrow becomes inadequate. The foremost of these is iron deficiency, estimated to involve some 500 million people in the world today (Finch and Cook, 1984). Although symptoms relate primarily to anemia, all tissues suffer. Too little available iron in the diet and/or excess blood loss are the usual causes. We are all familiar with the ways in which excess blood loss can occur, most importantly excessive menstruation in the female and hookworm disease in the tropics. Less apparent causes include hemosiderinuria and pulmonary siderosis. A variety of laboratory tests, including transferrin saturation, red cell protoporphyrin, plasma ferritin, and mean red cell volume, make detection easy; their respective value depends on the severity and duration of the deficiency (Cook, 1982).

The amount of iron available to body tissues at a specific time is most directly shown by transferrin iron saturation (Bainton and Finch, 1964). In low transferrin iron saturation, the most difficult differential is between iron deficiency and inflammation because iron supply to the erythron is deficient in both, in one because of a decrease in total body iron and in the other because of a block of iron release from the RE cell. The two causes are usually distinguished by the presence of a plasma ferritin level of less than 12 $\mu g/L$ in the former and over 100 $\mu g/L$ in the latter (Finch *et al.*, 1986). If both iron deficiency and inflammation are present, a ferritin level of as much as 50 to 60 $\mu g/L$ may still indicate iron deficiency, and a response to iron therapy may occur.

Other internal causes may cause a deficient iron supply. A hereditary defect in which transferrin is virtually absent illustrates the importance of that protein in providing iron to body tissues. This defect is associated with very severe hypochromic microcytic anemia that is typical of iron deficiency and, it may be assumed, with iron deficiency in many other tissues (Goya *et al.*, 1972). However, liver iron increases because this organ takes up absorbed iron from circulation. Thus, the transferrin pathway is not essential for iron absorption.

Another abnormality, as yet not demonstrated in humans, has been studied in the Belgrade rat. This animal has an hereditary abnormality in iron release from the transferrin iron–receptor complex within the cell (Edwards *et al.*, 1986). Normally, all iron taken into the cell is retained. In the Belgrade rat, most of the iron cycles through the cell but is released back into the plasma, resulting in hypochromic microcytic anemia despite a high plasma iron. Thus, a tissue iron deficiency can result from inadequate dietary iron, impaired absorption, excessive iron losses, inadequate transport protein, abnormal receptor behavior, or an RE blockade to iron release.

## B. Iron Overload

Humans also suffer from iron overload. In a number of conditions, the predominant iron deposits are either RE or parenchymal (Finch *et al.*, 1985). The most common is idiopathic hemochromatosis (Bothwell *et al.*, 1983). This genetic disorder is inherited as a recessive human leukocyte antigen-related trait. In its heterozygous form, it is benign and at present indistinguishable from normal, but in its homozygous form, it can lead to massive iron deposits, tissue damage, and death if not treated. The molecular abnormality in iron absorption in this disorder has not been determined. It appears to be more than an isolated mucosal defect because RE cells cannot store iron until the late stages of the disease (Brink *et al.*, 1977). The diagnosis depends on two screening tests, plasma ferritin and transferrin saturation, followed up, when positive, by a liver biopsy. In younger subjects who have not had time to accumulate large stores, the elevation of transferrin saturation over 70% is the more useful screen (Edwards *et al.*, 1977). The presence of normal erythropoiesis in these individuals permits effective iron removal by phlebotomy, with the red cell deficit being replaced by storage iron.

Certain types of anemia, particularly thalassemia and sideroblastic anemia, are also associated with excessive iron absorption. We postulated that the increased iron balance in anemia might be a function of the increased rate of erythropoiesis. However, when we compared absorption in thalassemia and hereditary spherocytosis, we found a marked difference in level of iron absorption between the two disorders, even though the rate of erythropoiesis was similar (unpublished observations). The finding that the increased absorption in thalassemia was reversed when the marrow was suppressed by transfusion suggested that the iron loading must not relate to red-cell turnover but perhaps to the degree of intravascular hemolysis or to some other special feature of red-cell destruction.

The inability to employ bleeding in most of the iron-loading anemias has led to the development of an alternative way to increase iron removal. Deferoxamine (DFO), because of its iron chelating ability, has prevented liver damage (Barry *et al.*, 1974) and heart failure (Wolfe *et al.*, 1985). In individuals with severe parenchymal iron overload, DFO causes iron loss in urine and bile, amounting to about 25 mg iron/g DFO. The urinary loss relates to the degree of erythroid activity (Pippard *et al.*, 1982), but the precise location from which the chelator obtains its iron is debated. Because studies indicate that the RE cell cannot donate iron, the hepatocyte is the likely source (Pippard *et al.*, 1982; Kim *et al.*, 1985). DFO penetrates the hepatocyte and chelates iron in transit within the cell. Once ferrioxamine is formed, the chelate cannot recross the hepatocyte membrane into the plasma but must be excreted in the bile. Other chelators, including some effective oral compounds, appear to act similarly in causing biliary excretion (Kim, 1987). Parenterally administered DFO also enters the intestinal mucosal cells and blocks iron absorption (unpublished observations).

## V. SUMMARY

Total body iron is regulated predominantly through absorption. The effectiveness of this regulation is frequently compromised by an inadequate amount of available food iron, rather than by dysregulation. From a nutritional standpoint, emphasis in recent years has been on the availability, rather than on the amount, of food iron. Normal individuals can effectively defend against excessive iron absorption with one apparent exception: excessive absorption is associated with certain alcoholic beverages. However, certain internal disorders—including increased erythropoiesis, liver disease, and genetic idiopathic hemochromatosis—are associated with dysregulation of iron absorption and iron overload. Fortunately, the largest group, the patients with hemochromatosis, can be effectively treated once the disease is detected, even though the nature of the abnormality is still unknown. The extensive use of screening tests for transferrin saturation and plasma ferritin have assisted greatly in detecting this disorder.

## REFERENCES


Bainton, D. F., and Finch, C. A. (1964). The diagnosis of iron deficiency anemia. *Amer. J. Med.* **37**, 62–70.

Barry, M., Flynn, D. M., Letsky, E. A., and Risdon, R. A. (1974). Long-term chelation therapy in thalassemia major: Effect on liver iron concentration, liver histology and clinical progress. *Brit. Med. J.* **1**, 16–20.

Bjorn-Rasmussen, E., Hallberg, L., Isaksson, B., and Arvidsson, B. (1974). Food iron absorption in man. *J. Clin. Invest.* **53**, 247–255.

Bothwell, T. H., Charlton, R. W., Cook, J. D., and Finch, C. A. (eds.) (1979). "Iron Metabolism in Man." Blackwell Scientific Publications, Oxford.

Bothwell, T. H., Charlton, R. W., and Motulsky, A. G. (1983). Idiopathic hemochromatosis. *In* "Metabolic Basis of Inherited Disease" (J. V. Stanbury, J. B. Wyngaarden, D. S. Fredrickson, and M. S. Brown, eds.), pp. 1269–1298. McGraw-Hill, New York.

Brink, B., Disler, P., Lynch, S., Jacobs, P., Charlton, R., and Bothwell, T. (1977). Patterns of iron storage in dietary iron overload and idiopathic hemochromatosis. *J. Lab. Clin. Med.* **88**, 725–731.

Brittin, G. M., and Raval, D. (1971). Duodenal ferritin synthesis in iron-replete and iron-deficient rats: Response to small doses of iron. *J. Lab. Clin. Med.* **77**, 54–58.

Cavill, I., and Ricketts, C. (1980). Human iron kinetics. *In* "Iron in Biochemistry and Medicine" (A. Jacobs and M. Worwood, eds.), Vol. II, pp. 573–604. Academic Press, New York.

Cazzola, M., Huebers, H. A., Sayers, M. H., MacPhail, A. P., Eng, M., and Finch, C. A. (1985). Transferrin saturation, plasma iron turnover, and transferrin uptake in normal humans. *Blood* **66**, 935–939.

Cazzola, M., Pootrakul, P., Huebers, H. A., Eng, M., Eschbach, J., and Finch, C. A. (1987). Erythroid marrow function in anemic man. *Blood* **69**, 296–301.

Conrad, M. E., and Crosby, W. H. (1963). Intestinal mucosal mechanisms controlling iron absorption. *Blood* **22**, 406–415.

Cook, J. D. (1982). Clinical evaluation of iron deficiency. *Sem. Hematol.* **19**, 6–18.

Cook, J. D., Brown, G. M., and Valberg, L. S. (1964). The effect of achylia gastrica on iron absorption. *J. Clin. Invest.* **43**, 1185–1191.

Cook, J. D., Marsaglia, G., Eschbach, J. W., Funk, D. D., and Finch, C. A. (1970). Ferrokinetics: A biologic model for plasma iron exchange in man. *J. Clin. Invest.* **49**, 197–205.

Cook, J. D., Layrisse, M., Martinez-Torres, C., Walker, R., Monsen, E., and Finch, C. A. (1972). Food iron absorption measured by an extrinsic tag. *J. Clin. Invest.* **51**, 805–815.

Crosby, W. H. (1963). The control of iron balance by the intestinal mucosa. *Blood* **22**, 441–449.

Dautry-Varsat, A., Ciechanover, A., and Lodish, H. F. (1983). pH and the recycling of transferrin during receptor-mediated endocytosis. *Proc. Nat. Acad. Sci. USA* **80**, 2258–2262.

Edwards, C. Q., Carroll, M., Bray, P., and Cartwright, G. E. (1977). Hereditary hemochromatosis. Diagnosis in siblings and children. *N. Engl. J. Med.* **297**, 7–13.

Edwards, J., Huebers, H. A., Kunzler, C., and Finch, C. A. (1986). Iron metabolism in the Belgrade rat. *Blood* **67**, 623–628.

Finch, C. A., and Cook, J. D. (1984). Iron deficiency. *Amer. J. Clin. Nutr.* **39**, 471–477.

Finch, C. A., and Huebers, H. A. (1982). Perspectives in iron metabolism. *N. Engl. J. Med.* **306**, 1520–1528.

Finch, C. A., Huebers, H. A., Cazzola, M., Bergamaschi, G., and Bellotti, V. (1985). Storage iron. *In* "Ferritins and Isoferritins as Biochemical Markers" (A. Albertini, *et al.*, eds.), pp. 3–21. Elsevier Science Publishers, Amsterdam.

Finch, C. A., Bellotti, V., Stray, S., Lipschitz, D. A., Cook, J. D., Pippard, M. J., and Huebers, H. A. (1986). Plasma ferritin determination as a diagnostic tool. *West. J. Med.* **145**, 657–663.

Goya, N., Miyazaki, S., Kodate, S., and Ushio, B. (1972). A family of congenital atransferrinemia. *Blood* **40**, 239–245.

Green, R., Charlton, R., Seftel, H., Bothwell, T., Mayet, F., Finch, C. A., and Layrisse, M. (1968). Body iron excretion in man. *Amer. J. Med.* **45**, 336–353.

Hallberg, L., and Bjorn-Rasmussen, E. (1972). Determination of iron absorption from whole diet. A new two-pool model using two radioiron isotopes given as haem and non-haem iron. *Scand. J. Haematol.* **9**, 193–197.

Haskins, D., Stevens, A. R., Jr., Finch, S., and Finch, C. A. (1952). Iron metabolism. Iron stores in man as measured by phlebotomy. *J. Clin. Invest.* **31**, 543–547.

Huebers, H., and Finch, C. A. (1987). The physiology of transferrin and transferrin receptors. *Physiol. Rev.* **67**, 520–582.

Huebers, H. A., Josephson, B., Huebers, E., Csiba, E., and Finch, C. A. (1984). Occupancy of the iron binding sites of human transferrin. *Proc. Nat. Acad. Sci. USA* **81**, 4326–4330.

Huebers, H., Csiba, E., Huebers, E., and Finch, C. A. (1985). Molecular advantage of diferric transferrin in delivering iron to reticulocytes: A comparative study. *Proc. Soc. Biol. Med.* **179**, 222–226.

Kim, B.K. (1987). Effectiveness of oral iron chelators demonstrated by a rat bioassay. *Amer. J. Hematol.* **24**, 277–282.

Kim, B.K., Huebers, H.A., Pippard, M.J., and Finch, C.A. (1985). Storage iron exchange in the rat as affected by deferoxamine. *J. Lab. Clin. Med.* **105**, 440–448.

Klausner, R.D., Ashwell, G., Van Renswoudf, J., Harford, J.B., and Bridges, K.R. (1983). Binding of apotransferrin to K562 cells: Explanation of the transferrin cycle. *Proc. Nat. Acad. Sci. USA* **80**, 2263–2266.

Kohgo, Y. (1986). Structure of transferrin and transferrin receptor. *Acta Haematol. Jap.* **49**, 1627–1634.

Kohgo, Y., Nishisato, T., Kondo, H., Tsushima, N., Niitsu, Y., and Urushizaki, I. (1986). Circulating transferrin receptor in human serum. *Brit. J. Haematol.* **64**, 277–281.

Layrisse, M., Cook, J.D., Martinez, D., Roche, M., Kuhn, I.N., Walker, R.B., and Finch, C.A. (1969). Food iron absorption: A comparison of vegetable and animal foods. *Blood* **33**, 430–443.

Magnusson, B., Faxen, A., Cederblad, A., Rosander, L., Kenwenter, J., and Hallberg, L. (1979). The effect of parietal cell vagotomy and selection vagotomy with pyloroplasty on iron absorption. A prospective, randomized study. *Scand. J. Gastroenterol.* **14**, 177–182.

Monsen, E.R., Hallberg, L., Layrisse, M., and Finch, C.A. (1978). Estimation of available dietary iron. *Amer. J. Clin. Nutr.* **31**, 134–141.

Monsen, E.R., Critchlow, C.W., Finch, C.A., and Donohue, D.M. (1983). Iron balance in superdonors. *Transfusion* **23**, 221–225.

Pippard, M.J., Callender, S.T., and Finch, C.A. (1982). Ferrioxamine excretion in iron-loaded man. *Blood* **60**, 288–294.

Wolfe, L., Olivieri, N., Sallan, D., Colan, S., Rose, V., Propper, R., Freedman, M.H., and Nathan, D.G. (1985). Prevention of cardiac disease by subcutaneous deferoxamine in patients with thalassemia major. *N. Engl. J. Med.* **312**, 1600–1603.

Wretlind, A. (1968). The supply of food iron. *In* ''Gastroenterology'' (G. Blix, ed.), pp. 73–91. Almqvist and Wiksell, Stockholm.

# 6

# Dietary Omega-3 Fatty Acids and the Regulation of Lipoproteins

William E. Connor

*Division of Endocrinology/Metabolism and Clinical Nutrition*
*Department of Medicine*
*Oregon Health Sciences University*
*Portland, Oregon*



## I. INTRODUCTION

The hypocholesterolemic effects of polyunsaturated fatty acids (PUFAs) in the diet were first recognized more than 30 years ago (Goodnight *et al.*, 1982). These effects were thought to result from the amount of polyunsaturation, irrespective of the structure of the specific fat. For many years, the possibility that different essential fatty acids (EFAs) might have different effects on plasma lipids, lipoproteins, and lipid metabolism received scant attention. Recently, however, distinctions have been made between EFAs of the omega-6 structure found in vegetable oils and those of the very long-chain omega-3 structure found in fish oils.

The omega-3 fatty acids constitute a unique group of PUFAs with important biological functions (Goodnight *et al.*, 1982; Prichette *et al.*, 1981; Karmali *et al.*, 1984; Neuringer and Connor, 1986). They are precursors and inhibitors of prostaglandins and leukotrienes. They exhibit antithrombotic effects by inhibiting platelet aggregation and hypolipidemic effects by inhibiting the synthesis of triglycerides, very low-density lipoproteins (VLDL), and low-density lipoproteins (LDL). Omega-3 fatty acids are essential constituents of neural cell membranes, especially in the brain, and are an important component of spermatozoa. Immunological and anticarcinogenetic effects have also been proposed.

## II. FATTY ACID STRUCTURE AND NOMENCLATURE

Each fatty acid consists of an even-numbered chain of 2 to 22 carbon atoms, with a methyl ($CH_3$) group attached to one end and a carboxyl (COOH) group attached to the other end. Attached to each carbon atom in the chain is one hydrogen atom (double bond) or two hydrogen atoms (single bond). PUFAs are long-chain fatty acids with 18 or more carbon atoms and two or more double bonds. Fig. 1 shows structural characteristics and dietary sources of three different fatty acids: omega-3, omega-6, and omega-9.

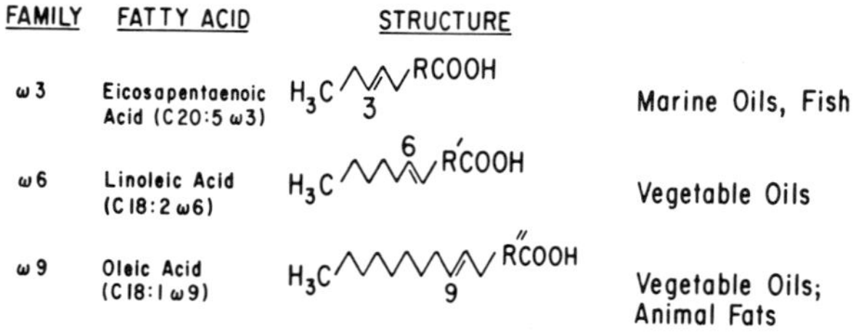


**Fig. 1.** The structure and dietary sources of common unsaturated fatty acids from three families are shown. Polyunsaturated fatty acids are long-chain fatty acids with 18 or more carbon atoms and two or more double bonds. The names of fatty acid families are derived from the position of the first double bond from the methyl or omega end of the carbon chain. Thus, omega-3 fatty acids have the first double bond at the third carbon. Within families, fatty acids are named by their chain length, followed by number of double bonds, as shown parenthetically above.

The names of fatty acid families are derived from the position of the first double bond from the methyl or omega end of the carbon chain. Omega-3 fatty acids, for example, have the first double bond at the third carbon. Within families, fatty acids are named by their chain length, followed by number of double bonds. Thus, the two major omega-3 fatty acids are referred to as 20:5 omega-3 (eicosapentaenoic acid or EPA) and 22:6 omega-3 (docosahexaenoic or DHA). An alternate system of nomenclature replaces the omega with an "n". Thus, EPA would be written as 20:5(n-3). Although members of one omega family may be metabolically interconverted, conversions from one family to another do not occur in mammals or birds.

## III. EFFECTS OF DIFFERENT FATTY ACIDS ON PLASMA LIPIDS

We have studied the hypolipidemic effects of dietary fish oil and vegetable oils on plasma lipids and lipoproteins in normal and hyperlipidemic subjects (Harris *et al.*, 1983; Phillipson *et al.*, 1985). We have also explored the mechanisms underlying these effects in human studies of VLDL and LDL turnover and of carbohydrate-induced hypertriglyceridemia (Harris *et al.*, 1984a; Harris *et al.*, 1984b).

### A. Studies in Normal Subjects

Our first study of normal subjects (Harris *et al.*, 1983) included 12 healthy adults (6 men and 6 women) with initial total plasma cholesterol levels ranging from 132 to 259 mg/dl (mean 192 ± 41) and initial total plasma triglyceride levels ranging from 41 to 162 mg/dl (mean 85 ± 36). To date, this is the only reported study using diets with controlled fatty acid compositions to compare fish oils with polyunsaturated vegetable oils and with saturated fats in the same subjects.

#### 1. *Composition of Test Diets*

Three diets differing only in fatty acid composition were consumed in random order for 4 weeks each—a control diet containing saturated fat, a vegetable-oil diet high in omega-6 fatty acids, and a salmon-oil diet high in omega-3 fatty acids. Each diet provided 40% of calories as fat, 15% as protein, and 45% as carbohydrate and about 500 mg/day cholesterol.

The control diet, which simulated a typical American diet (Ahrens and Boucher, 1978), consisted of whole fruits, vegetables, and grains and a liquid formula containing most of the fat and protein. Cholesterol was supplied as egg yolk, and fat as cocoa butter and peanut oil. The vegetable-oil diet was identical to the control diet, except that a mixture of safflower and corn oils, stripped to reduce the plant sterols from 1,000 to 300 mg/dl, provided the dietary fat. Use of liquid formulas was necessary in the saturated-fat and vegetable-oil diets in order to achieve a balance with the fat, cholesterol, and protein content of the salmon-oil diet. The salmon-oil diet contained the same carbohydrate sources as the other diets, but the liquid formula was replaced by salmon fillets and salmon oil. Salmon was chosen as the omega-3 fatty acid source because of its ready accessibility in the Pacific Northwest, its exceptionally good taste, and its high fat content. The control diet had a fatty acid pattern similar to that of the typical Western diet and virtually no omega-3 fatty acids, whereas the salmon-oil diet was greatly enriched with the two major omega-3 fatty acids (Table I). The omega-3 family provided about 20% of total fatty acids in the salmon-oil diet, which amounted to about 20–29 g/day. Although the salmon-oil diet supplied less linoleic acid than in the other two diets, it still provided an adequate quantity of this essential fatty acid.

**TABLE I**

**Major Fatty Acids in the Three Experimental Diets**[a]

| Fatty acid | Control | Vegetable oil | Salmon oil |
|---|---|---|---|
| Saturated | | | |
| 16:0 | 19 | 12 | 15 |
| 18:0 | 17 | 3 | 6 |
| Total | 36 | 15 | 21 |
| Monounsaturated | | | |
| 16:1 omega-7 | 1 | 0 | 6 |
| 18:1 omega-9 | 40 | 26 | 23 |
| 20:1 omega-9 | 0 | 0 | 10 |
| 22:1 omega-11 | 0 | 0 | 9 |
| Total | 41 | 26 | 48 |
| Polyunsaturated Omega-3 | | | |
| 20:5 omega-3 | <1 | <1 | 9 |
| 22:5 + 22:6 omega-3 | <1 | <1 | 11 |
| Total | <1 | <1 | 20 |
| Polyunsaturated Omega-6 | | | |
| 18:2 omega-6 | 18 | 54 | 3 |
| Total | 18 | 54 | 3 |
| Polyunsaturated/saturated ratio | 0.5 | 3.4 | 1.3 |

[a]All values stated as percentages of total fat. Dietary fat sources were cocoa butter and peanut oil in the control diet, safflower and corn oil in the vegetable-oil diet, and salmon oil and salmon fillets in the salmon-oil diet. (Modified from Harris *et al.*, 1983.)

All meals consumed during the study were prepared in the metabolic kitchens of our Clinical Research Center (CRC), and, except for an occasional weekend meal taken home, all meals were eaten at the CRC. None of the subjects had any difficulty in eating the test diets, some of which included up to 1 lb of salmon steak. The doses of 3–6 tablespoons/day of salmon oil were well tolerated by all subjects. No gastrointestinal discomfort was reported, and bowel habits remained regular. There were no significant weight changes during the study.

### 2. *Effects of the Diets on Plasma Lipid Levels*

Plasma lipid levels during the salmon-oil diet were compared to levels during the control diet in all 12 normal subjects. During the salmon-oil diet, the mean total plasma triglyceride level fell from 77 to 48 mg/dl ($p < 0.005$), and the mean total plasma cholesterol level fell from 188 to 162 mg/dl ($p < 0.001$). The mean VLDL cholesterol level fell from 13 to 8 mg/dl ($p < 0.001$), and the mean LDL cholesterol level fell from 128 to 108 mg/dl ($p < 0.005$). However, the mean high-density lipoprotein (HDL) cholesterol level, which was 50 mg/dl on the control diet, was unaffected by the salmon-oil diet.

An important difference between the salmon-oil and vegetable-oil diets was their content of omega-3 and omega-6 fatty acids: the salmon-oil diet contained about 8% of total calories as omega-3 fatty acids and less than 1% as omega-6, whereas the vegetable-oil diet contained about 21% of total calories as omega-6 fatty acids and less than 1% as omega-3. Therefore, we also compared plasma lipid levels during the salmon-oil diet to those during the vegetable-oil diet and the control diet in 7 study subjects.

Decreases in mean total cholesterol were similar, with declines of about 11% below control values during the salmon-oil diet ($p < .01$) and about 9% during the vegetable-oil diet ($p < .05$). However, the mean total triglyceride values, which fell by about 34% ($p < 0.01$) during salmon-oil diet, were unaffected by the vegetable-oil diet. Similarly, mean VLDL cholesterol, which fell by about 50% during the salmon-oil diet ($p < 0.01$), matched control values during the vegetable-oil diet. Mean LDL cholesterol fell by almost 13% on the salmon-oil diet ($p < 0.05$) and by about 9% on the vegetable-oil diet ($p < 0.05$). Neither diet affected mean HDL cholesterol.

The incorporation of omega-3 fatty acids into plasma lipids during the salmon-oil diet was compared to that during the control diet. Cholesterol esters, triglyceride, and phospholipids all contained 25–30% omega-3 fatty acids (20:5, 22:5, and 22:6) during the salmon-oil diet and less than 5% during the control diet (Fig. 2). Concurrently, 18:2 omega 6 (linoleic acid) levels decreased rapidly to about 50% of control values in most lipid

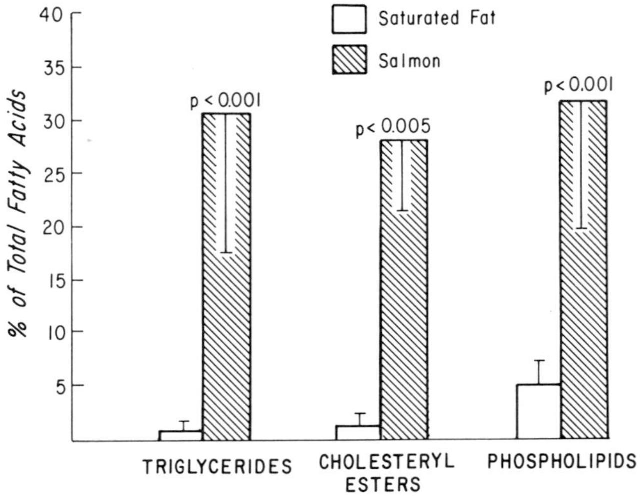


**Fig. 2.** The incorporation of omega-3 fatty acids into plasma lipids during a control diet was compared to that during a salmon oil diet in normolipidemic subjects. The omega-3 fatty acid content of three plasma lipid fractions is expressed as the percentage of total fatty acids from this family (20:5 + 22:5 + 22:6). Values for the same subjects during the vegetable oil diet matched control values. (From Harris *et al.*, 1983. Reprinted with permission.)

fractions, and 20:4 omega-6 (arachidonic acid) content fell by 23% in the phospholipid fraction (data not shown). Changes were detectable within 1 day, and peak concentrations were reached at 10 days.

Although the hypocholesterolemic effects of marine oils were appreciated as early as the 1950s (Bronte-Stewart *et al.*, 1956; Malmros and Wigand, 1957; Keys *et al.*, 1957; Ahrens *et al.*, 1959), their hypotriglyceridemic effects were not recognized for another 20 years (von Lossonczy *et al.*, 1978; Bronsgeest-Schoute *et al.*, 1981). Therefore, our most striking finding was the ability of salmon oil to lower plasma triglyceride levels as well as plasma cholesterol, VLDL, and LDL levels in normolipidemic subjects.

Previous studies of the effects of omega-6 PUFAs on total plasma triglyceride levels have produced inconclusive results. Triglyceride levels fell among normal and hypertriglyceridemic subjects in one study, but its 10-day duration probably allowed too little time for plasma lipids to stabilize (Chait *et al.*, 1974). Others have reported that these PUFAs lowered triglyceride levels by 14–15% (Nestel *et al.*, 1974; Shepherd *et al.*, 1980). Our study among normal subjects, which found no effects of vegetable oils on triglyceride levels (Harris *et al.*, 1983), supported similar findings in earlier studies (Nestel *et al.*, 1973; Turner *et al.*, 1981; Nestel *et al.*, 1975; Connor *et al.*, 1969).

Previous studies of the effects of omega-6 PUFAs on plasma HDL cholesterol levels have also produced inconclusive results. Although PUFAs in vegetable oils lowered HDL cholesterol levels in some studies (Shepherd *et al.*, 1978; Shepherd *et al.*, 1980; Turner *et al.*, 1981), our studies support the findings by others that vegetable-oil feeding has little effect on HDL cholesterol (Harris *et al.*, 1983; Phillipson *et al.*, 1985; Chait *et al.*, 1974; Nestel *et al.*, 1975). On the other hand, some have reported that omega-3 fish oils slightly elevated HDL cholesterol (von Lossonczy *et al.*, 1978; Sanders *et al.*, 1981), whereas others found no effect (Bronsgeest-Schoute *et al.*, 1981).

Based on our findings among normal subjects and on earlier studies, we concluded that only omega-3 fatty acids have significant hypotriglyceridemic effects and that omega-3 fatty acids are more hypocholesterolemic, gram-for-gram, than linoleic acid, the major omega-6 fatty acid. Clearly, omega-3 fatty acids produce different metabolic effects than omega-6 or saturated fatty acids.

Although the reasons for the greater hypolipidemic effects of omega-3 fatty acids are unclear, the higher polyunsaturation of the omega-3 fatty acids partly explains these effects. The primary omega-6 fatty acid, linoleic acid, contains only two double bonds per molecule, whereas the primary omega-3 fatty acids, EPA (20:5) and DHA (22:6), average 5.5 double bonds per molecule. Thus, gram for gram, omega-3 fatty acids are about 2.75 times more polyunsaturated than omega-6 fatty acids. In our study, the ratio of the omega-6 fatty acids in the vegetable-oil diet to the omega-3 fatty acids in the salmon-oil diet was about 2.7:1, which, considering the reverse ratio of double bonds per molecule, gave a similar amount of polyunsaturation in each diet. Our results, while confirming the frequently observed correlation between the amount of polyunsaturation and cholesterol levels (Goodnight *et al.*, 1982), did not show a correlation between the amount of polyunsaturation and triglyceride levels. We therefore concluded that some other structural characteristic may be responsible for the lower triglyceride levels observed during the salmon-oil diet.

## B. Studies in Hyperlipidemic Subjects

The hypolipidemic effects of omega-3 fatty acids observed in normal subjects led us to study their potential effects in hyperlipidemic patients (Phillipson *et al.*, 1985). We selected two groups of patients with hypertriglyceridemia and high VLDL levels for our study because depression of total plasma triglyceride and VLDL levels appeared to be unique benefits of fish oils.

### 1. *Characteristics of Study Volunteers*

Twenty hypertriglyceridemic patients (8 men and 12 women) volunteered for the study. All had normal thyroid, renal, and hepatic function. Special care was taken before entry to ensure that patients were in a steady-state condition, with constant body weight and diet and no residual hypolipidemic drug effects. Most patients had not taken hypolipidemic drugs immediately prior to the study. Drugs were discontinued for patients who had previously received them, and plasma lipid levels were monitored until pre-drug levels were attained.

The first group of 10 volunteers had a mean plasma level of 337 mg/dl for total cholesterol and 355 mg/dl for total triglyceride at entry into the study. These 10 patients had the high VLDL and LDL levels consistent with familial combined hyperlipoproteinemia Type IIb, a disorder characterized by a strong predisposition to coronary heart disease and by overproduction of lipoproteins, especially VLDL (Fredrickson and Levy, 1972). The genotype in these 10 volunteers was familial combined hyperlipoproteinemia in 7 patients and unknown in the other 3.

The second group of 10 volunteers had a mean plasma level of 514 mg/dl for total cholesterol and 2874 mg/dl for total triglyceride at entry. These patients had hyperlipoproteinemia Type V with high chylomicrons and very high VLDL levels in the fasting state. This phenotype is characterized by overproduction of VLDL and impaired clearance of chylomicrons, VLDL, and their remnant particles. Type V patients, many from families with combined familial hyperlipoproteinemia, suffer episodic abdominal pain caused by enlargement of abdominal viscera (hepatomegaly and splenomegaly), episodic acute pancreatitis, eruptive xanthomata, neuropathy, and lipemia retinalis. Although Type V patients have low LDL levels, the presence of atherogenic remnant particles and low HDL levels predisposes them to coronary artery disease and other atherosclerotic complications. The genotypes were combined familial hyperlipoproteinemia for one patient, Type III or dysbetalipoproteinemia (homozygous for apoprotein [apo]-E-2) for another, and undiagnosed for the other 8 patients. Four patients in this group had concomitant, noninsulin-dependent diabetes mellitus, and two had adult-onset, insulin-dependent diabetes. Their insulin doses and diabetic control remained constant throughout the study.

## 2. *Composition of Test Diets*

The study used six diets, all of which were eucaloric so that patients neither gained nor lost weight. Three diets (control, fish oil, and vegetable oil) were designed for the Type IIb volunteers, and another three (control, fish oil, and vegetable oil) were designed for the Type V volunteers (Table II). To achieve maximum lowering of plasma triglyceride levels in the Type V patients, the control diet was very low in cholesterol with only 5% of calories as fat (Connor and Connor, 1982). All patients participated in the control and fish-oil phases of the study, but only 4 Type IIb patients and 8 Type V patients participated in the vegetable-oil phase. Each dietary phase lasted 3–4 weeks, and all diets were prepared and consumed exactly as in the study of normal subjects (Harris *et al.*, 1983).

Each diet consisted of cereals, fruits, vegetables, and milk, plus fat. The fat in the control and vegetable-oil diets was provided via a liquid formula, and the fat in the fish-oil diet was provided via salmon or a commercial fish-oil preparation. Again, the fatty acid composition and the amount of total calories as fat were the principal differences among the diets. The two control diets contained relatively similar amounts of saturated, monounsaturated, and diunsaturated (linoleic) fatty acids.

Type V patients were monitored with special care during the fish-oil and vegetable-oil diets to minimize the risk of hepatosplenomegaly, abdominal pain, and acute pancreatitis.

**TABLE II**

**Design of Study of Effects of Omega-3 Fatty Acids in Hypertriglyceridemic Patients[a]**

| Dietary period | Percentage of total calories as fat | Cholesterol intake[b] |
|---|---|---|
| Control | | |
| Type IIb ($n$ = 10) | 20–30 | 150 |
| Type V ($n$ = 10) | 5 | <100 |
| Salmon or Fish Oil | | |
| Type IIb ($n$ = 10) | 30 | 325 |
| Type V ($n$ = 10) | 20–30 | 350 |
| Vegetable Oil | | |
| Type IIb ($n$ = 4) | 30 | 325 |
| Type V ($n$ = 8) | 20–30 | 350 |

[a]Modified from Phillipson *et al.*, 1985. Reprinted with permission.
[b]Values stated in mg/day. Cholesterol intakes varied with total calories. The values given represent the cholesterol intake of a subject consuming 2600 kcal/day.

### 3. *Effects of the Diets on Plasma Lipid Levels*

In Type IIb patients, the fish-oil diet lowered the mean total plasma cholesterol level by 27% from 324 to 236 mg/dl ($p < 0.001$). The most significant decline was observed in the mean VLDL cholesterol level, which fell from 62 to 17 mg/dl ($p < 0.001$), but a modest decline was also observed in the mean LDL cholesterol level, which fell from 220 to 194 mg/dl ($p < 0.05$), and in the mean HDL cholesterol level, which fell from 41 to 34 mg/dl ($p < 0.05$). Even more striking was the change in the mean total plasma triglyceride level, which fell by about 65%, from 334 to 118 mg/dl ($p < 0.001$). This decline was largely attributable to the fall in mean VLDL triglyceride, from 216 to 55 mg/dl ($p < 0.005$).

Table III compares mean changes in plasma lipids among the 4 Type IIb patients who consumed all three diets. Although mean plasma cholesterol and triglyceride levels dropped during both test diets, more marked declines in mean total cholesterol, total triglyceride, and VLDL cholesterol and triglyceride occurred during the fish-oil diet. Mean LDL values were similar during all three diets, whereas mean HDL cholesterol was higher after the vegetable-oil diet. Plasma apolipoprotein changes mirrored the lipoprotein changes. During the fish-oil phase, significant reductions and apo B and C-III levels paralleled the declines in LDL and VLDL levels (data not shown).

The effects of the fish-oil diet were even more striking in the 10 Type V patients. Plasma lipid levels remained greatly elevated even during the very low-fat control diet, even though this diet lowered plasma lipids considerably, and 5 patients continued to have milky-appearing plasma with chylomicrons present in the fasting state. The first dramatic change during the fish-oil diet was the virtual disappearance of fasting chylomicronemia as the mean triglyceride content of these chylomicron fractions declined from 443 $\pm$ 210 to 22 $\pm$ 31 mg/dl. The mean total plasma triglyceride level dropped 79% on the fish-oil diet, from 1,353 to 281 mg/dl (Fig. 3), while mean VLDL triglyceride decreased similarly from 1,087 to 167 mg/dl (data not shown). The mean total plasma cholesterol level declined into the normal range after the fish-oil diet, from 373 to 207 mg/dl (Fig. 4). Most of this decline resulted from the marked changes in mean VLDL cholesterol, which decreased from 270 to 70 mg/dl (data not shown). Of interest was the concomitant rise in mean LDL cholesterol from 84 to 125 mg/dl. As in the Type IIb patients, changes in apolipoprotein levels mirrored changes in lipoprotein levels. Apo A-1 levels did not change, but apo B, C-III, and E levels all decreased significantly.

When 8 of the Type V patients switched from the fish-oil diet to omega-6-rich vegetable-oil diet, their plasma triglyceride levels all rose within 3–4 days. As shown in Table IV, mean total plasma triglyceride and

**TABLE III**

**Plasma Lipid Changes in Four Patients With Hyperlipoproteinemia Type IIb After Control, Fish-Oil, and Vegetable-Oil Diets[a]**

| | | | | $p$ value | | |
|---|---|---|---|---|---|---|
| Plasma lipids | Control | Fish oil | Vegetable oil | Control vs. fish oil | Control vs. vegetable oil | Fish oil vs. vegetable oil |
| Cholesterol | | | | | | |
| Total | 285 ± 8 | 199 ± 12 | 235 ± 6 | <0.01 | <0.01 | <0.01 |
| VLDL | 80 ± 22 | 18 ± 6 | 46 ± 18 | <0.01 | <0.01 | <0.05 |
| LDL | 173 ± 25 | 156 ± 19 | 149 ± 16 | NS | <0.05 | NS |
| HDL | 36 ± 5 | 33 ± 7 | 44 ± 9 | NS | <0.05 | <0.01 |
| Triglyceride | | | | | | |
| Total | 374 ± 105 | 137 ± 26 | 258 ± 72 | <0.01 | <0.05 | <0.01 |
| VLDL | 304 ± 94 | 69 ± 21 | 177 ± 62 | <0.01 | <0.05 | <0.05 |
| LDL | 59 ± 16 | 64 ± 11 | 56 ± 9 | NS | NS | NS |

[a]Values are means ± SD, stated in mg/dl. To convert cholesterol from mg/dl, to m*M*, multiply by 0.026; to convert triglyceride from mg/dl to m*M*, multiply by 0.0113. (Modified from Phillipson *et al.*, 1985. Reprinted with permission.)

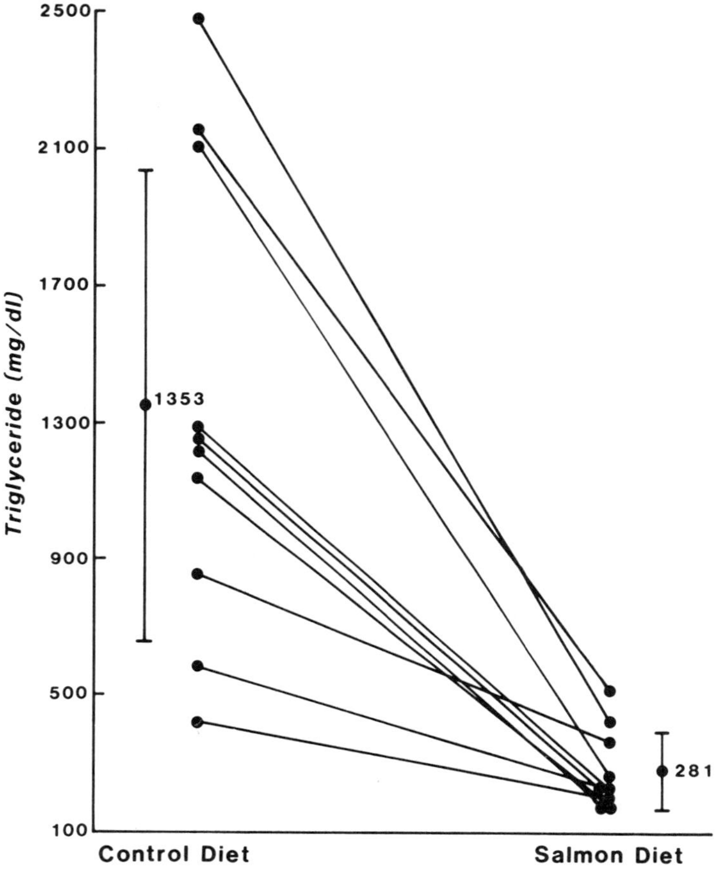


**Fig. 3.** Total plasma triglyceride changes were plotted for 10 patients with hyperlipoproteinemia Type V during control and salmon oil diets. The mean decrease was 1,072 mg/dl ($p < 0.001$). To convert triglyceride from mg/dl to m*M*, multiply by 0.0113. (From Phillipson *et al.*, 1985. Reprinted with permission.)

VLDL triglyceride levels more than tripled after 10–14 days of vegetable-oil feeding. The mean total plasma cholesterol showed a modest rise during the vegetable oil diet, while mean LDL cholesterol decreased. The vegetable-oil phase was prematurely discontinued after two weeks because all 8 patients experienced enhanced hypertriglyceridemia, and some developed abdominal symptoms.

The triglyceride responses of one Type V patient are of special interest. His total plasma triglyceride level, which fell from 2,130 to 516 mg/dl after switching from the control to the fish-oil diet, rose to 1,400 mg/dl after

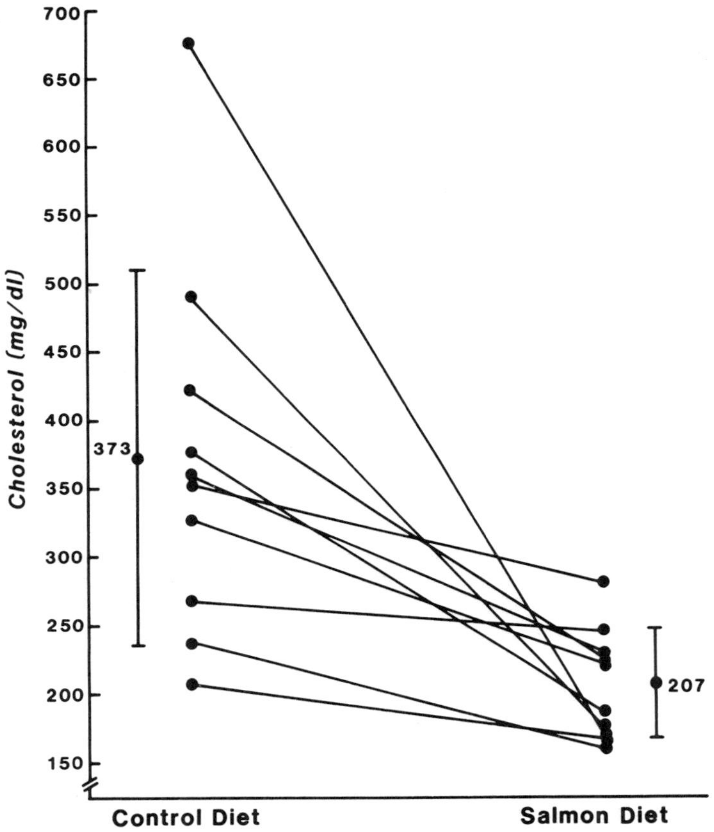


**Fig. 4.** Total plasma cholesterol changes were plotted for 10 patients with hyperlipoproteinemia Type V during control and salmon oil diets. The mean decrease was 166 mg/dl ($p < 0.01$). To convert cholesterol from mg/dl to m*M*, multiply by 0.026. (From Phillipson *et al.*, 1985. Reprinted with permission.)

only 10 days on the vegetable-oil diet. Because this increase was accompanied by abdominal discomfort and liver tenderness, he switched back to the fish-oil diet. After 12 days, his total plasma triglyceride level stabilized at 250 mg/dl, and his symptoms disappeared.

Our studies showed that the fish-oil diet had a more profound effect on the 20 hypertriglyceridemic patients than on the 12 normal patients (Phillipson *et al.*, 1985; Harris *et al.*, 1983). In the hypertriglyceridemic patients, the mean total plasma triglyceride level fell 79% in the 10 Type V patients and 65% in the 10 Type IIb patients, while the mean total plasma cholesterol level fell 45% in the Type V group and 27% in the Type IIb

TABLE IV

**Plasma Lipid Changes in 8 Patients With Hyperlipoproteinemia Type V After Control, Fish-Oil, and Vegetable-Oil Diets[a]**

| | | | | *p* value | |
|---|---|---|---|---|---|
| Plasma lipids | Control | Fish oil | Vegetable oil | Control vs. fish oil | Fish oil vs. vegetable oil |
| Cholesterol | | | | | |
| Total | 377 ± 155 | 195 ± 31 | 264 ± 97 | <0.01 | NS |
| VLDL | 251 ± 148 | 74 ± 67 | 216 ± 219 | <0.05 | <0.05 |
| LDL | 77 ± 55 | 110 ± 34 | 79 ± 30 | <0.05 | <0.05 |
| HDL | 31 ± 7 | 35 ± 12 | 31 ± 11 | NS | NS |
| Triglyceride | | | | | |
| Total | 1,432 ± 750 | 272 ± 120 | 841 ± 514 | <0.01 | <0.05 |
| VLDL | 1,249 ± 681 | 171 ± 119 | 550 ± 360 | <0.01 | NS |
| LDL | 70 ± 34 | 65 ± 18 | 71 ± 31 | NS | NS |

[a]Values are means ± SD, stated in mg/dl. To convert cholesterol from mg/dl, to m*M*, multiply by 0.026; to convert triglyceride from mg/dl to m*M*, multiply by 0.0113. Differences between the control and vegetable-oil diets were not significant. (Modified from Phillipson *et al.*, 1985. Reprinted with permission.)

group. In the 12 normal subjects, decreases were 38% for triglyceride and 14% for cholesterol. Therefore, dietary fish oil appears to produce greater reductions in plasma lipids, especially VLDL, as the severity of the hypertriglyceridemia increases.

These data may have considerable therapeutic importance for patients with moderate to severe hypertriglyceridemia. Up to now, the only dietary treatment for severely hyperlipoproteinemic Type V patients has been drastic restriction of dietary fat to 5–10% of total calories (Connor and Connor, 1982). Americans, who are accustomed to consuming almost 40% of calories as fat, find such restriction possible on a short-term basis but almost impossible on a long-term basis.

Our findings suggest that fish, shellfish, or other foods containing marine omega-3 fatty acids may lower plasma triglyceride more than a very low-fat diet in patients with hypertriglyceridemia Type IIb, IV, or V and high VLDL levels. Salmon, which contains 10% fat by weight and was previously contraindicated for severely hypertriglyceridemic patients, now appears to be appropriate. Also appropriate are the commonly consumed white fish, which contain 1–2% fat by weight and up to 48% of total fatty acids as omega-3 fatty acids. Type V patients may also consume shellfish, which, although high in cholesterol, are low in fat and high in omega-3 fatty acids.

The value of commercial fish-oil supplements in treating patients with hypertriglyceridemia remains uncertain. High doses were used in our studies to produce maximal effects, but these doses should still be considered experimental. Further studies will be required to establish the minimum amounts of fish or fish oils that will produce optimum results in hyperlipidemic patients.

The reduction of chylomicrons observed in the Type V patients during the fish-oil diet also raised a number of unanswered questions. We had previously reported that fish oils improve fat tolerance by markedly decreasing the usual chylomicronemia that follows fatty meals (Goodnight *et al.*, 1982). This improvement could result from diminished absorption, decreased synthesis, and slower transport of chylomicrons into the systemic circulation, or, alternatively, from more rapid removal of chylomicrons that reach the circulation. No evidence of diminished absorption exists, and fat balance studies did not show increased fat excretion in stools during consumption of fish-oil-enriched diets (Connor and Connor, 1982). The role of reduced chylomicron production or enhanced chylomicron removal has not yet been examined.

## IV. MECHANISMS OF THE HYPOLIPIDEMIC EFFECTS OF FISH OILS

We designed two further experiments to explore how omega-3 fatty acids may exert their effects on plasma triglyceride and cholesterol levels. The first study examined how fish oil inhibits the usual hypertriglyceridemia that follows ingestion of a high-carbohydrate meal. The second assessed the effects of fish oil on VLDL and LDL synthesis and turnover.

### A. Effects of Fish Oil on Carbohydrate-Induced Hypertriglyceridemia

Carbohydrate-induced hypertriglyceridemia is a well-known physiological response to abrupt increases in carbohydrate intake. In this model, an abrupt increase in carbohydrate intake stimulates VLDL triglyceride synthesis and leads to hypertriglyceridemia, which may persist for many weeks (Ahrens *et al.*, 1961; Ruderman *et al.*, 1971; Mancini *et al.*, 1973; Witztum and Schonfeld, 1978). We postulated that incorporation of fish oil into a high-carbohydrate diet would inhibit VLDL synthesis and the consequent hypertriglyceridemia. We tested this hypothesis in seven mildly hypertriglyceridemic but otherwise healthy subjects, whose ages ranged from 22 to 54 years (Harris *et al.*, 1984b).

### 1. *Composition of Test Diets*

The seven subjects were fed three experimental diets, each composed of a liquid formula plus three bran muffins per day to supply fiber. The baseline diet contained 45% of calories as carbohydrate. The high-carbohydrate control diet and the high-carbohydrate/fish-oil diet each contained 15% of calories as fat, 10% as protein, and 75% as carbohydrate. A blend of peanut oil and cocoa butter provided the fat in the baseline and high-carbohydrate control diets. About 3.5 tablespoons of a commercial marine-lipid concentrate provided the 50 g of fat per 3000 kcal/day in the high-carbohydrate/fish-oil diet. This diet contained 32% of fat as omega-3 fatty acids and included 8.5 g of EPA and 5.5 g of DHA.

After 7 days of the baseline diet, subjects consumed the experimental diets in three sequences in the CRC. In the first and second sequences, the high-carbohydrate control diet preceded the high-carbohydrate/fish-oil diet (Figs. 5A and 5B). The control diet was fed for 10 days in the first sequence and 20 days in the second sequence to ensure that the hypertriglyceridemia did not resolve spontaneously after 10 days. In the third sequence, the high-carbohydrate/fish oil diet was fed for 25 days, followed by the high-carbohydrate control diet for 15 days (Fig. 5C). The first sequence included 3 subjects, and the second and third sequences each included 2 subjects.

An additional study in 3 of the subjects tested a high-carbohydrate/corn-oil regimen. This diet was similar to the high-carbohydrate/fish-oil diet, except that corn oil replaced the fish oil. Linoleic acid (18:2 omega-6) provided 57% of the fatty acids in the high-carbohydrate/corn-oil diet. The high-carbohydrate control diet preceded the corn-oil phase exactly as in the first two fish-oil studies.

### 2. *Effects of the Diets on Plasma Lipid Levels*

During the first sequence, the mean total plasma triglyceride level rose from 105 mg/dl during the baseline diet to 194 mg/dl during the high-carbohydrate control diet ($p < 0.01$). The magnitude of the increase in triglyceride level correlated directly with the baseline triglyceride level in each subject. The rise in the mean total plasma triglyceride level, which peaked within 5 days, resulted almost entirely from the mean increase in the VLDL triglyceride fraction, which more than doubled from 69 to 156 mg/dl ($p < 0.01$) during the high-carbohydrate control diet (Fig. 6). Although the mean total plasma cholesterol level declined only slightly, the mean VLDL cholesterol level nearly doubled, from 18 to 34 ($p < 0.01$). LDL cholesterol fell from 125 to 106 mg/dl ($p < 0.01$), and HDL cholesterol decreased from 49 to 41 mg/dl ($p < 0.05$).

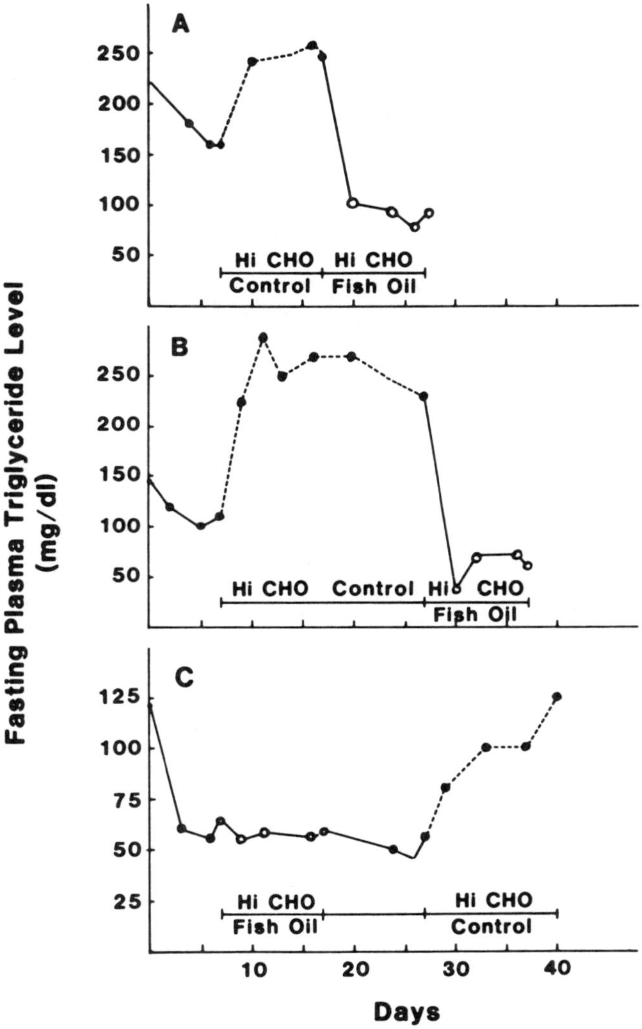


**Fig. 5.** The effects of the baseline (o———o) diet, the high-carbohydrate control (Hi CHO Control) diet (o— — —o) and the high-carbohydrate/fish-oil (Hi CHO Fish Oil) diet (o———o) on fasting total plasma triglyceride level was studied in seven mildly hypertriglyceridemic but otherwise healthy subjects. **5A.** Carbohydrate-induced hypertriglyceridemia decreased when three subjects consuming the Hi CHO Control diet for 10 days were switched to the Hi CHO Fish Oil diet. **5B.** Carbohydrate-induced hypertriglyceridemia, which persisted through 20 days on the Hi CHO Control diet, was reversed by the Hi CHO Fish Oil diet in two subjects. **5C.** The Hi CHO Fish Oil diet prevented carbohydrate-induced hypertriglyceridemia in two subjects. (From Harris *et al.*, 1984b). Reprinted with permission.)

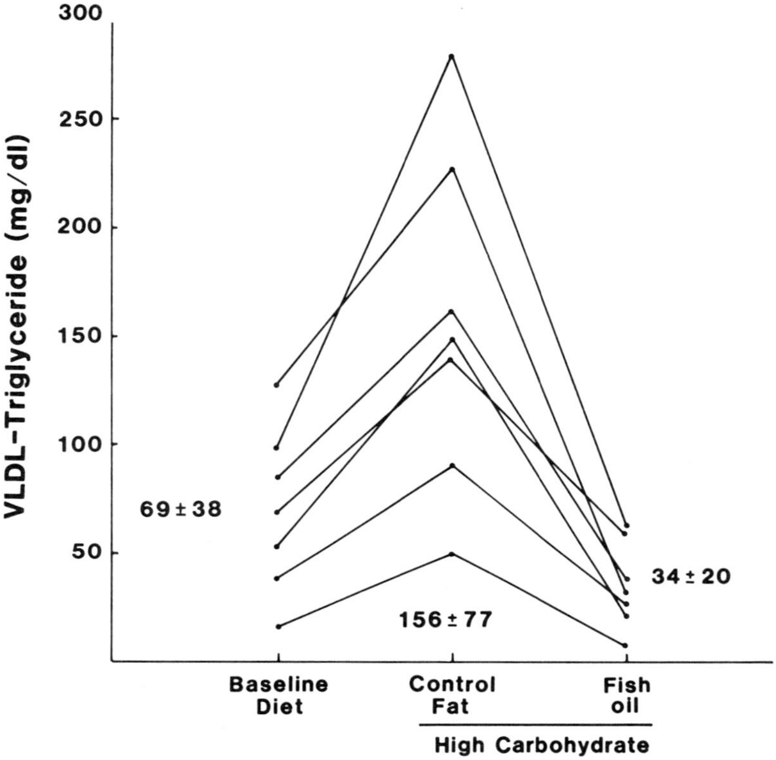


**Fig. 6.** The effects of the baseline diet, the high-carbohydrate control diet and the high-carbohydrate/fish-oil diet on VLDL triglyceride level were studied in seven mildly hypertriglyceridemic but otherwise healthy subjects. (From Harris *et al.*, 1984b. Reprinted with permission.)

When the high-carbohydrate diet was isocalorically replaced by the high-carbohydrate/fish oil diet 10 days later, the elevated mean total plasma triglyceride concentration dropped 61% from 194 to 75 mg/dl ($p < 0.01$). This decrease occurred within 3 days (Fig. 5A). Once again, the mean decrease in VLDL triglyceride from 156 to 34 mg/dl ($p < 0.01$) was largely responsible for this effect. The mean total plasma cholesterol level also decreased significantly from 172 to 153 mg/dl ($p < 0.01$), primarily because of the mean decrease in VLDL cholesterol from 34 to 12 mg/dl ($p < 0.01$).

In the second sequence, the hypertriglyceridemia persisted when the high-carbohydrate diet phase was increased from 10 to 20 days, and no significant decreases were observed until the high-carbohydrate/fish-oil diet was introduced (Fig. 5B). In the third sequence, when the high-carbohydrate/fish-oil diet followed the baseline diet, the mean total plasma triglyceride level fell and remained low until the fish oil was removed from the high-carbohydrate diet. Then the triglyceride level promptly increased (Fig. 5C).

In the related study, the high-carbohydrate/corn-oil regimen did not affect carbohydrate-induced hypertriglyceridemia, as evidenced by mean total plasma triglyceride levels measured during the baseline diet (93 mg/dl), the high-carbohydrate control diet (196 mg/dl), the high-carbohydrate/corn-oil diet (215 mg/dl), and the high-carbohydrate/fish-oil diet (86 mg/dl).

Apolipoprotein changes were also measured. The high-carbohydrate control diet lowered apo B levels ($p < 0.01$) and raised apo C-III concentrations ($p < 0.01$), but apo A-1 and apo E levels did not change. The high-carbohydrate/fish-oil diet decreased levels of apo A-1 ($p < 0.05$) and apo C-III ($p < 0.01$) but did not affect apo B and apo E concentrations.

These data indicated that dietary fish oil not only prevented but also rapidly reversed carbohydrate-induced elevations in total triglyceride and VLDL triglyceride levels. Because the primary difference between the high-carbohydrate/fish-oil and high-carbohydrate/corn-oil diets was their fatty acid composition, the differences in their effects were probably attributable to the omega-3 fatty acids in the fish-oil diet. This finding implied an inhibitory effect of omega-3 fatty acids on hepatic VLDL production.

## B. Effects of Fish Oils on VLDL and LDL Synthesis and Turnover

The hypothesis that omega-3 fatty acids reduce VLDL levels by inhibiting VLDL synthesis and turnover was further supported in another study of the hypotriglyceridemic effects of these fatty acids. In this experiment, we injected [$^3$H]glycerol into subjects who had consumed control and fish-oil diets and measured the rates of synthesis and turnover of VLDL triglyceride (Harris *et al.*, 1984a).

Because we wanted to study these mechanisms in subjects with greatly different pool sizes of plasma triglyceride, we selected 10 male subjects whose fasting plasma triglyceride concentrations ranged from 34 to 4,180 mg/dl. Three subjects had normal triglyceride levels, and 7 were hypertriglyceridemic.

### 1. *Composition of Test Diets*

Two liquid formula diets were used in the study—a fish-oil diet and a control diet containing fats found in the typical American diet. Both contained 15–20% of calories as fat, 65–75% as carbohydrate, and 10–15% as protein. Once more, the only difference between the two diets was the fat source: The control diet was high in linoleic acid (18:2 omega-6) and contained virtually no omega-3 fatty acids, and the fish-oil diet provided about 17 g of omega-3 fatty acids per day. Fat in the control diet was administered as a 1:2 blend of cocoa butter and peanut oil incorporated into the liquid formula, whereas fat in the fish oil diet was a commercial preparation given separately and divided into three doses per day.

Each experimental diet was consumed for 3–5 weeks to allow plasma triglyceride levels to stabilize, particularly in the hypertriglyceridemic patients, before VLDL turnover was measured. Seven subjects consumed the control diet first, and three consumed the fish-oil diet first.

### 2. *Effects of the Diets on Plasma Lipid Levels*

The isocaloric substitution of fish oil for the control vegetable fat produced the expected reductions in total and lipoprotein lipid levels in all 10 subjects, irrespective of the order in which the diets were consumed. The mean total plasma cholesterol level fell 26% from 195 to 144 mg/dl ($p < 0.005$) during the fish-oil diet, largely as a result of the mean decrease in VLDL cholesterol from 83 to 21 mg/dl ($p < 0.005$). Although LDL cholesterol did not change significantly, HDL cholesterol fell from 31 to 24 mg/dl ($p < 0.005$). Similarly, the fish-oil regimen resulted in a significant decrease in mean total triglyceride from 442 to 150 mg/dl ($p < 0.025$) and in mean VLDL triglyceride from 398 to 87 mg/dl ($p < 0.005$). The normal and hypertriglyceridemic subjects responded similarly.

After the [$^3$H]glycerol was administered and incorporated into VLDL triglyceride, kinetic decay curves were analyzed via a computer model system, and VLDL synthesis and turnover were calculated (Zech *et al.*, 1979). The incorporation of omega-3 fatty acids into the diet caused a 72% decrease ($p < 0.025$) in the mean VLDL triglyceride pool size (Table V). This decrease was associated with a 45% reduction in the rate of VLDL triglyceride synthesis ($p < 0.005$) and a 45% decrease in the residence time of VLDL triglyceride in plasma ($p < 0.005$). The reciprocal of the residence time is the fractional catabolic rate (FCR), which increased 65% ($p < 0.005$). The VLDL cholesterol/triglyceride ratio also rose significantly during the fish-oil diet ($p < 0.05$). Finally, the ratio of the fast to the slow synthesis pathway remained unchanged during fish-oil feeding. The same trends were seen in the 3 normal and 7 hypertriglyceridemic patients studied.

Similar results were also found in a somewhat different dietary study, in which the apo B of VLDL was labeled (Nestel *et al.*, 1984). In the third experiment, LDL turnover was measured in normal subjects. The production of LDL apo B diminished significantly during fish-oil consumption, and the fractional catabolic rate for LDL increased (Illingworth *et al.*, 1983). Because VLDL apo B is the precursor of LDL apo B in normal humans

**TABLE V**

**The Effects of Dietary Fish Oil on VLDL Metabolism**[a]

| | VLDL Lipids | | VLDL Triglyceride | | | | | |
|---|---|---|---|---|---|---|---|---|
| | Triglyceride[b] (mg/dl) | Rate of Cholesterol/ triglyceride | Pool size (g) | Synthesis (mg/hr) | Synthesis (mg/kg ideal weight/hr) | Fractional catabolic rate ($hr^{-1}$) | Residence time in plasma (hr) | Ratio of fast/ slow synthesis pathways |
| Control diet[c] | 398 ± 317 | 0.18 ± 0.03 | 11.4 ± 10.2 | 1,685 ± 1,073 | 23.0 ± 14.3 | 0.23 ± 0.12 | 5.8 ± 3.4 | 2.3 ± 0.79 |
| Fish-oil diet[c] | 87 ± 77 | 0.25 ± 0.08 | 3.2 ± 2.5 | 918 ± 563 | 12.6 ± 7.5 | 0.38 ± 0.16 | 3.2 ± 1.6 | 2.4 ± 1.34 |
| *p* value | $<0.005$ | $<0.05$ | $<0.025$ | $<0.005$ | $<0.005$ | $<0.005$ | $<0.005$ | NS |
| Change | −78% | +39% | −72% | −46% | −45% | +65% | −45% | +4% |
| Normal values[d] | 113 ± 10 | 0.21 ± 0.01 | — | 806 ± 123 | 11.5 ± 1.8 | 0.19 ± 0.01 | 5.2 ± 0.4 | 2.7 ± 0.36 |

[a]Modified from Harris *et al.*, 1984a. Reprinted with permission.
[b]Data represent the average VLDL triglyceride concentration during the 48-hour turnover study.
[c]Values represent the means ± SD for 10 male subjects who consumed this diet.
[d]Normal values represent the means ± SD for 13 normal subjects.

(Sigurdsson *et al.*, 1975), these additional data support the hypothesis that omega-3 fatty acids reduce the rate of VLDL secretion from the liver.

Three *in vitro* studies provide direct evidence that omega-3 fatty acids from fish oil suppress hepatic synthesis of triglyceride and VLDL. These were carried out in the perfused rat liver and in rat and rabbit liver cells in primary culture (Wong *et al.*, 1983; Wong *et al.*, 1985; Benner *et al.*, 1985). In each study, triglyceride synthesis decreased. In one, production of ketone bodies increased, and in the other two, omega-3 fatty acids were diverted from triglyceride synthesis to phospholipid synthesis. Taken together, all of these studies offer very strong evidence that suppression of VLDL and triglyceride synthesis is a primary mechanism by which omega-3 fatty acids exert their hypolipidemic effects.

## V. SUMMARY

The studies described here show that dietary omega-3 fatty acids from fish and fish oil have profound hypolipidemic effects in normal subjects and in hypertriglyceridemic patients with combined hyperlipoproteinemia Type IIb and hyperlipoproteinemia Type V. A total of 68 adults participated in these carefully controlled metabolic experiments. In each study participant, marked reductions in plasma cholesterol and triglyceride concentrations were observed, and the drop in triglyceride was especially significant. Decreases in VLDL, chylomicrons, chylomicron remnants, LDL, apo B, and apo E were also seen. Changes in HDL were inconsistent and varied from subject to subject.

Whereas the mechanisms underlying the hypolipidemic action of corn, safflower, or other omega-6-rich vegetable oils containing linoleic acid remains unclear, the mechanisms by which the omega-3-rich fish oils exert these effects is well documented. Omega-3 fatty acids lower triglyceride and VLDL synthesis in the liver; they shorten the turnover rate of VLDL in plasma; and they decrease LDL production.

The use of omega-3 fatty acids, combined with such other dietary measures as reduction of saturated fat and cholesterol, to treat some hypertriglyceridemic patients and especially Type V hypertriglyceridemic patients appears to rest on a well-supported rationale. Further studies are needed to determine the precise doses and indications for treatment of hyperlipidemia and to determine any differences in the effects of EPA and DHA, the two major omega-3 fatty acids in fish oil. These data, coupled with the known antithrombotic effects of omega-3 fatty acids on prostaglandin secretion and platelet function, suggest an important potential role for omega-3 fatty acids in coronary heart disease and other atherosclerotic disorders.

## ACKNOWLEDGMENTS

The work reported here was supported by research grants from the National Heart, Lung, and Blood Institute (No. HL25687) and from the General Clinical Research Center (No. RR00334).

## REFERENCES

Ahrens, E. H., and Boucher, C. A. (1978). The composition of a simulated American diet. *J. Amer. Diet. Assn.* **73**, 613–620.

Ahrens, E. H., Insull, W., Hirsch, J., Stoffel, W., Peterson, M., and Farquhar, J. (1959). The effect on human serum lipids of a dietary fat, highly unsaturated, but poor in essential fatty acids. *Lancet* **1**, 115–119.

Ahrens, E. H., Hirsch, J., Oette, K., Farquhar, J. W., and Stein, Y. (1961). Carbohydrate-induced and fat-induced lipemia. *Trans. Assn. Amer. Physicians* **74**, 134–146.

Benner, K. G., Connor, W. E., and Sasaki, A. (1985). Omega-3 fatty acid suppression of triglyceride synthesis and secretion by isolated rabbit hepatocytes [Abstract]. *Clin. Res.* **33**, 567A.

Bronsgeest-Schoute, H. C., van Gent, C. M., Luten, J. B., and Ruiter, A. (1981). The effects of various intakes of omega-3 fatty acids on the blood lipid composition in healthy human subjects. *Amer. J. Clin. Nutr.* **34**, 1752–1757.

Bronte-Stewart, B., Antonis, A., Eales, L., and Brock, J. F. (1956). Effects of feeding different fats on serum cholesterol levels. *Lancet* **2**, 521–526.

Chait, A., Onitiri, A., Nicoll, A., Rabaya, E., Davies, J., and Lewis, B. (1974). Reduction of serum triglyceride levels by polyunsaturated fat. Studies on the mode of action and on very low density lipoprotein composition. *Atherosclerosis* **20**, 347–364.

Connor, W. E., and Connor, S. L. (1982). The dietary treatment of hyperlipidemia: rationale, technique and efficacy. *Med. Clin. N. Amer.*, **66**, 485–518.

Connor, W. E., Witiak, D. T., Stone, O. B., and Armstrong, M. L. (1969). Cholesterol balance and fecal neutral steroid and bile acid excretion in normal men fed dietary fats of different fatty acid composition. *J. Clin. Invest.* **48**, 1363–1375.

Fredrickson, D. S., and Levy, R. I. (1972). Familial hyperlipoproteinemia. *In* "Metabolic Basis of Inherited Disease" (J. B. Stanbury, J. B. Wyngaarden, and D. S. Fredrickson, eds.), 3rd ed., p. 545. McGraw-Hill, New York.

Goodnight, S. H., Harris, W. S., Connor, W. E., and Illingworth, D. R. (1982). Polyunsaturated fatty acids, hyperlipidemia and thrombosis. *Arteriosclerosis* **2**, 87–113.

Harris, W. S., Connor, W. E., and McMurry, M. P. (1983). The comparative reduction of the plasma lipids and lipoproteins by dietary polyunsaturated fats: salmon oil vs. vegetable oils. *Metabolism* **32**, 179–184.

Harris, W. S., Connor, W. E., Illingworth, D. R., Rothrock, D. W., and Foster, D. M. (1984a). The mechanism of the hypotriglyceridemic effects of dietary omega-3 fatty acids in man [Abstract]. *Clin. Res.* **32**, 560A.

Harris, W. S., Connor, W. E., Inkeles, S. B., and Illingworth, D. R. (1984b). Dietary omega-3 fatty acids prevent carbohydrate-induced hypertriglyceridemia. *Metabolism* **33**, 1016–1019.

Illingworth, D. R., Harris, W. S., and Connor, W. E. (1983). Inhibition of low density lipoprotein synthesis by dietary omega-3 fatty acids in humans. *Arteriosclerosis* **4**, 270–275.

Karmali, R. H., Marsh, J., and Fuchs, C. (1984). Effect of omega-3 fatty acids on growth of a mammary rat tumor. *J. Nat. Cancer Inst.* **73**, 457–461.

Keys, A., Anderson, J. T., and Grande, F. (1957). "Essential" fatty acids, degree of unsaturation and effects of corn (maize) oil on the serum cholesterol level in man. *Lancet* **1**, 66–68.

Malmros, H., and Wigand, G. (1957). The effect on serum cholesterol of diets containing different fats. *Lancet* **1**, 1–7.

Mancini, M., Mattock, M., Rabaya, E., Chait, A., and Lewis, B. (1973). Studies on the mechanisms of carbohydrate-induced lipemia in normal man. *Atherosclerosis* **17**, 445–454.

Nestel, P. J., Havenstein, N., Whyte, H. M., Scott, T. W., and Cook, L. J. (1973). Lowering of plasma cholesterol and enhanced sterol excretion with the consumption of polyunsaturated ruminant fats. *N. Engl. J. Med.* **288**, 379–382.

Nestel, P. J., Havenstein, N., Scott, T. W., and Cook, L. J. (1974). Polyunsaturated ruminant fats and cholesterol metabolism in man. *Aust. NZ J. Med.* **4**, 497–501.

Nestel, P. J., Havenstein, N., Homma, Y., Scott, T. W., and Cook, L. J. (1975). Increased sterol excretion with polyunsaturated-fat, high-cholesterol diets. *Metabolism* **24**, 189–198.

Nestel, P. J., Connor, W. E., Reardon, M. R., Connor, S., Wong, S., and Boston, R. (1984). Suppression by diets rich in fish oil of very low density lipoprotein production in men. *J. Clin. Invest.* **74**, 82–89.

Neuringer, M., and Connor, W. E. (1986). N-3 fatty acids in the brain and retina. Evidence for their essentiality. *Nutr. Rev.* **44**, 285–294.

Phillipson, B. E., Rothrock, D. W., Connor, W. E., Harris, W. S., and Illingworth, D. R. (1985). The reduction of plasma lipids, lipoproteins, and apoproteins in hypertriglyceridemic patients by dietary fish oils. *N. Engl. J. Med.* **312**, 1210–1216.

Prichette, J. D., Robinson, D. R., and Seinberg, A. D. (1981). Dietary enrichment with the polyunsaturated fatty acid eicosapentaenoic acid prevents proteinuria and prolongs survival in NZB X NZW $F_1$ mice. *J. Clin. Invest.* **68**, 556–559.

Ruderman, N. B., Jones, A. L., Krauss, R. M., and Shafrir, E. (1971). A biochemical and morphologic study of very low density lipoproteins in carbohydrate-induced hypertriglyceridemia. *J. Clin. Invest.* **50**, 1355–1368.

Sanders, T. A. B., Vickers, M., and Haines, A. P. (1981). Effect on blood lipids and haemostasis of a supplement of cod liver oil, rich in eicosapentaenoic and docosahexaenoic acids in healthy young men. *Clin. Sci.* **61**, 317–324.

Shepherd, J., Packard, C. J., Patsch, J. R., Gotto, A. M., and Taunton, O. D. (1978). Effects of dietary polyunsaturated and saturated fat on the properties of high density lipoproteins and metabolism of apolipoprotein A-2. *J. Clin. Invest.* **61**, 1582–1592.

Shepherd, J., Packard, C. J., Grundy, S. M., Yeshurun, D., Gotto, A. M., and Taunton, O. D. (1980). Effects of saturated and polyunsaturated fat diets on the chemical composition and metabolism of low density lipoproteins in man. *J. Lipid Res.* **21**, 91–99.

Sigurdsson, G., Nicoll, A., and Lewis, B. (1975). Conversion of very low density lipoprotein to low density lipoprotein. A metabolic study of apolipoprotein B kinetics in human subjects. *J. Clin. Invest.* **56**, 1481–1490.

Turner, J. D., Le, N.-A., and Brown, W. V. (1981). Effect of changing dietary fat saturation on low density lipoprotein metabolism in man. *Amer. J. Physiol.* **241**, E57–E63.

von Lossonczy, T. O., Ruiter, A., Bronsgeest-Schoute, H. C., van Gent, C. M., and Hermus, R. J. (1978). The effect of a fish diet on serum lipids in healthy human subjects. *Amer. J. Clin. Nutr.* **31**, 1340–1346.

Witztum, J. L., and Schonfeld, G. (1978). Carbohydrate diet-induced changes in very low density lipoprotein composition and structures. *Diabetes* **27**, 1215–1229.

Wong, S. H., Nestel, P. J., Trimble, R. P., Storer, B. G., Illman, R. J., and Topping, D. L. (1984). The adaptive effects of dietary fish and safflower oil on lipid and lipoprotein metabolism in perfused rat liver. *Biochim. Biophys. Acta* **792**, 103–109.

Wong, S., Reardon, M., and Nestel, P. (1985). Reduced triglyceride formation from long chain polyenoic fatty acids in rat hepatocytes. *Metabolism* **34**, 900–905.

Zech, L., Grundy, S. M., Steinberg, D., and Berman, M. (1979). Kinetic model for production and metabolism of very low density lipoprotein triglycerides. Evidence for a slow production pathway and results for normolipidemic subjects. *J. Clin. Invest.* **63**, 1262–1273.

# 7

# Regulation of Carbohydrate Homeostasis in Diabetes Mellitus

Thomas T. Aoki, Robert M. Walter, and Michael C. Okimura

*Division of Endocrinology*
*University of California, Davis*
*School of Medicine*
*Davis, California*





Nutrition and the Origins of Disease

## I. INTRODUCTION

Conventional, subcutaneously administered insulin therapy often fails to restore normal dietary glucose processing and homeostasis in patients with diabetes mellitus. Today, 65 years following the introduction of insulin for treatment of diabetic patients, the problem remains. This lack of progress is primarily attributable to use of the control theory of treatment: administration of insulin when blood glucose is high and withholding of insulin or administration of glucose when blood glucose is low. Over the past several years, a growing number of investigators, perplexed by this lack of progress, have begun to reexamine the basic tenets underlying current insulin therapy. From this reappraisal has evolved a better appreciation of the important metabolic role the liver plays in fuel homeostasis, a process that functions abnormally in diabetic individuals.

This presentation describes the ''sleeping liver'' hypothesis, which, in addition to providing physiological and biochemical bases for both the inherent strengths and weaknesses of conventional insulin therapy, opens up major new areas of research with definable and clinically testable endpoints. The ''sleeping liver'' model evolved from the following observations.

## II. DISPOSITION OF A 100-g GLUCOSE MEAL IN NORMAL AND DIABETIC HUMANS

Shortly after a normal subject ingests a 100-g glucose meal, absorption of this fuel from the stomach and small intestine commences (20 g/30 cm small intestine/hour) (Holdsworth and Dawson, 1964), insulin levels rise markedly, and large quantities of glucose are transported via the portal vein to the liver. Hepatic glucose production (gluconeogenesis and glycogenolysis), which proceeds at the rate of approximately 2 mg/kg/min (DeFronzo *et al.*, 1981; DeFronzo *et al.*, 1982; Waldhausl *et al.*, 1982; Pilo *et al.*, 1981) to meet total body glucose requirements (*ca* 202 g/day), is promptly suppressed (Waldhausl *et al.*, 1982; Pilo *et al.*, 1981). In the postabsorptive state, exogenous glucose is used to meet energy requirements of the brain (20 g) and is also taken up by muscle (25 g) and stored as fat (5 g). The body oxidizes about 20–25 g of glucose above basal (Foss *et al.*, 1982), most likely in the liver (Meistas and Aoki, 1983), and approximately 25 g of exogenous carbohydrate is retained within the splanchnic bed as glycogen. These calculations, summarized in Table I, support those of other investigators (Meistas and Aoki, 1983; Bjornthorp and Sjöstrom, 1978; Bratusch-Marrain *et al.*, 1980; Costill *et al.*, 1973; Felig and Wahren, 1971; Felig *et al.*, 1975; Perley and Kipnis, 1967; Wahren *et al.*, 1972).

**TABLE I**

**Disposition of a 100-g Glucose Meal by Normal and Type I Diabetic Subjects[a]**

| | | Diabetic Patients | |
|---|---|---|---|
| | Normal Control[b] | Conventional Therapy[b] | Artificial Beta-Cell Therapy[b] |
| Oxidized | 25 | 10 | 100 |
| Stored as hepatic glycogen | 25 | 0 | 24 |
| Glucose transported to: | | | |
| Fat | 5 | 5 | 5 |
| Brain | 20 | 20 | 20 |
| Muscle | 25 | 25 | 25 |
| Glucose space: | | | |
| Left in extracellular fluid | 0 | 29 | 0 |
| Lost in urine | 0 | 22 | 0 |
| TOTAL | 100 | 111[c] | 100 |
| Change in serum glucose[d] | 0 | +150 | 0 |

[a]Data from Aoki *et al.*, 1983; Bjornthorp *et al.*, 1971; Foss *et al.*, 1982; Kety, 1957; Meistas and Aoki, 1983; Reinmuth *et al.*, 1965; Sokoloff, 1960.

[b]Values are given in g/3 hrs.

[c]An additional 11 g of glucose represent endogenous glucose production.

[d]Values are given in mg/dl above baseline after 3 hrs.

In contrast, in conventionally treated Type I insulin-dependent diabetic patients, much more exogenous carbohydrate is thought to pass through the splanchnic bed into the systemic circulation (Perley and Kipnis, 1967). Table I summarizes glucose extraction/deposition during a 3-hour test period in Type I diabetic patients who took their usual insulin injections 30 minutes before ingesting a 100-g glucose meal. The total amount of glucose entering the systemic circulation from the splanchnic bed is approximately 101 g. If an additional 10 g of glucose is oxidized over basal amounts (Foss *et al.*, 1982), a total of 111 g is obtained. These numbers suggest that exogenous glucose is not retained as glycogen on first or multiple passes in the splanchnic bed. To balance these numbers, 11 g of endogenously produced glucose must be postulated even though endogenous hepatic glucose production in Type I diabetic patients is promptly and easily inhibited (Rizza *et al.*, 1981) by moderate increases in systemic (compared to portal) insulin concentrations (50–100 microunits/ml). Furthermore, DeFronzo and associates (1982) reported endogenous glucose production of 14.7 g/hour (44 g/3 hours) in Type I diabetic patients who took their last insulin injection 24 hours before the study. If partial suppression of this extraordinarily large endogenous glucose production ($>350$ g/day) is assumed, so that only 22 g of glucose is produced in the 3-hour test period, then the liver retains 11 g of glucose as glycogen.

Glucose remaining in the glucose space above basal at the end of the 3-hour period may eventually be taken up in part by the gastrointestinal tract, a tissue that is not insulin-dependent, and processed to lactate on second pass, which, in turn, is oxidized or converted by the liver to glycogen or fat. We and others (Jackson *et al.*, 1973a; Jackson *et al.*, 1973b) have not found significant lactate production from muscle following glucose ingestion, which suggests that the gastrointestinal tract must be the primary source of lactate (Boyd *et al.*, 1981) synthesized into glycogen. In addition, because arterial lactate concentrations increase in normal subjects after ingestion of a glucose meal, hepatic lactate extraction (via portal vein, hepatic artery) and hence hepatic gluconeogenesis must be inhibited secondary to the marked increase in portal and systemic insulin concentrations. Thus, glycogen synthesis from lactate must be modest during the glucose meal study. However, when insulin levels fall to basal values, gastrointestinal lactate production may become more important in ongoing gluconeogenesis and glycogen synthesis.

These observations underscore the central role of the liver in dietary glucose processing and homeostasis in humans. Unfortunately, conventional insulin regimens do not restore to normal the demonstrably metabolically dormant ("sleeping") glucose-processing capability of the liver characteristic of insulin-dependent diabetes. In contrast, this can be achieved with two to three days of artificial Beta-cell-directed insulin therapy, a process in which insulin is infused under computer control to achieve and/or maintain predetermined measured circulating blood glucose concentrations within normal limits (Albisser *et al.*, 1974).

Surprisingly, although techniques required to test the "sleeping liver" hypothesis (indirect calorimetry, forearm procedure) have been available for the past 80 years, such studies were not performed until recently. Therefore, support for the "sleeping liver" hypothesis is now largely inferential. Ultimately, direct corroboration (liver biopsy with glycogen staining and appropriate enzymatic studies) is required. Nevertheless, this model appears to have broad implications with respect to the pathophysiology of Type I diabetes mellitus and to restatement of the primary objective of therapy of Type I diabetic patients—from simple control of circulating blood glucose to reestablishment of the metabolic competency of hepatic dietary glucose processing (oxidation, storage, conversion to fat).

## III. THE PROPOSED BIOCHEMICAL DEFECT IN HEPATIC GLUCOSE PROCESSING IN TYPE I DIABETES MELLITUS

Because insulin is not required for glucose entry into the hepatocyte (Cahill *et al.*, 1958), the next most likely rate-limiting site is the conversion of glucose to glucose 6-phosphate, a step mainly mediated by insulin-dependent glucokinase, and, to a lesser extent, by hexokinase, and perhaps by the phosphotransferase of glucose 6-phosphatase (Nordlie, 1974; Arion *et al.*, 1975).

The glucokinase enzyme in normal human liver appears to initiate phosphorylation of glucose (Storer and Cornish-Bowden, 1976; Pilkis, 1968). Its activity increases in the presence of insulin (Cahill *et al.*, 1959) and decreases in its absence (Cahill *et al.*, 1959; Ruderman and Lauris, 1968). In addition, its high $K_m$ (10–20 m$M$ glucose) (Storer and Cornish-Bowden, 1976; Pilkis, 1968) gives it an important regulatory role vis-a-vis portal glucose concentrations after a glucose meal. Indeed, presumably due in part to this enzyme, nondiabetic dog livers can autoregulate glucose concentrations to a degree (Soskin and Levine, 1937). In contrast, livers of diabetic animals lack significant glucokinase activity (Cahill *et al.*, 1958; Cahill *et al.*, 1959) and are thus unable to participate in processing the elevated portal venous glucose concentration after glucose ingestion. In contrast to glucokinase, hepatic hexokinase activity is low even in normal liver (Nordlie, 1974; Nordlie, 1976) and is not increased by insulin. In addition, due to its very low $K_m$ ($10^{-5}$ m$M$ glucose), this enzyme cannot have an important role in regulating glucose concentrations in human portal or systemic arterial or venous blood.

Glucose 6-phosphatase was once thought to be a hydrolase found only in liver and kidney (Anchors and Karnovsky, 1975). However, this enzyme has also been found in small intestinal mucosa, pancreas, adrenals, testes, brain, spleen, and lung (Nordlie, 1974; Anchors and Karnovsky, 1975; Lygre and Nordlie, 1968; Colilla *et al.*, 1975). In liver, 80–85% of this enzyme's activity is found in the endoplasmic reticulum and 15–20% in the nuclear membrane (Gunderson and Nordlie, 1975). This unique enzyme not only degrades glucose 6-phosphate, but has also been reported to have the capacity to synthesize glucose 6-phosphate in amounts that exceed by more than 50% its capacity to degrade glucose 6-phosphate (Nordlie, 1974; Nordlie, 1976; Lygre and Nordlie, 1968; Colilla *et al.*, 1975; Alvares and Nordlie, 1975; Alvares and Nordlie, 1976). The importance of this alternate enzymatic pathway remains to be determined.

It now appears that in normal liver, insulin-dependent glucokinase and, to a lesser extent, hexokinase, and possibly glucose 6-phosphatase all contribute to formation of glucose 6-phosphate. Experimental and clinical observations suggest that glucokinase activity is markedly decreased in poorly regulated insulin-dependent diabetic patients. Primarily because of this diminished glucokinase activity, incoming portal vein glucose surges through the liver on first and multiple passes following glucose ingestion. In the near absence of glucokinase, a small amount (10%) of glucose is apparently phosphorylated by insulin-independent hexokinase and possibly via the phosphotransferase activity of glucose 6-phosphatase.

When poorly regulated diabetic patients are placed on artificial Beta-cell therapy for three days, net synthesis and activation of glucokinase may be responsible for the observed restoration of dietary glucose processing and homeostasis (Foss *et al.*, 1982). In addition, we recently found that Type I diabetic subjects manifest net positive nitrogen balance (12 g protein/day × 4 days) while on artificial Beta-cell therapy, without any change in urinary 3-methylhistine excretion. This observation suggests that resynthesis of multiple enzymes, not just glucokinase, may be involved in carbohydrate and protein processing (Foss *et al.*, 1982).

## IV. CLINICAL OBSERVATIONS AND IMPLICATIONS

The ''sleeping liver'' model appears to reconcile a number of apparently disparate clinical observations:

1. Clinicians have long known that 4–7 days of aggressive pursuit of elevated glucose levels, with large and frequent subcutaneous, intramuscular, or intravenous insulin injections, are required to regulate Type I diabetic subjects (control theory). It is reasonable to expect a somewhat longer clinical course, culminating in partial activation of hepatic dietary glucose processing, if insulin is given subcutaneously.

2. Clinicians have long noted a diminution in the amount of insulin required to maintain this degree of control after ''regulation'' of circulating blood glucose is achieved. This latter observation correlates well with the biphasic insulin curve observed in insulin-dependent subjects under artificial Beta-cell therapy.

3. Once partial activation of hepatic dietary glucose processing has been achieved using aggressive subcutaneous, intramuscular, and/or intravenous insulin administration, placement of the now partially regulated/metabolically restored diabetic patient on a single or split (NPH + CZI) dose of insulin results in gradual (7–10 days) deterioration of the liver's ability to process dietary glucose.

4. Multiple episodes of hypoglycemia are seen in Type I diabetic subjects attempting to achieve physiological control of their diabetes by means of multiple injections and strict adherence to dietary guidelines. Because

the diabetic liver does not participate to any appreciable extent in the processing of dietary carbohydrate, the patient on conventional insulin therapy, must, in order to approach euglycemia, administer precisely the amount of insulin that will sequester both exogenous and endogenous glucose in muscle over and above that required by brain and other glucose-consuming tissues—a most difficult, if not impossible, task.

In summary, the "sleeping liver" hypothesis, derived from a substantial body of clinical observations and based on physiologically and biochemically testable theory, has far-reaching implications with respect to understanding the pathophysiology and treatment of Type I diabetes mellitus. Its verification by appropriate studies, some presented here, could ultimately lead to reestablishment of normal fuel processing and glucose homeostasis in insulin-dependent diabetic outpatients.

## V. FUEL PROCESSING IN NORMAL AND INSULIN-DEPENDENT HUMANS

We have reported (Foss *et al.*, 1982) that restoration of glucose processing in insulin-dependent diabetic patients is inducible by several days of artificial Beta-cell therapy. This metabolic feat has yet to be accomplished by any other treatment modality, including single or multiple preprandial insulin administration, the insulin pump, or infusion of exogenous insulin into the portal vein. It is likely that the artificial Beta-cell makes possible the net synthesis and activation of hepatic dietary fuel-processing enzymes, including glucokinase, by providing large, rapid increases in systemic insulin concentrations through intravenous insulin administration, by making insulin available throughout the basal period, and by sensitive, near-physiologic timing of insulin administration.

Several observations support the hypothesis that the dietary glucose-processing defect characteristic of conventionally insulin-treated diabetic subjects can largely be attributed to a marked reduction of hepatic glucose oxidation and storage. After several days of euglycemic control with the artificial Beta-cell, we observed a marked and progressive increase in the amount of dietary carbohydrate oxidized by the liver and a marked diminution of the calculated amount of both exogenous and endogenous glucose delivered into systemic circulation following oral glucose administration (Table I). Thus, restoration of hepatic glucose processing appears responsible for the improved glucose control that occurs with artificial Beta-cell treatment. By contrast, conventional subcutaneous insulin administration results only in an augmentation of peripheral, but not hepatic, glucose uptake.

## VI. FUEL PROCESSING IN TYPE I DIABETES MELLITUS

Our initial study to test the "sleeping liver" hypothesis involved five insulin-dependent diabetic patients and five normal controls (Foss *et al.*, 1982). Subjects assumed the recumbent position, and catheters were inserted into an antecubital vein. Following a 45-minute equilibration period, diabetic participants received their usual insulin injections, and baseline blood samples and respiratory exchange data were collected. Thirty minutes later, subjects ingested 100 g of glucose. Blood samples and respiratory gas-exchange measurements were performed at 30-minute intervals throughout the 3-hour study. Confirming original observations of Benedict and Joslin (1910), the Type I diabetic patients had minimal ability to oxidize glucose.

Diabetic participants were subsequently placed on artificial Beta-cell therapy for 72 hours, and the above protocol was repeated. The ability of these diabetic patients to oxidize and store carbohydrate was found to be nearly indistinguishable from that of normal subjects. Virtually all measured substrates (glucose, free fatty acids, glycerol, lactate, pyruvate, $\beta$-hydroxybutyric acid, acetoacetic acid, citrate, $\alpha$-ketoglutarate), hormones (C-peptide, glucagon), and calculated ratios (lactate/pyruvate and $\beta$-hydroxybutyric acid/acetoacetic acid) were indistinguishable from those of controls. Although this study suggested that the artificial Beta-cell could restore to normal glucose oxidation and storage in diabetic patients, it did not allow for determination of the actual time needed to accomplish this.

To address the time issue, participants in the above protocol were asked to ingest a daily mixed meal containing 100 g of dietary carbohydrate (50 g sucrose and 50 g starches), 30 g protein, and 30 g fat. This meal was ingested at noon, and the experimental format was the same as that for the glucose meal. The study revealed modest improvement in carbohydrate processing within 24 hours and further improvement after 48 and 72 hours of artificial Beta-cell therapy. Not surprisingly, as with the 100-g glucose meal, levels of substrates and hormones were similarly normalized. These data taken *in toto* suggest that restoration of dietary carbohydrate processing is inducible and requires several days on the artificial Beta-cell unit to achieve. This may explain why no others have reported the normalization of both oxidation and storage of dietary carbohydrate in Type I diabetic subjects despite clinical use of the artificial Beta-cell since 1975.

## VII. MUSCLE FUEL PROCESSING IN TYPE I DIABETES MELLITUS

Although attention here has been directed primarily toward elucidating the role of the liver in fuel processing in Type I diabetic patients, the contribution of muscle glucose processing has also been evaluated. A study of nine Type I diabetic patients, ranging in age from 21–35 years and with an average duration of diabetes of 13 years, was carried out on an outpatient basis (Aoki *et al.*, 1983). Participants arrived at 7:30 a.m. and assumed a recumbent position. Catheters for the forearm study were placed, and basal respiratory gas-exchange data were obtained. Thirty minutes prior to a 100-g glucose meal, all diabetic participants took their usual morning insulin injections. Respiratory gas-exchange data were again obtained before and after ingestion of the glucose meal and at 60 and 120 minutes. Forearm blood flow was measured by capacitance plethysmography.

As expected, basal blood-glucose determinations were markedly elevated in the conventionally treated Type I diabetic patients, and their forearm glucose-extraction rates increased significantly during the study. Several weeks later, the same nine diabetic patients were placed on artificial Beta-cell therapy for 72 hours. Glucose flux data across the forearm muscle bed of these patients are shown in Table II. Although blood-glucose concentrations were much lower during and after artificial Beta-cell therapy, net glucose flux across forearm muscle bed did not differ significantly from that seen in the same subjects while on conventional insulin therapy. As expected, the respiratory quotient (RQ) increased significantly (Table II).

If 3 micromoles glucose/100 ml/forearm/min is used as an average forearm extraction rate and extrapolated to a total body muscle mass of 25 kg, glucose extraction in diabetics by total body muscle would be approximately 25 g/3 hours both with or without artificial Beta-cell therapy. These data are comparable to those obtained by Jackson and associates (1973a) on 25 normal subjects undergoing a 100-g glucose-tolerance test. We also performed similar studies ($n = 6$) on a slightly older (age 36 $\pm$ 2 years) group of normal male subjects (100 $\pm$ 4% of ideal body weight, based on Metropolitan Life tables) and found comparable forearm glucose-extraction rates (Table II). Thus, total muscle glucose extraction after a 100-g glucose meal is the same in conventionally or artificial Beta-cell-treated Type I diabetic patients and normal subjects. These data support our hypothesis that the marked improvement in glucose homeostasis manifested by patients on the artificial Beta-cell for 72 hours is primarily attributable to improved hepatic processing and not muscle glucose processing. The study also suggested that essentially normal muscle glucose extraction was achieved in conventionally treated diabetic patients with circulating free insulin concentrations of 10–30 microunits/ml (Table II). Coincident with these relatively low levels of free insulin were markedly elevated glucose concentrations. However, because the same glucose flux into muscle was seen in these patients after 72 hours on the artificial Beta-cell (at a time when circulating blood-glucose concentrations were within the normal range), comparable muscle glucose extraction was achieved in the latter

**TABLE II**

**Comparison of Forearm Glucose Extraction Rates In Type I Diabetic and Normal Subjects[a]**

| | Minutes After Glucose Ingestion | | | |
|---|---|---|---|---|
| | 0 | 30 | 60 | 120 |
| Conventional insulin therapy | | | | |
| Forearm blood flow (ml/100 ml/forearm/min) | 2.6 ± 0.5 | 2.7 ± 0.6 | 2.6 ± 0.4 | 2.4 ± 0.4 |
| Arterial glucose (mg/dl) | 246 ± 22 | 339 ± 50 | 388 ± 24 | 406 ± 30 |
| Free insulin (microU/ml) | 13 ± 2 | — | 21 ± 3 | 24 ± 4 |
| Forearm glucose extraction (micromoles/100 ml/forearm/min) | −0.36 ± 0.90 | 5.49 ± 2.20 | 2.48 ± 1.20 | 1.97 ± 1.70 |
| Respiratory quotient | 0.778 ± 0.01 | 0.775 ± 0.02 | 0.776 ± 0.01 | 0.780 ± 0.01 |
| Artificial beta-cell therapy | | | | |
| Forearm blood flow (ml/100 ml/forearm/min) | 2.1 ± 0.3 | 2.3 ± 0.4 | 2.0 ± 0.2 | 2.2 ± 0.2 |
| Arterial glucose (mg/dl) | 65 ± 6 | 110 ± 11 | 167 ± 15 | 153 ± 15 |
| Free insulin (microU/ml) | 67 ± 23 | — | 189 ± 15 | 227 ± 53 |
| Forearm glucose extraction (micromoles/100 ml/forearm/min) | 0.87 ± 0.37 | 2.42 ± 0.32 | 3.45 ± 0.86 | 1.55 ± 1.04 |
| Respiratory quotient | 0.810 ± 0.01 | 0.813 ± 0.01 | 0.883 ± 0.02 | 0.924 ± 0.01 |
| Normal control | | | | |
| Forearm glucose extraction (micromoles/100 ml/forearm/min) | 0.40 ± 0.12 | 2.48 ± 0.34 | 2.47 ± 0.48 | 2.10 ± 0.62 |

[a]Data from Aoki *et al.*, 1983.

instance without the aid of glucose mass action but with significantly higher concentrations of insulin.

We measured total muscle $CO_2$ production as well as total body $CO_2$ production following ingestion of a 100-g glucose meal by six normal subjects (Meistas *et al.*, 1985). Total muscle (*ca* 25 kg) $CO_2$ production at rest was approximately one-seventh of that of the whole body. Following ingestion of the glucose meal, a marked increase in total body $CO_2$ production and only a very slight increase in muscle $CO_2$ production were observed. Thus, the marked increase in $CO_2$ production evident in normal subjects and absent in diabetic subjects following ingestion of a glucose meal was not attributable to muscle. We also measured $CO_2$ production during a 100-g glucose meal in two Type I diabetic subjects before and after artificial Beta-cell therapy (unpublished observations). Again, only a small increase in muscle $CO_2$ production was observed. Because the gastrointestinal tract does not oxidize carbohydrate to any appreciable extent, and because the amount of glucose oxidized by the brain, the major consumer of glucose, is not appreciably affected by changes in glucose and insulin concentrations, the increase in $CO_2$ production must, by exclusion, be by the liver. These data provide further support for the hypothesis that the liver plays the central role in processing dietary carbohydrate.

## VIII. COMBINED FOREARM/EUGLYCEMIC CLAMP/INDIRECT CALORIMETRY STUDIES IN NORMAL SUBJECTS

In the conventionally treated diabetic patient, glucose levels are very high and insulin levels low, and in the Beta-cell treated patient, glucose levels are normal and insulin levels are high. Therefore, the issue of peripheral tissue sensitivity to insulin was examined in baseline forearm/euglycemic clamp studies in normal subjects at insulin concentrations of 50, 100, 200, and 500 microunits/ml over basal levels (Brooks *et al.*, 1984). As expected, the amount of glucose needed to maintain euglycemia increased as circulating insulin concentrations were raised. However, the fraction of total infused glucose removed by muscle in the face of rising insulin levels was relatively constant, about 32 to 49%, independent of the method used to calculate total muscle mass. These data showed that extraction of glucose by both muscle and nonmuscle tissues increased absolutely as a function of increasing insulin concentrations. It remains to be determined if similar observations hold for Type I diabetic subjects.

In euglycemic clamp studies, DeFronzo and associates (1982) and others have reported increases in total body carbohydrate oxidation, with insulin levels reaching 100–125 microunits/ml over basal. To identify the source of increased $CO_2$ production, especially at lower insulin concentrations, six normal subjects underwent combined forearm/euglycemic clamp/indirect calorimetry studies in which circulating insulin levels were maintained at 40 and 100 microunits/ml. Although total body $CO_2$ production increased, muscle $CO_2$ production did not change significantly (Meistas *et al.*, 1983). Thus, the observed increment in total body carbohydrate oxidation with the euglycemic clamp is apparently not attributable to muscle but most likely to liver.

## IX. MARKED CHANGES IN INSULIN REQUIREMENTS OF INSULIN-DEPENDENT DIABETIC PATIENTS DURING ARTIFICIAL BETA-CELL REGULATION

We measured insulin requirements of six insulin-dependent diabetic patients being regulated by the artificial Beta-cell over a 7-day period (unpublished observations) (Table III). To maintain euglycemia on days 2–4, the amount of insulin infused by the artificial Beta-cell unit increased significantly over day 1. A marked decrease in insulin delivery occurred on days 6–7. This observation suggested that the marked decrease in insulin requirements might be attributable to further activation of mechanisms involved in maintaining glucose homeostasis.

We then studied another group of five Type I diabetic subjects to document the changes in insulin requirements during artificial Beta-cell therapy

**TABLE III**

**Insulin Requirements During Artificial Beta-Cell Therapy**[a]

| Day | Insulin required[b] |
|---|---|
| 1 | 48 ± 3 |
| 2 | 77 ± 4[c] |
| 3 | 69 ± 8[c] |
| 4 | 58 ± 4[c] |
| 5 | 46 ± 5 |
| 6 | 38 ± 3 |
| 7 | 33 ± 2 |

[a]Data from unpublished observations.
[b]Values are given in Units/day.
[c]$p$ = or $<0.05$, paired t, two-tailed, day 1 vs. other days.

(Wesson *et al.*, 1988). Subjects were placed on individualized diets that met their calculated caloric needs. Each meal (breakfast, lunch, dinner, and snack) during the 8-day study period (4-day control period, followed by 4-day artificial Beta-cell therapy) was the same calorically and compositionally. On days 1–4 of hospitalization, patients received their usual insulin doses at their usual times. On days 5–8, patients were placed on the artificial Beta-cell. The total insulin infused for each meal was timed from the preprogrammed level of glucose to the time after meal ingestion that the blood glucose returned to the preprogrammed level. During days 2–3, as expected, the amount of insulin infused in response to a given meal gradually increased, followed by a decline. This pattern appeared to hold for all four meals.

The above observations suggest that the lower insulin requirement on day 1 may be attributable to lingering effects of the NPH insulin. By days 2–3, fast-acting crystalline zinc insulin, infused by the artificial Beta-cell, was the primary means by which normal blood-glucose concentration was maintained. However, because the livers in these patients were only partially activated by day 2, large amounts of ingested carbohydrate still passed through or were not retained by the splanchnic bed and hence entered and remained in systemic circulation. When glucose enters the systemic circulation, the artificial Beta-cell responds by infusing large quantities of insulin, leading to sequestering of glucose in peripheral tissues, primarily muscle. With gradual restoration of the liver's metabolic integrity, less glucose escapes into the systemic circulation, the artificial Beta-cell responds to progressively smaller quantities of glucose, and insulin requirements fall (e.g., to 33 Units/day by day 7).

This biphasic insulin pattern implies that accomplishing the same task in Type I diabetic subjects using a conventional subcutaneous crystalline zinc insulin regimen would be difficult. However, it must be noted that the artificial Beta-cell delivers insulin intravenously and that the amount infused is probably not the amount actually required to restore normal liver activity; indeed, the amount required may be smaller. However, daily pancreatic Beta-cell secretion of insulin in normal humans has been estimated to range from 40–60 Units/day, the amount infused toward the end of the study (Meistas *et al.*, 1981).

## X. SUMMARY

The "sleeping liver" hypothesis appears uniquely capable of unifying disparate clinical, physiological, and biochemical observations. Verification of this hypothesis could result in a new objective for treating the Type I diabetic subject: Instead of directing treatment toward simple control of circulating blood glucose (control theory), we could direct treatment at reactivating the dormant dietary glucose-processing system in the liver.

Although this presentation has focused on changes in carbohydrate metabolism, equally significant changes in hepatic processing, synthesis, and degradation of amino acids, proteins, free fatty acids, and triglycerides may also occur. Because abnormal concentrations of these compounds have been persuasively implicated in development of complications in diabetes mellitus (Raskin and Rodenstock, 1986), and because evidence indicates that processing of some of these fuels is normalized in artificial Beta-cell-treated diabetic subjects (Foss *et al.*, 1982), it appears reasonable to expect that a significant salutary impact on the development of diabetic complications might follow long-term restoration and normalization of hepatic glucose processing.

## REFERENCES

Albisser, A. M., Liebel, B. S., Ewart, T. G., Davidovec, Z., Botz, C. K., and Zingg, W. (1974). An artificial endocrine pancreas. *Diabetes* **23**, 389–396.

Alvares, F. L., and Nordlie, R. C. (1975). Glucose uptake by perfused livers from fed and fasted normal rats: Involvement of phosphotransferase activities of glucose 6-phosphatase in regulation of blood glucose levels [Abstract]. *Fed. Proc.* **34**, 881.

Alvares, F. L., and Nordlie, R. C. (1976). Glucose uptake and phosphorylation by livers isolated from alloxan-diabetic rats and perfused in the presence of 3-mercaptopicolinate; involvement of synthetic activities of glucose 6-phosphatase [Abstract]. *Fed. Proc.* **35**, 1397.

Anchors, J. M., and Karnovsky, M. L. (1975). Purification of cerebral glucose 6-phosphatase. An enzyme involved in sleep. *J. Biol. Chem.* **250**, 6408–6416.

Aoki, T. T., Vlachokosta, F. V., Foss, M. C., and Meistas, M. T. (1983). Evidence for restoration of hepatic glucose processing in Type I diabetes mellitus. *J. Clin. Invest.* **71**, 837–839.

Arion, W. J., Wallin, B. K., Lange, A. J., and Ballas, L. M. (1975). On the involvement of a glucose 6-phosphate transport system in the function of microsomal glucose 6-phosphatase. *Mol. Cell Biochem.* **6**, 75–83.

Benedict, F. G., and Joslin, E. P. (1910). ''Metabolism in Diabetes Mellitus,'' Publ. 136, p. 213. Carnegie Institution of Washington, Washington.

Bjornthorp, P., and Sjöstrom, L. (1978). Carbohydrate storage in man: Speculations and some quantitative considerations. *Metabolism* **27**, 1853–1865.

Bjornthorp, P., Berchtold, P., Holm, J., and Larsson, B. (1971). The glucose uptake of human adipose tissue in obesity. *Eur. J. Clin. Invest.* **1**, 480–485.

Boyd, M. E., Albright, E. B., Foster, D. W., and McGarry, J. D. (1981). *In vitro* reversal of the fasting state of liver metabolism in the rat. Re-evaluation of the roles of insulin and glucose. *J. Clin. Invest.* **68**, 142–152.

Bratusch-Marrain, P. R., Waldhausl, W. K., Gasic, S., Korn, A., and Nowotny, P. (1980). Oral glucose tolerance test: Effect of different glucose loads on splanchnic carbohydrate and substrate metabolism in healthy man. *Metabolism* **29**, 289–295.

Brooks, D. C., Bessey, P. Q., Black, P. R., Aoki, T. T., and Wilmore, D. W. (1984). Post-traumatic insulin resistance in uninjured forearm tissue. *J. Surg. Res.* **37**, 100–107.

Cahill, G. F., Jr., Ashmore, J., Earle, A. S., and Zottu, S. (1958). Glucose penetration into liver. *Amer. J. Physiol.* **192**, 491–496.

Cahill, G. F., Jr., Ashmore, J., Renold, A. E., and Hastings, A. B. (1959). Blood glucose and the liver. *Amer. J. Med.* **26**, 264–282.

Colilla, W., Jorgenson, R. A., and Nordlie, R. C. (1975). Mammalian carbamyl phosphate: Glucose phosphotransferase and glucose 6-phosphate phosphohydrolase: Extended tissue distribution. *Biochim. Biophys. Acta* **377**, 117–125.

Costill, D. L., Bennett, A., Branam, G., and Eddy, D. (1973). Glucose ingestion at rest and during prolonged exercise. *J. Appl. Physiol.* **34**, 764–769.

DeFronzo, R. A., Jacot, E., Jequier, E., Maeder, E., Wahren, J., and Felber, J. P. (1981). The effect of insulin on the disposal of intravenous glucose: Results from indirect calorimetry and hepatic and femoral venous catheterization. *Diabetes* **30**, 1000–1007.

DeFronzo, R. A., Simonson, D., and Ferrannini, E. (1982). Hepatic and peripheral insulin resistance: A common feature of Type 2 (non-insulin-dependent) and Type 1 (insulin-dependent) diabetes mellitus. *Diabetologia* **23**, 313–319.

Felig, P., and Wahren, J. (1971). Influence of endogenous insulin secretion on splanchnic glucose and amino acid metabolism in man. *J. Clin. Invest.* **50**, 1702–1717.

Felig, P., Wahren, J., and Hendler, R. (1975). Influence of oral glucose ingestion on splanchnic glucose and gluconeogenic substrate metabolism in man. *Diabetes* **24**, 468–475.

Foss, M. C., Vlachokosta, F. V., Cunningham, L., and Aoki, T. T. (1982). Restoration of glucose homeostasis in insulin-dependent diabetic subjects: An inducible process. *Diabetes* **31**, 46–52.

Gunderson, H. M., and Nordlie, R. C. (1975). Carbamyl phosphate: glucose phosphotransferase and glucose 6-phosphate phosphohydrolase of nuclear membrane. Interrelationships between membrane integrity, enzymic latency, and catalytic behavior. *J. Biol. Chem.* **250**, 3552–3559.

Holdsworth, C. D., and Dawson, A. M. (1964). The absorption of monosaccharides in man. *Clin. Sci.* **27**, 371–379.

Jackson, R. A., Peters, N., Advani, U., Perry, G., Rogers, J., Brough, W. H., and Pilkington, T. R .E. (1973a). Forearm glucose uptake during oral glucose tolerance test in normal subjects. *Diabetes* **22**, 442–458.

Jackson, R. A., Perry, G., Rogers, J., Advani, U., and Pilkington, T. R. E. (1973b). Relationship between the basal glucose concentration, glucose tolerance, and forearm glucose uptake in maturity-onset diabetes. *Diabetes* **22**, 751–761.

Kety, S. S. (1957). The general metabolism of the brain *in vivo*. *In* "The Metabolism of the Nervous System" (D. Richter, ed.), 2nd International Neurochemical Symposium, p. 221. Pergamon Press, London.

Lygre, D. G., and Nordlie, R. C. (1968). Phosphohydrolase and phosphotransferase activities of intestinal glucose 6-phosphatase. *Biochem.* **7**, 3219–3226.

Meistas, M. T., and Aoki, T. T. (1983). Hepatic $CO_2$ production following oral glucose administration in man [Abstract]. *Clin. Res.* **31**, 504A.

Meistas, M. T., Zadik, Z., Margolis, S., and Kowerski, A. A. (1981). Correlation of urinary excretion of C-peptide with the integrated concentration and secretion rate of insulin. *Diabetes* **30**, 639–643.

Meistas, M. T., Bessey, P. Q., Vlachokosta, F. V., and Aoki, T. T. (1983). Euglycemic clamp and forearm glucose metabolism [Abstract]. *Diabetes* **32** (Suppl. 1), 163A.

Meistas, M. T., Vlachokosta, F. V., Gleason, R. E., Arcangeli, M., and Aoki, T. T. (1985). Role of muscle in $CO_2$ production after oral glucose administration in man. *Diabetes* **34**, 960–963.

Nordlie, R. C. (1974). Metabolic regulation by multifunctional glucose 6-phosphatase. *In* "Current Topics in Cellular Regulation," vol. 8, pp. 33–117. Academic Press, New York.

Nordlie, R. C. (1976). Multifunctional hepatic glucose 6-phosphatase and the "tuning" of blood glucose levels. *Trends Biol. Sci.* **I**, 199–202.

Perley, M. J., and Kipnis, D. M. (1967). Plasma insulin responses to oral and intravenous glucose: Studies in normal and diabetic subjects. *J. Clin. Invest.* **46**, 1954–1962.

Pilkis, S. J. (1968). Identification of human hepatic glucokinase and some properties of the enzyme (33396). *Proc. Soc. Exper. Biol. Med.* **129**, 681–684.

Pilo, A., Ferrannini, E., Biorkman, O., Wahren, J., Reichard, G. A., Felig, P., and DeFronzo, R.A. (1981). Analysis of glucose production and disappearance rates following an oral glucose load in normal subjects: A double tracer approach. *In* "Carbohydrate Metabolism" (C. Cobelli and R. N. Bergman, eds.), pp. 221–238. John Wiley and Sons, Ltd., New York.

Raskin, P., and Rodenstock, J. (1986). Blood glucose control and complications. *Ann. Int. Med.* **105**, 254–263.

Reinmuth, O. M., Scheinberg, P., and Bourne, B. (1965). Total cerebral blood flow and metabolism. A new method for the repeated serial measurement of the total cerebral blood flow using iodoantipyrine ($^{131}I$) with a report of determination in normal human beings of blood flow, oxygen consumption, glucose utilization and respiratory quotient of the whole brain. *Arch. Neurol.* **12**, 49–66.

Rizza, R. A., Mandarino, L. J., and Gerich, J. E. (1981). Dose-response characteristics for effects of insulin on production and utilization of glucose in man. *Amer. J. Physiol.* **240**, E630–E639.

Ruderman, N. B., and Lauris, V. (1968). Effect of acute insulin deprivation on rat liver glucokinase. *Diabetes* **17**, 611–617.

Sokoloff, L. (1960). Metabolism of the central nervous system *in vivo*. *In* "Handbook of Physiology" (Field, J., Magoun, and Hall, K. E., eds.), p. 1843. Waverly Press, Inc., Baltimore.

Soskin, A., and Levine, R. (1937). A relationship between the blood sugar level and the rate of sugar utilization affecting the theories of diabetes. *Amer. J. Physiol.* **120**, 761–770.

Storer, A. C., and Cornish-Bowden, A. (1976). Kinetics of rat liver glucokinase. *Biochem. J.* **159**, 7–14.

Wahren, J., Felig, P., Cerasi, E., and Luft, R. (1972). Splanchnic and peripheral glucose and amino acid metabolism in diabetes mellitus. *J. Clin. Invest.* **51**, 1870–1878.

Waldhausl, W., Bratusch-Marrain, P., Gasic, S., Korn, A., and Nowotny, P. (1982). Insulin production rate, hepatic insulin retention and splanchnic carbohydrate metabolism after oral glucose ingestion in hyperinsulinaemic Type 2 (non-insulin-dependent) diabetes mellitus. *Diabetologia* **23**, 6–15.

Wesson, D. E., Black, P. R., Vlachokosta, F. V., Aoki, T. T., and Wilmore, D. W. (1988). Artificial Beta-cell promotes positive nitrogen balance and whole body protein synthesis in insulin-dependent diabetic subjects. *JPEN* **12**, 237–243.

# 8

# Vitamin D, Calcium, and Metabolic Bone Disease

Hector F. DeLuca

*Department of Biochemistry*
*College of Agricultural and Life Sciences*
*University of Wisconsin-Madison*
*Madison, Wisconsin*



## I. INTRODUCTION

The fat-soluble vitamins represent a unique group, characterized not only by their lipid solubility but also by their mode of action. Unlike water-soluble vitamins, fat-soluble vitamins carry out specialized functions in highly differentiated animals. Water-soluble vitamins, present in both simple and complex organisms, function largely as cofactors in metabolic reactions.

Vitamin D is a fat-soluble vitamin with several important functions. It is required for normal mineralization of the skeleton. Its absence leads to rickets in the young and osteomalacia in adults. These diseases are characterized by a failure to mineralize the organic matrix elaborated by osteoblasts and chondrocytes in the bone-forming systems (DeLuca, 1967; Hess, 1929). Vitamin D does not play a direct role in synthesizing new organic matrix or in mineralization, but it is required to provide adequate calcium and phosphorus in circulating fluids to support normal skeletal mineralization (Underwood and DeLuca, 1984; Weinstein *et al.*, 1984). Because calcium has important functions elsewhere, especially in neuromuscular activity, the absence of vitamin D often brings about low calcium concentrations in plasma and extracellular fluids, resulting in hypocalcemic tetany (Hess, 1929). Vitamin D prevents this disorder by elevating plasma calcium concentration.

Vitamin D elevates plasma calcium and phosphorus concentrations by three mechanisms. First, it is the only substance known to stimulate intestinal transport or absorption of dietary calcium (DeLuca *et al.*, 1982). It also stimulates the enterocytes of the small intestine to transport phosphorus into the plasma compartment (DeLuca, 1981a; DeLuca, 1981b; DeLuca *et al.*, 1982). Vitamin D is also required for the organism to use bone calcium for soft tissue needs (DeLuca, 1981b). Thus, in hypocalcemia, the active form of vitamin D stimulates mobilization of both calcium and phosphorus from bone into plasma, which requires the presence of parathyroid hormone (PTH) (DeLuca, 1974). The third site of action in raising blood calcium and phosphorus is the distal renal tubule, where the vitamin D hormone acts with PTH to increase renal reabsorption of calcium (Yamamoto *et al.*, 1984). On the other hand, the small intestine responds only to the active form of vitamin D, and this response does not require PTH. This regulation of intestinal calcium absorption plays an important role in maintaining mineral balance and a major role in preventing skeletal losses that result in thin bones or osteoporosis (Boyle *et al.*, 1972). By these mechanisms, vitamin D increases plasma calcium and phosphorus concentrations required to mineralize the skeleton and prevent hypocalcemic tetany.

In another important calcium-related function, the active form of vitamin D plays a role in suppressing PTH synthesis, thus preventing secondary hyperparathyroidism (Russell *et al.*, 1986).

## II. METABOLISM OF VITAMIN D REQUIRED FOR CARRYING OUT ITS FUNCTIONS

Although two different investigators concluded that vitamin D acts directly to carry out the above functions (Haussler and Norman, 1967; Kodicek, 1960), work in the mid-to-late 1960s demonstrated conclusively that vitamin D must be metabolized to an active form before becoming functional (DeLuca, 1974; DeLuca, 1981a; DeLuca, 1981b). It first must be hydroxylated on carbon-25 to produce the major circulating form of vitamin D, 25-hydroxyvitamin D (25-OH-D). This compound does not act directly in any target tissue under physiologic circumstances and must be hydroxylated on carbon-1 to produce the final vitamin D hormone, 1$\alpha$,25-dihydroxyvitamin $D_3$ (1,25-$(OH)_2D_3$) or calcitriol (DeLuca, 1974; DeLuca, 1981a). 25-hydroxylation is largely carried out in the liver, whereas 1$\alpha$-hydroxylation in the normal nonpregnant mammal is carried out exclusively in the proximal renal tubule (Brunette *et al.*, 1978). Both enzyme reactions are cytochrome P-450 dependent (DeLuca and Schnoes, 1983). The more critical enzyme is 1$\alpha$-hydroxylase, a three-component, mixed-function monooxygenase that is very tightly regulated by the need for calcium and phosphorus.

Acute nephrectomy eliminates any significant production of 1,25-$(OH)_2D_3$ in the nonpregnant mammal (Reeve *et al.*, 1983; Shepard *et al.*, 1979). However, abnormal production of 1,25-$(OH)_2D_3$ can take place in other tissues, such as the granuloma tissue in patients with sarcoidosis or undetermined sites of long-term anephric subjects (Barbour *et al.*, 1981; Koeffler *et al.*, 1985). In both man and animals, 1,25-$(OH)_2D_3$ stimulates intestinal calcium absorption whether kidneys are present or not, whereas its precursor, 25-OH-$D_3$, cannot stimulate these functions except at very large, pharmacologic doses (DeLuca, 1974; DeLuca, 1981a; DeLuca, 1981b). Thus, 1,25-$(OH)_2D_3$ or a further metabolite must be the active form of vitamin D that mobilizes calcium from bone and stimulates intestinal calcium and phosphorus transport.

This demonstrates that 1,25-$(OH)_2D_3$ or a further metabolite must be a true hormone, because it is synthesized in the proximal renal convoluted tubule and functions in the enterocytes in the small intestine, in osteoblasts, in bone-lining cells, and in distal renal tubule cells (DeLuca, 1974; DeLuca, 1981a; DeLuca, 1981b). Further metabolism of 1,25-$(OH)_2D_3$ is not completely understood. Certainly this compound is rapidly converted to 1,24,25-$(OH)_3D_3$ (Castillo *et al.*, 1978) or 1,25,26-$(OH)_3D_3$ (Tanaka *et al.*, 1981b) and ultimately is excreted, primarily in bile as calcitroic acid, a biologically inactive metabolite (Esvelt *et al.*, 1979). Of the known metabolites of 1,25-$(OH)_2D_3$, none approaches the biological activity of 1,25-$(OH)_2D_3$ itself, providing strong evidence that 1,25-$(OH)_2D_3$, and not a further metabolite, is the active form of vitamin D in intestine, bone, and kidney.

25-hydroxyvitamin D is metabolized to a variety of other metabolites, primarily in the kidney but also in other tissues. Figure 1 illustrates the pathways of physiologic vitamin D metabolism. Although some 33 vitamin D metabolites are known, the above represents the only truly known physiological metabolism. 25-OH-$D_3$, if not hydroxylated in the

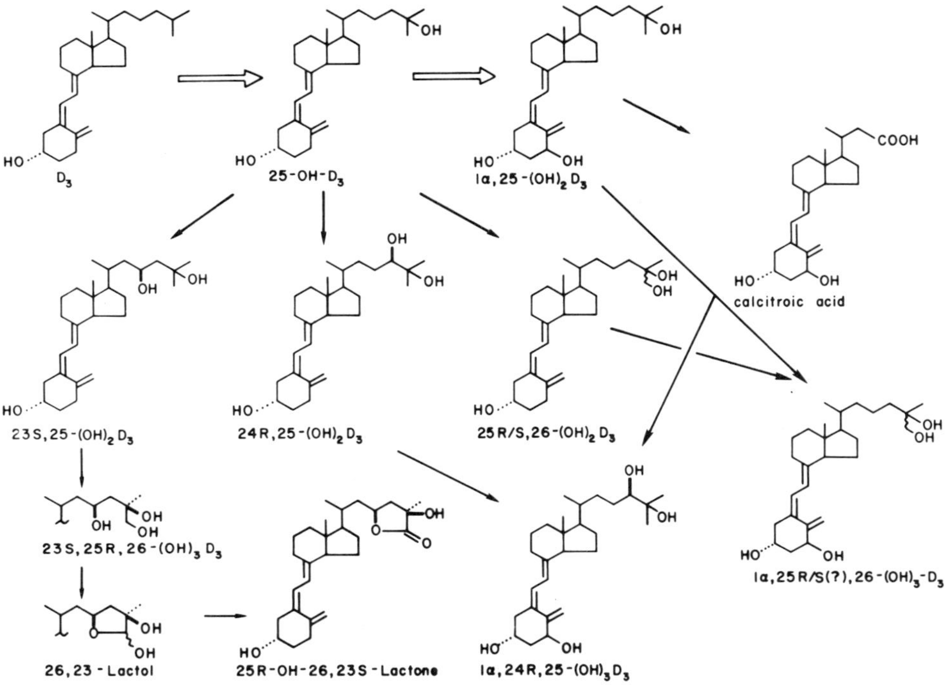


**Fig. 1.** Physiological metabolism of vitamin D is diagrammed. Large arrows indicate activation of vitamin D to its final active form, 1α,25-$(OH)_2D_3$. Other arrows indicate physiological metabolism to metabolites likely for degradation and excretion.

1 position, is hydroxylated in either the 23 or 24 position. If it is 23*S*-hydroxylated, it proceeds to further oxidation of carbon-26 and ultimately converts to the 25-OH-$D_3$-26,23-lactone (Tanaka *et al.*, 1981a; Yamada *et al.*, 1984). If it is 24-hydroxylated, it may be further converted to 24-oxo-25-OH-$D_3$ (Takasaki *et al.*, 1982), the fate of which remains unknown. One other pathway discovered under physiologic circumstances is 26-hydroxylation to form 25,26-$(OH)_2D_3$ (DeLuca and Schnoes, 1983).

Conversion to 24*R*,25-$(OH)_2D_3$ has been suggested to be another functionally active pathway (Brommage and DeLuca, 1985). Thus, it has been suggested that 24,25-$(OH)_2D_3$ is required for mineralizing the skeleton (Ornoy *et al.*, 1978; Rasmussen and Bordier, 1978), for hatching in birds (Henry and Norman, 1978) and for regulating plasma calcium concentration (Norman *et al.*, 1980). By using fluoro derivatives that block hydroxylation at these sites, it has been shown that these pathways do not provide for functions of vitamin D (Brommage and DeLuca, 1985). Thus, 26,27-$F_6$-25-OH-$D_3$, 24,24-$F_2$-25-OH-$D_3$, and 23,23-$F_2$-25-OH-$D_3$ are fully active in carrying out the functions of vitamin D (Brommage and DeLuca, 1985). Furthermore, animals have been grown for two generations on 24,24-$F_2$-25-OH-$D_3$ without adverse effects or impairment of skeletal mineralization. Finally, the idea that 24-hydroxylation is required for development in birds has been quite thoroughly disproved (Hart *et al.*, 1984; Hart *et al.*, 1986). We can, therefore, focus on 25-hydroxylation and 1$\alpha$-hydroxylation as the known functional pathways of vitamin D metabolism. The remaining metabolic processes probably involve excretion and degradation of this very potent vitamin.

Vitamin $D_2$, the alternate and more synthetic form of vitamin D, is metabolized in a similar series of reactions, but very little is known of metabolic pathways other than 24-hydroxylation (DeLuca and Schnoes, 1983).

## III. REGULATION OF PRODUCTION OF THE VITAMIN D HORMONE, 1,25-$(OH)_2D_3$

Low blood calcium stimulates PTH secretion, which, in turn, stimulates production of 1,25-$(OH)_2D_3$ in the renal proximal convoluted tubules (DeLuca, 1974; DeLuca, 1981a; DeLuca, 1981b). 1,25-$(OH)_2D_3$ then stimulates intestinal calcium transport, bone mobilization, and renal reabsorption of calcium. The latter two functions require the presence of PTH. Action at these sites results in elevation of plasma calcium and suppression of PTH secretion, which, in turn, suppress production of the vitamin D hormone. Figure 2 illustrates this regulation (DeLuca, 1974; DeLuca, 1981a; DeLuca, 1981b).

Plasma phosphorus concentration also regulates production of 1,25-$(OH)_2D_3$ (DeLuca, 1981a; DeLuca and Schnoes, 1983). By a poorly understood mechanism, low blood phosphorus brings about elevated

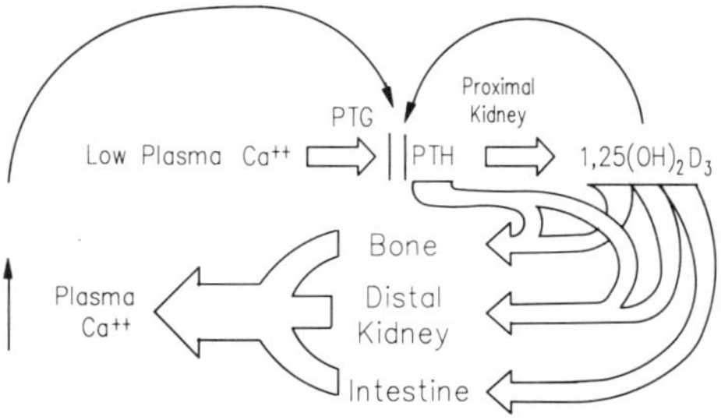


**Fig. 2.** Role of the vitamin D endocrine system in regulating plasma calcium concentration is shown.

plasma levels of 1,25-$(OH)_2D_3$, leading to increased phosphorus absorption and suppressed PTH production and thereby to reduced PTH-dependent phosphorus excretion. Determining whether phosphorus levels have other sites of regulation of vitamin D metabolism will require additional investigation.

1,25-$(OH)_2D_3$ suppresses production of itself and increases production of 24*R*,25-$(OH)_2D_3$ (DeLuca, 1981a; DeLuca and Schnoes, 1983). Thus 24-hydroxylase is turned on by the vitamin D hormone (Tanaka and DeLuca, 1984). In addition, the absence of PTH or the presence of high blood phosphorus stimulates 24-hydroxylation and suppresses 1$\alpha$-hydroxylase by a nuclear-mediated mechanism (Larkins *et al.*, 1974). How phosphorus regulates this process remains unknown. How PTH regulates it is not entirely known, although it is mediated by a cyclic-AMP (cAMP) mechanism (Horiuchi *et al.*, 1977).

An important aspect of regulation is the role of the vitamin D hormonal system in intestinal calcium absorption. When calcium is required to maintain plasma calcium concentration, it is to the advantage of the organism to use dietary calcium if at all possible. Thus, hypocalcemia stimulates PTH secretion and 1,25-$(OH)_2D_3$ production in the normal animal, bringing about a marked increase in the efficiency of calcium absorption. The efficiency of intestinal calcium transport system rises markedly in animals deprived of calcium (Ribovich and DeLuca, 1978). If calcium is not needed in the extracellular fluid compartment, PTH secretion and 1,25-$(OH)_2D_3$ production are suppressed, and fecal excretion of calcium is increased. This system prevents the loss of skeleton when calcium is needed. To illustrate: if an animal is fed a low-calcium diet, no calcium is available to be absorbed from the small intestine, even though the intestine is stimulated to absorb calcium with maximum efficiency. Inadequate dietary calcium brings about increased PTH production, which, together with 1,25-$(OH)_2D_3$, mobilizes skeletal calcium and increases the efficiency of renal conservation of calcium. However, this correction of hypocalcemia is at the expense of the skeleton. Continued reliance on skeletal calcium for soft tissue needs causes loss of bone mass and ultimately gives rise to symptomatic osteoporosis (DeLuca, 1981a; DeLuca, 1981b). Thus, dietary calcium and the vitamin D system are required to prevent skeletal calcium loss. This relationship is important in considering osteoporosis and other bone-loss diseases.

## IV. MECHANISM OF ACTION OF THE VITAMIN D HORMONE, 1,25-$(OH)_2D_3$

When radiolabeled 1,25-$(OH)_2D_3$ is given intravenously to a vitamin D-deficient animal, it rapidly localizes in cell nuclei of such target tissues as intestine, bone and distal renal tubule (Stumpf *et al.*, 1979; Stumpf *et al.*,

1981). This specific nuclear localization, which has been clearly demonstrated, provides an important line of evidence supporting a nuclear action of 1,25-$(OH)_2D_3$. Nuclear localization has not been found in non-target tissues such as skeletal and heart muscle, spleen, liver, gastric mucosa, or smooth muscle (Stumpf *et al.*, 1979; Stumpf *et al.*, 1981), but it has been found in tissues not previously appreciated as target organs, including skin keratinocytes and fibroblasts, endocrine cells of stomach, pancreatic islet cells, parathyroid cells, and certain brain and reproductive cells. Recent evidence in some of these tissues suggests that the vitamin D hormone may have other, previously unappreciated biochemical functions.

Of systems responsive to the vitamin D hormone, enterocytes of the small intestine have been the most widely studied. Intestinal response to 1,25-$(OH)_2D_3$ is blocked by inhibitors of RNA and protein synthesis (Franceschi and DeLuca, 1981; Kendrick *et al.*, 1981). The reported rapid effect of 1,25-$(OH)_2D_3$ in the small intestine (Nemere *et al.*, 1984) has not been confirmed by others and is doubted by this author. Because 1,25-$(OH)_2D_3$ is a steroid hormone that localizes in nuclei of target cells before it functions, its mechanism of action is probably similar to that of other steroids. Thus, a specific nuclear receptor for 1,25-$(OH)_2D_3$ has been identified in intestinal and other target cells (Link and DeLuca, 1985). This receptor, which has a molecular weight of 55,000 in mammals (Dame *et al*; 1985; Pierce *et al.*, 1988) and approximately 63,000 in birds (Pike *et al.*, 1987), binds 1,25-$(OH)_2D_3$ quite specifically with a $K_d$ of $5 \times 10^{-11} M$. Although the receptor appears to be almost entirely nuclear, it is unclear whether it is totally absent in the cytoplasm (Nakada *et al.*, 1984). The receptor for 1,25-$(OH)_2D_3$ recognizes other vitamin D metabolites. The closest neighbor is 1,24,25-$(OH)_3D_3$, which binds at approximately one-tenth the affinity of 1,25-$(OH)_2D_3$ (Link and DeLuca, 1985), and 25-hydroxyvitamin $D_3$ binds at 1/20 the affinity of 1,25-$(OH)_2D_3$. Thus, high serum concentrations of 25-OH-$D_3$ may act without 1-hydroxylation as an analog of 1,25-$(OH)_2D_3$. This may account for the effectiveness of large amounts of 25-OH-$D_3$ or vitamin $D_3$ in treating metabolic bone disease.

The mammalian receptor has been purified to 24% purity, and 24 monoclonal antibodies have been raised to it (Dame *et al.*, 1986). Similar purification of the chicken receptor has been achieved, and two monoclonal antibodies to this receptor have been prepared (Pike *et al.*, 1983). Immunoblots of one-dimensional gels of fresh tissue reveal the largest molecular weight to be 55,000, providing no evidence for a precursor protein of higher molecular weight. However, two-dimensional electrophoretic blots illustrate the charge heterogeneity of the receptor, demonstrating the presence of three forms (Pierce *et al.*, 1988) (Fig. 3). Which of these three is the functional receptor remains unknown. 1,25-$(OH)_2D_3$ appears to upregulate the receptor in cell cultures (Mangelsdorf *et al.*, 1987), but this has not been shown *in vivo*. Monoclonal antibodies have been used to

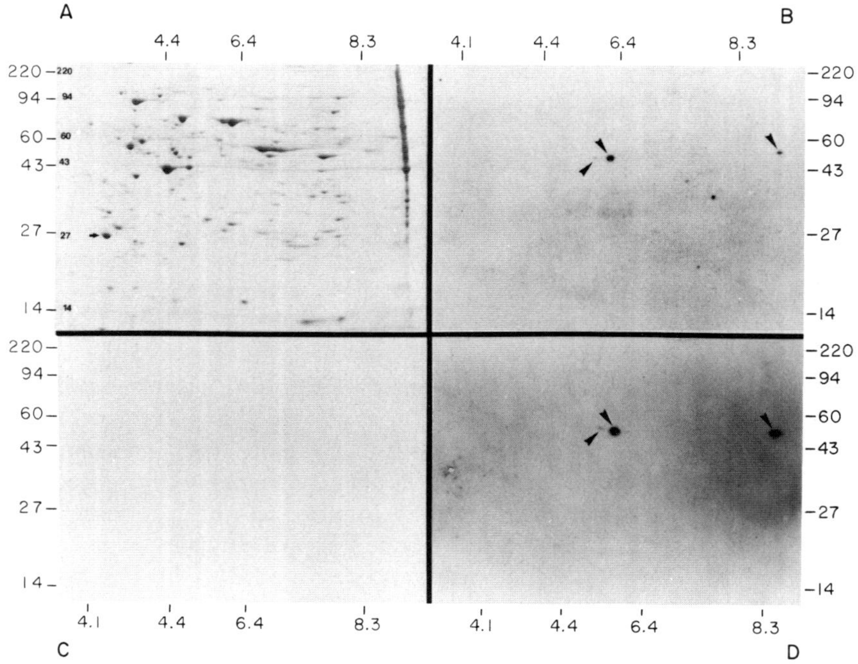


**Fig. 3.** Immunoblots show whole-pig intestinal enterocytes using two monoclonal antibodies directed to the 1,25-$(OH)_2D_3$ receptor. Panel A represents Coomassie stain two-dimensional gel electrophoresis of pig intestinal mucosa. Panels B, C, and D represent immunoblots. Fresh pig intestinal mucosa were solubilized in sodium dodecyl sulfate buffer and subjected to two-dimensional gel electrophoresis. The proteins were transferred to nitrocellulose paper by an electrotransfer and the blots were then probed with antibody. Panel C was probed with an antibody directed to an irrelevant substance; Panel B was probed with IVG8Cll, an antibody that cross-reacts with receptor for many species; and Panel D was probed with IVIE6, an antibody directed to the pig receptor. Both IVG8Cll and XVIE6 detect three forms of the receptor, all having molecular weights of 55,000. No higher molecular weight protein were detected by the immunoblots; thus, the molecular weight of the porcine receptor is 55,000. Three distinct spots were detected, one at pI 5.9, another at pI 6.1, and still another that did not enter the electrofocusing gel. The small fragments in Panel B are probably degradation products of the receptor (From Pierce *et al.*, 1988. Reprinted with permission.)

isolate the cDNA of the receptor for the chicken (McDonnell *et al.*, 1987) and for the rat (Burmester *et al.*, 1988). The cDNA clone has been totally sequenced, and the amino acid structure of the receptor will soon be largely revealed. Rapidly accumulating data on the receptor will help unravel the mechanisms of some vitamin D-resistant diseases.

The generally accepted mechanism of action of 1,25-$(OH)_2D_3$ in the intestine is diagrammed in Fig. 4. The nature of calcium and phosphorus transport proteins produced in response to the hormone is not fully defined. However, the calcium-binding protein originally discovered by

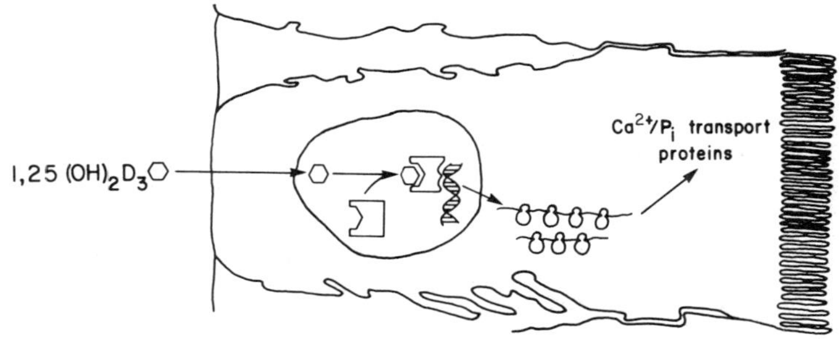


**Fig. 4.** The diagram represents the expected molecular mechanism of action of 1,25-$(OH)_2D_3$ in inducing intestinal calcium and phosphorus transport. Exactly what proteins are induced to carry out the transport are unknown. The detailed mechanism whereby 1,25-$(OH)_2D_3$, through its receptor, turns on the genes expressing these proteins is also unknown.

Wasserman and Taylor (1966) has been cloned in the rat, and its full-length cDNA and entire structure are known. The gene has also been isolated from a rat genomic library, and the entire system is encased in a 4.1 kb genomic fragment that also contains the regulatory regions (Darwish *et al.*, 1987). The binding sites for the vitamin D hormone and its receptor will probably be discovered on the regulatory regions of the calcium-binding protein gene. However, other genes regulated by the vitamin D hormone are currently under study to determine their nature. Molecular biology techniques and two-dimensional gel electrophoresis double-labeling experiments have great promise in elucidating the proteins involved in the calcium-transport system.

The receptor mechanism is clearly essential for the function of the vitamin D hormone. In vitamin D-dependent rickets Type II, for example, a target-organ form of vitamin D resistance results in part from a defective receptor (Eil *et al.*, 1986). Furthermore, in neonatal rats, intestinal calcium absorption and responsiveness to vitamin D correlate exactly with developmental appearance of the receptor (Halloran and DeLuca, 1981). Thus, evidence strongly suggests that the vitamin D hormone functions almost entirely through a receptor mechanism involving regulation of gene expression. Reports of nongenomic functions of the vitamin D hormone have yet to receive adequate support.

## V. DISEASES RESULTING FROM A DEFECT IN VITAMIN D METABOLISM

A defect in vitamin D metabolism results in vitamin D-dependent rickets Type I, renal osteodystrophy and other diseases. Vitamin D-dependent rickets Type I is an autosomal recessive disorder characterized by rickets and hypocalcemia in the face of normal intakes of vitamin D. Because it can be corrected by administering large doses of vitamin D, it has been termed "vitamin D-dependent rickets" (Prader *et al.*, 1961). This disease is clearly a defect in the 1$\alpha$-hydroxylase system for vitamin D (Fraser *et al.*, 1973). 1,25-dihydroxyvitamin $D_3$ is vanishingly low in untreated patients (Scriver *et al.*, 1978). Although physiologic doses of 1,25-$(OH)_2D_3$ will cure this disorder, pharmacologic amounts of 25-OH-$D_3$ or vitamin D are needed. Cure is achieved because 25-hydroxylation of vitamin D is not tightly regulated, and high serum concentrations result when large amounts of vitamin D are given. 25-hydroxyvitamin $D_3$ interacts with the receptor when it is present at 20 times the level of 1,25-$(OH)_2D_3$ (unpublished observations). Thus, it acts as analog to provide functional receptor binding to regulatory regions of the genome. Therefore, this disease clearly represents a metabolic defect that is cured by administering the vitamin D hormone.

Renal osteodystrophy is an example of an induced metabolic defect in which kidney disease results in failure to produce the vitamin D hormone (DeLuca and Avioli, 1979). This failure prevents both calcium absorption and normal suppression of PTH production. Intravenous administration of the vitamin D hormone is extremely effective in shutting down PTH production and secretion, allowing adequate calcium absorption (Slatopolsky *et al.*, 1984). Renal osteodystrophy, especially in children, is treated with the 1$\alpha$-hydroxylated form of vitamin D.

X-linked hypophosphatemic vitamin D-resistant rickets is not a primary defect in vitamin D metabolism but in renal transport of phosphorus (Glorieux and Scriver, 1972). However, a secondary defect exists in production of the vitamin D hormone (Scriver *et al.*, 1978). Thus, in X-linked hypophosphatemic vitamin D-resistant rickets, oral administration of large amounts of inorganic phosphorus results in increased healing of the skeleton. However, because production of the vitamin D hormone is suppressed, secondary hyperparathyroidism occurs unless exogenous 1,25-$(OH)_2D_3$ or an analog is provided. Thus, frequent administration of phosphorus plus vitamin D hormone or an analog provides the best treatment for this disorder (Glorieux *et al.*, 1980).

Vitamin D-dependent rickets Type II was discovered after high circulating blood levels of 1,25-$(OH)_2D_3$ were found in patients presenting with severe rickets (Bell *et al.*, 1978; Rosen *et al.*, 1979). This disease proved to be an autosomal recessive disorder in which target organs of intestine, bone, and kidney do not respond to the vitamin D hormone. Thus it is not treatable with any of the new active forms of vitamin D. In subjects studied thus far, some appear to have a defect in the receptor for 1,25-$(OH)_2D_3$; others appear to have a normal receptor but may have a dysfunction either in gene expression or in expressed structural genes that provide the cell components needed for calcium and phosphorus transport

(Eil *et al.*, 1986). Treatment of this disorder rests on important basic scientific discovery: vitamin D compounds are not directly required for normal bone growth and mineralization, provided that serum calcium and phosphorus are normal (Underwood and DeLuca, 1984; Weinstein *et al.*, 1984). Thus, satisfactory skeletal mineralization in patients with vitamin D-dependent rickets Type II has been achieved by night-time infusion of calcium and phosphorus through indwelling catheters (Balsan *et al.*, 1986).

## VI. DISEASES OF THE VITAMIN D REGULATORY SYSTEM

Perhaps the most notable disease of the vitamin D regulatory system is hypoparathyroidism, in which parathyroid glands are absent as a result of surgery, autoimmune disease, or birth defect. Without the parathyroid glands to recognize hypocalcemia, there is no signal to produce the vitamin D hormone. This double deficiency of vitamin D hormone and PTH results in hypocalcemia and hence convulsive tetany. Pseudohyperparathyroidism is a disease in which PTH secretion occurs along with PTH resistance in target organs. This results in a deficiency of 1,25-$(OH)_2D_3$ and a defect in the PTH-activated mechanisms. Both hypoparathyroidism and pseudohypoparathyroidism are nicely treated with about 1–2 g/day of elemental dietary calcium plus about 1 $\mu$g 1,25-$(OH)_2D_3$ or an equivalent amount of an analog such as 1$\alpha$-OH-$D_3$ (Kooh *et al.*, 1975; Neer *et al.*, 1975).

Osteoporosis is the most interesting and prevalent disorder that may involve vitamin D metabolism. It is beyond the scope of this presentation to discuss all aspects of osteoporosis. However, in this disorder, skeletal calcium is used as the primary source of calcium to support soft tissue needs. In postmenopausal women, the primary defect results from a lack of estrogen and progesterone. In these women, withdrawal of estrogen and progesterone increases the lability of skeletal calcium, thus increasing circulating calcium. Delivery of calcium from bone to the circulation suppresses PTH secretion, resulting in decreases in vitamin D hormone production (Gallagher *et al.*, 1979) and intestinal calcium absorption. Thus, the calcium source for soft tissue needs shifts from the intestine to the skeleton, with a continuous loss of skeleton and a negative calcium balance of about 100 mg/day. Clearly, the primary defect in this disorder is not vitamin D metabolism but withdrawal of estrogen. Thus, estrogen treatment effectively and safely prevents this bone loss if progesterone is also administered (Lindsay *et al.*, 1976). However, 1,25-$(OH)_2D_3$ can also be administered to stimulate intestinal calcium absorption and bone remodeling. Thus 1,25-$(OH)_2D_3$ appears to be beneficial in treating osteoporosis in postmenopausal women (Aloia *et al.*, 1987; Gallagher *et al.*, 1982).

Age-related decreases in intestinal calcium absorption correlate with declining levels of 1,25-$(OH)_2D_3$ (Gallagher *et al.*, 1979). Unlike their younger counterparts, healthy elderly subjects do respond to PTH by producing 1,25-$(OH)_2D_3$ (Slovik *et al.*, 1981). The intestine of elderly subjects also responds to exogenous 1,25-$(OH)_2D_3$. Thus, hip fractures in the elderly, which probably result from age-related bone loss, may be caused by age-related decline in 1$\alpha$-hydroxylation of 25-OH-$D_3$. The efficacy of 1,25-$(OH)_2D_3$ administration in preventing hip fracture in the elderly has not been tested in clinical trials.

Glucocorticoid-induced osteoporosis is a more complex disease involving a defect in calcium absorption unrelated to the vitamin D hormone and a secondary interference with production of this hormone. No clinical trials to test the possible benefits of the vitamin D hormone in this disorder have been completed.

## VII. NEW SITES OF ACTION OF VITAMIN D

The specific binding of the vitamin D hormone in cells not previously thought to be targets of vitamin D raises the possibility that the vitamin D hormone may play significant roles in the function of many tissues (Stumpf *et al.*, 1979; Stumpf *et al.*, 1981). Thus, it has been suggested that the vitamin D hormone may be required for normal insulin secretion in the islets of the pancreas (Kadowaki and Norman, 1985). Although this is debated, some function of the vitamin D hormone in the islets will probably be found. Certainly, the vitamin D hormone plays a major role in regulating PTH production. Russell and associates (1986) have shown that the vitamin D hormone suppresses expression of the parathyroid gene.

Approximately 60% of all cancer cell lines have receptors to 1,25-$(OH)_2D_3$ (Frampton *et al.*, 1982). At low concentrations, 1,25-$(OH)_2D_3$ may stimulate growth of these cells, whereas, at high concentrations, 1,25-$(OH)_2D_3$ suppresses growth and causes these cells to differentiate into benign or nonmalignant cells (Frampton *et al.*, 1983). Suda and his group made the important discovery that addition of the vitamin D hormone to promyelocyte cultures (M1 mouse cultures or human HL-60 cultures) causes them to differentiate into benign monocytes or macrophages (Abe *et al.*, 1981; Tanaka *et al.*, 1982). Superphysiological concentrations were required for this differentiation, raising the question of whether differentiation occurs *in vivo*. Of interest, the monocyte is a precursor of the osteoclast or the bone-resorbing cell (Ash *et al.*, 1980). 1,25-dihydroxyvitamin $D_3$ induces osteoclast-mediated bone resorption in culture (Raisz *et al.*, 1972; Reynolds *et al.*, 1973). Whether this phenomenon, which occurs *in vivo* as part of the bone-remodeling system, results from

$1,25\text{-}(OH)_2D_3$ recruitment of monocytes for osteoclast formation or from indirect activation of osteoclasts remains to be seen. More important, could vitamin D compounds be used to treat acute myelocytic leukemias? At the concentrations currently needed, the vitamin D hormone clearly could not be used because it would induce severe hypercalcemia—the patient would die of hypercalcemia rather than malignancy. However, analogs that would show preferential activity in causing promyelocyte differentiation could possibly be synthesized. We have studied the effect of a number of side chain analogs of the vitamin D hormone on cell differentiation (Fig. 5). Lengthening the side chain by one carbon preferentially increases the action of the vitamin D hormone in causing differentiation of HL-60 cells over its action in raising blood calcium (Ostrem *et al.*, 1987a; Ostrem *et al.*, 1987b). Shortening the side chain reduces activity in both systems, but substituting a short hydrocarbon side chain for the side chain of $1,25\text{-}(OH)_2D_3$ produces compounds with no calcium activity but with only one-twentieth the activity of $1,25\text{-}(OH)_2D_3$ in causing HL-60 differentiation. Thus, these compounds might well be considered for treating acute myelocytic leukemia and should be prepared for clinical trials.

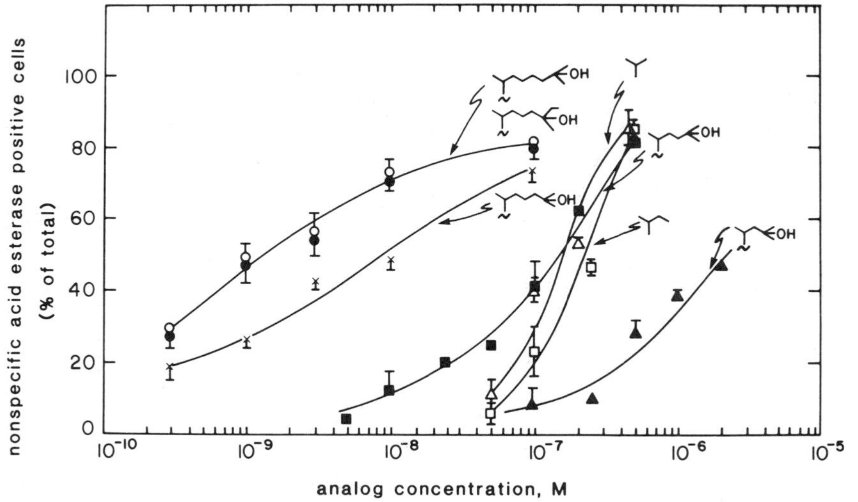


**Fig. 5.** Log dose curves show analogs of $1,25\text{-}(OH)_2D_3$ that induce differentiation of the human HL-60 promyelocyte line to monocytes. Monocytes are detected by measuring nonspecific acid esterase microscopically or by other methods of detecting the phenotype. $1,25\text{-}(OH)_2D_3$ activity is denoted by the curved line with X's. Vertical bar represents SEM of 6 determinations. Note the surprising activity of the $1,25\text{-}(OH)_2D_3$ analog in which the side chain is replaced with the small isobutyl or isopropyl side chain.

Skin fibroblasts and keratinocytes have been shown to contain receptor to 1,25-$(OH)_2D_3$ (Feldman *et al.*, 1980; Simpson and DeLuca, 1980). Because addition of 1,25-$(OH)_2D_3$ to keratinocytes causes them to differentiate, it was thought that the vitamin D hormone or its analogs might be used to treat proliferative skin disorders such as psoriasis or contact dermatitis (Smith *et al.*, 1986; Takamoto *et al.*, 1986). These compounds, given systemically or topically, have markedly improved the condition of psoriatic patients. Thus, new uses of vitamin D compounds in disease can be anticipated.

## VIII. CALCIUM NUTRITION, VITAMIN D, AND BONE DISEASE

Calcium is a popular supplement now being championed in the United States. Its addition to a number of foods is being used as a selling point. Certainly, a normal calcium intake is essential for normal bone growth and development and for normal nerve and muscle function. An intake of 800 mg calcium/day should be strongly encouraged for people of all ages. The question of whether extra calcium can prevent serious bone disease is an entirely different matter. It has been suggested that the RDA be increased for postmenopausal women and for the elderly, despite the lack of evidence that these groups can utilize extra dietary calcium. In fact, recent evidence suggests that providing additional calcium to postmenopausal women does not prevent skeletal loss (Nilas *et al.*, 1984; Riggs *et al.*, 1982). If a defect in production of the vitamin D hormone exists in older people, calcium administration cannot correct it. It is, therefore, misleading to increase the RDA for these groups when additional calcium not only fails to provide any benefit but might discourage them from seeking other treatment for bone disease. In postmenopausal women, treatment with estrogen plus progesterone effectively prevents bone loss; this treatment, rather than an increased level of dietary calcium, should be used (Lindsay *et al.*, 1976).

## IX. SUMMARY

Much has been learned in the last two decades about vitamin D, calcium, and metabolic bone disease. Vitamin D, which is converted to a hormone in a series of reactions in the kidney, functions in intestine, bone, and kidney. Administration of the vitamin D hormone and measurements of this hormone and its precursor are effective new tools in diagnosing and treating metabolic bone disease. Among diseases that have been diagnosed and treated are hypoparathyroidism, pseudohyperparathyroidism, vitamin D-resistant rickets, vitamin D-dependent rickets, renal osteodystrophy, and osteoporosis. New sites of action of the vitamin D hormone are being discovered, and its use to treat disorders of these organs is now indicated. For example, the vitamin D hormone or its analogs are being used to treat psoriasis. Some vitamin D compounds may also be useful adjuncts to treatment of certain malignancies.

## ACKNOWLEDGMENTS

This work was supported in part by a program project grant DK-14881 and by the Harry Steenbock Fund of the Wisconsin Alumni Research Foundation.

## REFERENCES

Abe, E., Miyaura, C., Sakagami, H., Takeda, M., Konno, K., Yamazaki, T., Yoshiki, S., and Suda, T. (1981). Differentiation of mouse myeloid leukemia cells induced by 1α,25-dihydroxyvitamin $D_3$. *Proc. Nat. Acad. Sci. USA* **78**, 4990–4994.

Aloia, J., Vasawi, A., Yeh, J., Allis, K. and Cohn, S. (1987). Calcitriol in the treatment of postmenopausal osteoporosis. *In* "Calcium Regulation and Bone Metabolism. Basic and Clinical Aspects" (D. V. Cohn, T. J. Martin, and P. J. Muenier, eds.), Vol. 9, pp. 113–118. Excerpta Medica, Amsterdam.

Ash, P., Loutit, J. F. and Townsend, M. M. S. (1980). Osteoclasts derived from haematopoietic stem cells. *Nature* **283**, 669–670.

Balsan, S., Garabedian, M., Larchet, M., Groski, A. M., Cournot, G., Tau, C., Bordeau, A., Silve, C., and Ricour, C. (1986). Long-term nocturnal calcium infusions can cure rickets and promote normal mineralization in hereditary resistance to 1,25-dihydroxyvitamin D. *J. Clin. Invest.* **77**, 1661–1666.

Barbour, G. L., Coburn, J. W. Slatopolsky, E. Norman, A. W., and Horst, R. L. (1981). Hypercalcemia in an anephric patient with sarcoidosis: Evidence for extrarenal generation of 1,25-dihydroxyvitamin D. *N. Engl. J. Med.* **305**, 440–443.

Bell, N. H., Hamstra, A. J., and DeLuca, H. F. (1978). Vitamin D-dependent rickets type II: Resistance of target organs to 1,25-dihydroxyvitamin D. *N. Engl. J. Med.* **298**, 996–999.

Boyle, I. T., Gray, R. W., Omdahl, J. L , and DeLuca, H. F. (1972). Calcium control of the *in vivo* biosynthesis of 1,25-dihydroxyvitamin $D_3$: Nicolaysen's Endogenous Factor. *In* "Endocrinology 1971" (S. Taylor, ed.), pp. 468–476. Wm. Heinemann Medical Books, Ltd., London.

Brommage, R., and DeLuca, H. F. (1985). Evidence that 1,25-dihydroxyvitamin $D_3$ is the physiologically active metabolite of vitamin $D_3$. *Endocrine Rev.* **6**, 491–511.

Brunette, M. G., Chan, M., Ferriere, C., and Roberts, K. D. (1978). Site of 1,25-dihydroxyvitamin $D_3$ synthesis in the kidney. *Nature* **276**, 287–289.

Burmester, J. K., Maeda, N., and DeLuca, H. F. (1988). Isolation and expression of rat 1,25-dihydroxyvitamin $D_3$ receptor cDNA. *Proc. Nat. Acad. Sci. USA* **85**, 1005–1009.

Castillo, L., Tanaka, Y., DeLuca, H. F., and Ikekawa, N. (1978). On the physiological role of 1,24,25-trihydroxyvitamin $D_3$. *Min. Electrol. Metab.* **1**, 198–207.

Dame, M. C., Pierce, E. A., and DeLuca, H. F. (1985). Identification of the porcine intestinal 1,25-dihydroxyvitamin $D_3$ receptor on sodium dodecyl sulfate-polyacrylamide gels by renaturation and immunoblotting. *Proc. Nat. Acad. Sci. USA* **82**, 7825–7829.

Dame, M. C., Pierce, E. A., Prahl, J. M., Hayes, C. E., and DeLuca, H. F. (1986). Monoclonal antibodies to the porcine intestinal receptor for 1,25-dihydroxyvitamin $D_3$: Interaction with distinct receptor domains. *Biochemistry* **25**, 4523–4534.

Darwish, H. M., Krisinger, J., Strom, M., and DeLuca H. F. (1987). Molecular cloning of the cDNA and chromosomal gene for vitamin D-dependent calcium-binding protein of rat intestine. *Proc. Nat. Acad. Sci. USA* **84**, 6108–6111.

DeLuca, H. F. (1967). Mechanism of action and metabolic fate of vitamin D. *Vitamins Hormones* **25**, 315–367.

DeLuca, H. F. (1974). Vitamin D: The vitamin and the hormone. *Fed. Proc.* **33**, 2211–2219.

DeLuca, H. F. (1981a). The transformation of a vitamin into a hormone: The vitamin D story. *In* "The Harvey Lectures," Series 75, pp. 333–379. Academic Press, New York.

DeLuca, H. F. (1981b). The vitamin D system: A view from basic science to the clinic. *Clin. Biochem.* **14**, 213–222.

DeLuca, H. F., and Avioli, L. V. (1979). Renal osteodystrophy. *In* "Renal Disease" (S. D. Black and N. F. Jones. eds.), pp. 766–803. Blackwell Scientific Publications, London.

DeLuca, H. F., and Schnoes, H. K. (1983). Vitamin D: Recent advances. *Ann. Rev. Biochem.* **52**, 411–439.

DeLuca, H. F., Franceschi, R. T., Halloran, B. P., and Massaro, E.R. (1982). Molecular events involved in the 1,25-dihydroxyvitamin $D_3$ stimulation of intestinal calcium transport. *Fed. Proc.* **41**, 66–71.

Eil, C., Liberman, U. A. and Marx, S. J. (1986). The molecular basis for resistance to 1,25-dihydroxyvitamin-D—Studies in cells cultured from patients with hereditary hypocalcemic 1,25-$(OH)_2D_3$-resistant rickets. *In* "Steroid Hormone Resistance" (G. P. Chrousos, D. L. Loriaus, and M. B. Lipsett, eds.), pp. 407–418. Plenum Press, New York.

Esvelt, R. P., Schnoes, H. K., and DeLuca, H. F. (1979). Isolation and characterization of 1$\alpha$-hydroxy-tetranorvitamin D-23-carboxylic acid: A major metabolite of 1,25-dihydroxyvitamin $D_3$. *Biochemistry* **18**, 3977–3983.

Feldman, D., Chen, T., Hirst, M. Colston, K., Karasek, M., and Cone, C. (1980). Demonstration of 1,25-dihydroxyvitamin $D_3$ receptors in human skin biopsies. *J. Clin. Endocrinol. Metab.* **51**, 1463–1465.

Frampton, R. J., Suva, L. J., Eisman, J. A., Findlay, D. M., Moore, G. E., Moseley, J. M., and Martin. T. J. (1982). Presence of 1,25-dihydroxyvitamin $D_3$ receptors in established human cancer cell lines in culture. *Cancer Res.* **42**, 1116–1119.

Frampton, R. J., Osmond, S. A., and Eisman, J. A. (1983). Inhibition of human cancer cell growth by 1,25-dihydroxyvitamin $D_3$ metabolites. *Cancer Res.* **43**, 4443–4447.

Franceschi, R. T., and DeLuca, H. F. (1981). The effect of inhibitors of protein and RNA synthesis on 1$\alpha$,25-dihydroxyvitamin $D_3$ dependent calcium uptake in cultured embryonic chick duodenum. *J. Biol. Chem.* **256**, 3848–3852.

Fraser, D., Kooh, S. W., Kind, H. P., Holick, M. F., Tanaka, Y., and DeLuca, H.F. (1973). Pathogenesis of hereditary vitamin D dependent rickets: An inborn error of vitamin D metabolism involving defective conversion of 25-hydroxyvitamin D to 1$\alpha$,25-dihydroxyvitamin D. *N. Engl. J. Med.* **289**, 817–822.

Gallagher, J. C., Riggs, B. L. Eisman, J., Hamstra, A., Arnaud, S. B., and DeLuca, H. F. (1979). Intestinal calcium absorption and serum vitamin D metabolites in normal subjects and osteoporotic patients. Effect of age and dietary calcium. *J. Clin. Invest.* **64**, 729–736.

Gallagher, J. C., Jerpbak, C. M., Jee, W. S. S., Johnson, K. A., DeLuca, H.F., and Riggs, B. L. (1982). 1,25-dihydroxyvitamin $D_3$: Short- and long-term effects of bone and calcium metabolism in patients with postmenopausal osteoporosis. *Proc. Nat. Acad. Sci.* **79**, 3325–3329.

Glorieux, F., and Scriver, C. V. (1972). Loss of a parathyroid-sensitive component of phosphate transport in X-linked hypophosphatemia. *Science* **175**, 997–1000.

Glorieux, F. H., Marie, P. J., Pettifor, J. M.. and Delvin, E. E. (1980). Bone response to phosphate salts, ergocalciferol, and calcitriol in hypophosphatemic vitamin D-resistant rickets. *N. Engl. J. Med.* **303**, 1023–1031.

Halloran, B. P., and DeLuca, H. F. (1981). Appearance of the intestinal cytosolic receptor for 1,25-dihydroxyvitamin $D_3$ during neonatal development in the rat. *J. Biol. Chem.* **256**, 7338–7342.

Hart, L. E., DeLuca, H. F., Yamada, S., and Takayama, H. (1984). Hydroxylation of carbon-24 of 25-hydroxycholecalciferol is not necessary for normal embryonic development in chickens. *J. Nutr.* **114**, 2059–2065.

Hart, L. E., Schnoes, H. K., and DeLuca, H. F. (1986). Studies on the role of 1,25-dihydroxyvitamin D in chick embryonic development. *Arch. Biochem. Biophys.* **250**, 426–434.

Haussler, M. R., and Norman, A .W. (1967). The subcellular distribution of physiological doses of vitamin $D_3$. *Arch. Biochem. Biophys.* **118**, 145–153.

Henry, H. L., and Norman, A. W. (1978). Vitamin D: two dihydroxylated metabolites are required for normal chicken egg hatchability. *Science* **201**, 835–837.

Hess, A. (1929). The history of rickets. *In* ''Rickets, Including Osteomalacia and Tetany'' (A. Hess, ed.), pp. 22–37. Lea & Febiger, Philadelphia.

Horiuchi, N., Suda, T., Takahashi, H., Shimazawa, E., and Ogata, E. (1977). *In vivo* evidence for the intermediary role of 3′,5′-cyclic AMP in parathyroid hormone-induced stimulation of 1$\alpha$,25-dihydroxyvitamin $D_3$ synthesis in rats. *Endocrinology* **101**, 969–974.

Kadowaki, S., and Norman, A. W. (1985). Demonstration that the vitamin D metabolite 1,25$(OH)_2$-vitamin $D_3$ and not 24R,25$(OH)_2$-vitamin $D_3$ is essential for normal insulin secretion in the perfused rat pancreas. *Diabetes* **34**, 315–320.

Kendrick, N. C., Kabakoff B., and DeLuca, H. F. (1981). Oxygen-dependent 1,25-dihydroxycholecalciferol-induced calcium ion transport in rat intestine. *Biochem. J.* **194**, 178–186.

Kodicek, E. (1960). The metabolism of vitamin D. *In* ''Proceedings of the Fourth International Congress of Biochemistry'' (W. Umbreit and H. Molitor, eds.), vol. XI, pp. 198–208. Pergamon Press, London.

Koeffler, H. P., Reichel H., Bishop, J. E., and Norman, A. W. (1985). Gamma-interferon stimulates production of 1,25-dihydroxyvitamin $D_3$ by normal human macrophages. *Biochem. Biophys. Res. Commun.* **127**, 596–603.

Kooh, S. W., Fraser, D., DeLuca, H. F., Holick, M. F., Belsey, R. E., Clark, M. B., and Murray, T. M. (1975). Treatment of hypoparathyroidism and pseudohypoparathyroidism with metabolites of vitamin D: Evidence for impaired conversion of 25-hydroxyvitamin D to 1$\alpha$,25-dihydroxyvitamin D. *N. Engl. J. Med.* **293**, 840–844.

Larkins, R. G., MacAuley, S. J., and MacIntyre, I. (1974). Feedback control of vitamin D metabolism by nuclear action of 1,25-dihydroxyvitamin $D_3$ on the kidney. *Nature* **252**, 412–414.

Lindsay, R., Hart, D. M., Aitken, J. M., MacDonald, E. B., Anderson, J. B., and Clarke, A. C. (1976). Long-term prevention of postmenopausal osteoporosis by estrogen. *Lancet* **1**, 1038–1039.

Link, R., and DeLuca, H. F. (1985). The vitamin D receptor. *In* ''The Receptors'' (P. M. Conn, ed.), vol. II, pp. 1–35. Academic Press, New York.

Mangelsdorf, D. J., Pike, J. W., and Haussler, M. R. (1987). Avian and mammalian receptors for 1,25-dihydroxyvitamin $D_3$: *In vitro* translation to characterize size and hormone-dependent regulation. *Proc. Nat. Acad Sci. USA* **84**, 354–358.

McDonnell, D. P., Mangelsdorf, D. J., Pike J. W., Haussler, M. R., and O'Malley, B. W. (1987). Molecular cloning of complementary DNA encoding the avian receptor for vitamin D. *Science* **235**, 1214–1217.

Nakada, M., Simpson, R. U., and DeLuca, H. F. (1984). Subcellular distribution of DNA and non-DNA-binding 1,25-dihydroxyvitamin D receptors in chick intestine. *Proc. Nat. Acad. Sci. USA* **81**, 6711–6713.

Neer, R. M., Holick, M. F., DeLuca, H. F., and Potts, J. T., Jr. (1975). Effects of 1α-hydroxyvitamin $D_3$ and 1,25-dihydroxyvitamin $D_3$ on calcium and phosphorus metabolism in hypoparathyroidism. *Metabolism* **24**, 1403–1413.

Nemere, I., Yoshimoto, Y., and Norman, A. W. (1984). Calcium transport in perfused duodena from normal chicks. Enhancement within fourteen minutes of exposure to 1,25-dihydroxyvitamin $D_3$. *Endocrinology* **115**, 1476–1483.

Nilas, L., Christiansen, C., and Rodbro, P. (1984). Calcium supplementation and postmenopausal bone loss. *Brit. Med. J.* **289**, 1093–1096.

Norman, A. W., Henry, H. L., and Malluche, H. H. (1980). 24*R*,25-dihydroxyvitamin $D_3$ and 1α-25-dihydroxyvitamin $D_3$ are both indispensable for calcium and phosphorus homeostasis. *Life Sci.* **27**, 229–327.

Ornoy, A., Goodwin, D., Noff, D., and Edelstein, S. (1978). 24,25-dihydroxyvitamin D is a metabolite of vitamin D essential for bone formation. *Nature* **276**, 517–519.

Ostrem, V. K., Lau, W. F., Lee, S. H., Perlman, K., Prahl, J., Schnoes, H. K., DeLuca, H. F., and Ikekawa, N. (1987a). Induction of monocytic differentiation of HL-60 cells by 1,25-dihydroxyvitamin D analogs. *J. Biol. Chem.* **262**, 14164–14171.

Ostrem, V. K., Tanaka, Y., Prahl, J., and DeLuca, H. F. (1987b). 24- and 26-homo-1,25-dihydroxyvitamin $D_3$: Preferential activity in inducing differentiation of human leukemia cells H-60 *in vitro*. *Proc. Nat. Acad. Sci. USA* **84**, 2610–2614.

Pierce, E. A., Dame, M. C., and DeLuca, H. F. (1988). Size and charge of the functional 1,25-dihydroxyvitamin D receptor in porcine intestine. *J. Biol. Chem.* (In press.)

Pike, J. W., Marion, S. L., Donaldson, C. A., and Haussler, M. R. (1983). Serum and monoclonal antibodies against the chick intestinal receptor for 1,25-dihydroxyvitamin $D_3$. *J. Biol. Chem.* **258**, 1289–1296.

Pike, J. W., Sleator, N. M., and Haussler, M. R. (1987). Chicken intestinal receptor for 1,25-dihydroxyvitamin $D_3$. Immunologic characterization and homogeneous isolation of a 60,000 dalton protein. *J. Biol. Chem.* **262**, 1305–1309.

Prader, A., Illig, R. and Heierli, E. (1961). Eine besondere form der vitamin D-resistenten rachitis mit hypocalcamie und autosomal-dominantem erbgang: Die hereditare pseudomangelrachitis. *Helv. Paediat. Acta* **16**, 452–468.

Raisz, L. G., Trummel, C. L., Holick, M. F., and DeLuca, H. F. (1972). 1,25-dihydroxycholecalciferol: A potent stimulator of bone resorption in tissue culture. *Science* **175**, 768–769.

Rasmussen, H., and Bordier, P. (1978). Vitamin D and bone. *Metab. Bone Dis. Related Res.* **1**, 7–13.

Reeve, L., Tanaka, Y., and DeLuca, H. F. (1983). Studies on the site of 1,25-dihydroxyvitamin $D_3$ synthesis *in vivo*. *J. Biol. Chem.* **258**, 3615–3617.

Reynolds, J. J., Holick, M. F., and DeLuca, H. F. (1973). The role of vitamin D metabolites in bone resorption. *Calcif. Tissue Res.* **12**, 295–301.

Ribovich, M. L., and DeLuca, H. F. (1978). Effect of dietary calcium and phosphorus on intestinal calcium absorption and vitamin D metabolism. *Arch. Biochem. Biophys.* **188**, 145–156.

Riggs, B. L., Seemone, E., Hodgson, S. F., Tavers, D. R., and O'Fallon, W. M. (1982). The effect of fluoride/calcium regimen on vertebral fracture occurrence in postmenopausal osteoporosis: Comparison with conventional therapy. *N. Engl. J. Med.* **306**, 446–450.

Rosen, J. F., Fleischman, A. R., Finberg, L., Hamstra, A., and DeLuca, H. F. (1979). Rickets with alopecia: An inborn error of vitamin D metabolism. *J. Pediat.* **94**, 729–735.

Russell, J., Lettieri, D., and Sherwood, L. M. (1986). Suppression by $1,25(OH)_2D_3$ of transcription of the pre-proparathyroid hormone gene. *Endocrinology* **119**, 2864–2868.

Scriver, C. R., Reade, T. M., DeLuca, H. F., and Hamstra, A. J. (1978). Serum $1,25\text{-}(OH)_2D$ levels in normal subjects and in patients with hereditary rickets or bone disease. *N. Engl. J. Med.* **299**, 976–979.

Shepard, R. M., Horst, R. L., Hamstra, A. J., and DeLuca, H. F. (1979). Determination of vitamin D and its metabolites in plasma from normal and anephric man. *Biochem. J.* **182**, 55–69.

Simpson, R. U., and DeLuca, H. F. (1980). Characterization of a receptor like protein for 1,25-dihydroxyvitamin $D_3$ in rat skin. *Proc. Nat. Acad. Sci. USA* **77**, 5822–5826.

Slatopolsky, E., Weerts, C., Thieland, J., Horst, R., Harter, H., and Martin, K. (1984). Marked suppression of secondary hyperparathyroidism by i.v. administration of 1,25-dihydroxycholecalciferol in uremic patients. *J. Clin. Invest.* **74**, 2136–2139.

Slovik, D. M., Adams, J. S., Neer, R. M., Holick, M. F., and Potts, J. T., Jr. (1981). Deficient production of 1,25-dihydroxyvitamin D in elderly osteoporotic patients. *N. Engl. J. Med.* **305**, 372–376

Smith, E. L., Walworth, N. C., and Holick, M. F. (1986). Effect of 1$\alpha$,25-dihydroxyvitamin $D_3$ on the morphologic and biochemical differentiation of cultured human epidermal keratinocytes grown in serum-free conditions. *J. Invest. Dermatol.* **86**, 709–711.

Stumpf, W. E., Sar, M., Reid, F. A., Tanaka, Y., and DeLuca, H. F. (1979). Target cells for 1,25-dihydroxyvitamin $D_3$ in intestinal tract, stomach. kidney, skin, pituitary and parathyroid. *Science* **206**, 1188–1190.

Stumpf, W. E., Sar, M., and DeLuca, H. F. (1981). Sites of action of 1,25$(OH)_2$ vitamin $D_3$ identified by thaw-mount autoradiography. *In* ''Hormonal Control of Calcium Metabolism'' (D. V. Cohn, R. V. Talmage, and J. L. Matthews, eds.) pp. 222–229. Excerpta Medica, Amsterdam.

Takamoto, S., Onishi, T., Morimoto S., Imanaka, S., Yukawa, S., Kozuka, T., Kitano, Y., Seino, Y., and Kumahara, Y. (1986). Effect of 1$\alpha$-hydroxycholecalciferol on psoriasis vulgaris: a pilot study. *Calcif. Tissue Int.* **39**, 360–366.

Takasaki, Y., Suda, T., Yamada, S., Ohmori, M., Takayama, H., and Nishii, Y. (1982). Chemical synthesis, biological activity, and metabolism of 25-hydroxy-24-oxovitamin $D_3$. *J. Biol. Chem.* **257**, 3732–3738.

Tanaka, H., Abe, E., Miyaura, C., Kuribayashi, T., Konno, K., Nishii, Y., and Suda, T. (1982). 1$\alpha$,25-dihydroxycholecalciferol and a human myeloid leukaemia cell line (HL-60). The presence of a cytosol receptor and induction of differentiation. *Biochem. J.* **204**, 713–719.

Tanaka, Y., and DeLuca, H. F. (1984). Rat renal 25-hydroxyvitamin $D_3$-1- and 24-hydroxylases: Their *in vivo* regulation. *Amer. J. Physiol.* **246**, E168–E173.

Tanaka, Y., DeLuca, H. F., Schnoes, H. K., Ikekawa, N., and Eguchi, T. (1981a). 23,25-dihydroxyvitamin $D_3$: A natural precursor in the biosynthesis of 25-hydroxyvitamin $D_3$-26,23-lactone. *Proc. Nat. Acad. Sci. USA* **78**, 4805–4808.

Tanaka, Y., Schnoes, H. K., Smith, C. M., and DeLuca, H. F. (1981b). 1,25,26-trihydroxyvitamin $D_3$: isolation, identification, and biological activity. *Arch. Biochem. Biophys.* **210**, 104–109.

Underwood, J. L., and DeLuca, H. F. (1984). Vitamin D is not directly necessary for bone growth and mineralization. *Amer. J. Physiol.* **246**, E493–E498.

Wasserman, R. H., and Taylor, A. N. (1966). Vitamin $D_3$-induced calcium-binding protein in chick intestinal mucosa. *Science* **152**, 791–793.

Weinstein, R. S., Underwood, J. L., Hutson, M. S., and DeLuca, H. F. (1984). Bone histomorphometry in vitamin D-deficient rats infused with calcium and phosphorus. *Amer. J. Physiol.* **246**, E499–E505.

Yamada, S., Nakayama, K., Takayama, H., Shinki, T., Takasaki, Y., and Suda, T. (1984). Isolation, identification, and metabolism of (23*S*,25*R*)-25-hydroxyvitamin $D_3$ 26,23-lactol. (A biosynthetic precursor of (23*S*25*R*)-25-hydroxyvitamin $D_3$ 26,23-lactone). *J. Biol. Chem.* **259**, 884–889.

Yamamoto, M., Kawanobe, Y., Takahashi, H., Shimazawa, E., Kimura, S., and Ogata, E. (1984). Vitamin D deficiency and renal calcium transport in the rat. *J. Clin. Invest.* **74**, 507–513.

# 9

# The Pathogenesis of Obesity

George A. Bray

*Los Angeles County/USC Medical Center*
*Division of Diabetes and Clinical Nutrition*
*Department of Medicine*
*University of Southern California*
*School of Medicine*
*Los Angeles, California*



## I. INTRODUCTION

Obesity is an outward reflection of increased nutrients stored as fat. Body fat above 25% of body weight in young men and 30% in young women defines obese. This positive nutrient balance implies a disturbance in a system that is normally regulated. The regulatory system for body weight has several features: a controlled nutrient system of food intake, storage, and metabolism; a controller located in the brain; feedback elements that tell the controller about the controlled system; and efferent control mechanisms.

The regulatory system for body weight is often considered a controller of energy balance *per se* (Woo *et al.*, 1985; Garrow, 1978). However, more detailed analysis suggests that each macronutrient is regulated separately. Although species variations obviously exist, the basic neurochemical and physiological mechanisms regulating energy and nutrient balance appear to apply to most mammalian species (Bray, 1987).

To analyze a controlled or regulated system, we can begin with the controlled system, the controller, the feedback signals, or the efferent controls. This analysis begins with the controlled system and ends with the efferent controls.

## II. CONTROLLED NUTRIENT SYSTEM

The controlled or regulated system for nutrient balance is concerned with maintaining appropriate stores of each macronutrient. In addition to water, which is the major constituent of all living cells and is closely regulated, the controlled system for macronutrients regulates intake, storage, and disposal of protein, carbohydrate, and fat.

### A. Nutrient Intake and Storage

In a normal human, total body fat stores are approximately 140,000 kcal (Garrow, 1978; Bray, 1976). This is about six times the energy stored as protein (24,000 kcal). Carbohydrate stores, available as glycogen from liver, kidney, muscle, and other tissues and as circulating blood glucose, are minute, equivalent to only 800 kcal. Figure 1 shows the distribution of a typical intake of 2,000 kcal. Carbohydrate intake at 800 kcal/day (200 g) is equal to 100% of total body carbohydrate, whereas protein intake is only a little over 1% of body protein, and fat intake is less than 1% of body fat. Studies of nutrient balance in experimental animals (Flatt, 1987) have noted that changes in carbohydrate balance on one day influence carbohydrate intake on the subsequent day. On the other hand, one day's intake of fat has much less effect on subsequent fat intake.

### B. Energy Expenditure

Basal or resting energy use by muscle, viscera, and brain is a second feature of the nutrient regulatory system (Fig. 2). Muscle and skin account

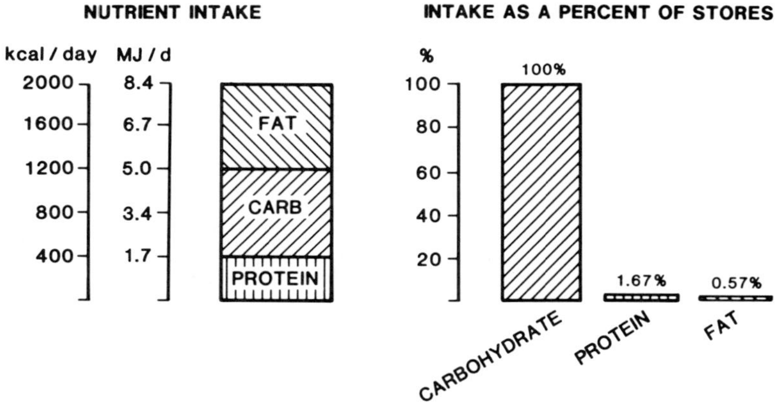


**Fig. 1.** Typical intake of 2,000 kcal includes 20% protein, 40% carbohydrate, and 40% fat. Adjacent bars represent the percentage of daily nutrient intake in relation to the quantities of each nutrient already in body stores. (Copyright 1987, George A. Bray. Reprinted with permission.)

for about 18% of energy expenditure at rest and for as much as 50% or more during locomotion or other physical activity (Garlson and Hsieh, 1970). Brain and visceral metabolism account for a much larger, more stable fraction of resting energy expenditure. The brain primarily oxidizes glucose and accounts for 20% of total daily energy expenditure. Visceral tissues predominantly use fatty acids or ketones and only small quantities of carbohydrate; amounts vary slightly with diet or exercise. Muscle, depending on its state of training and on the intensity and duration of exercise, utilizes variable quantities of carbohydrate and fat. A major difference between physically trained and untrained muscle is that trained muscle can oxidize fatty acids during exercise and at rest. During short bouts of intense exercise, carbohydrate, mobilized largely from muscle glycogen stores, provides the major fuel. During more prolonged aerobic exercise, muscle oxidizes a larger percentage of fatty acids, and its respiratory quotient falls.

## C. Nutrient Control Equation

Basic facts about the nutrient control system can be summarized in the following equation (Reaction 1):

$$\text{NUTRIENT BALANCE} = \sum[(\Delta\,\text{CARB BALANCE}) + (\Delta\,\text{FAT BALANCE}) + (\Delta\,\text{PROTEIN BALANCE})] \quad (1)$$

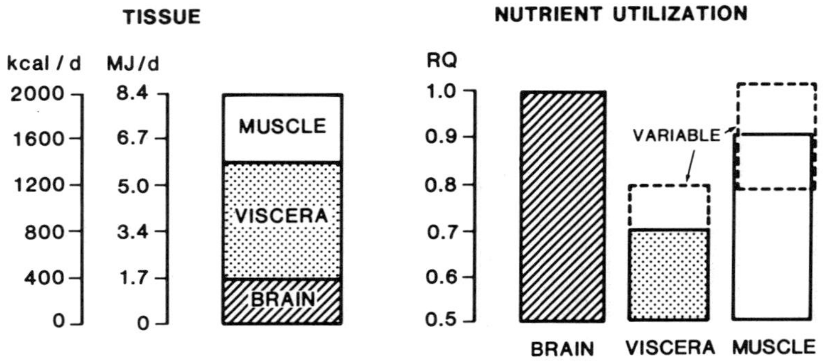


**Fig. 2.** Resting energy utilization by tissues is shown on the left, and the relative contribution of each tissue to oxidation of carbohydrate and fat, expressed as the respiratory quotient (RQ), is shown on the right. The RQ is the ratio of carbon-dioxide production to oxygen consumption. A tissue with an RQ of 1 oxidizes 100% carbohydrate, and a tissue with an RQ of 0.7 oxidizes 100% fat. The brain burns 100% carbohydrate and has an RQ of 1. Viscera and muscle show some adaptability in their use of carbohydrate or fat, represented by broken lines above, with muscle showing greater variation. (Copyright 1987, George A. Bray. Reprinted with permission.)

This equation suggests several hypotheses:

1. The balance of each major nutrient may be regulated separately.
2. The time required to achieve balance varies for each nutrient as a function of the amount ingested each day in relation to total body stores. Because body storage systems for carbohydrate are limited, a high-carbohydrate diet would appear to be less likely to cause obesity than a high-fat diet (Donato and Hegsted, 1985). Although excess carbohydrate can be converted to fatty acids, this is energetically expensive. Body fat stores, however, are many times larger than fat intake, implying a much greater fat storage capacity and a much longer time constant to achieve balance.
3. Achievement of nutrient balance requires that the net oxidation of each nutrient equals the average composition of dietary nutrients.
4. A high-fat diet requires greater fat oxidation than a low-fat diet.
5. Because physical training can increase oxidation of fatty acids by muscle, regular aerobic exercise might reduce the tendency to become obese on a higher fat diet.
6. Finally, positive and negative feedback elements, operating through the central controller, regulate nutrient stores for each component.

## D. Animal Models of Obesity

Nutrient intake plays a variable role in the development of obesity in experimental animals (Bray and York, 1979; Sclafani, 1984) and thus

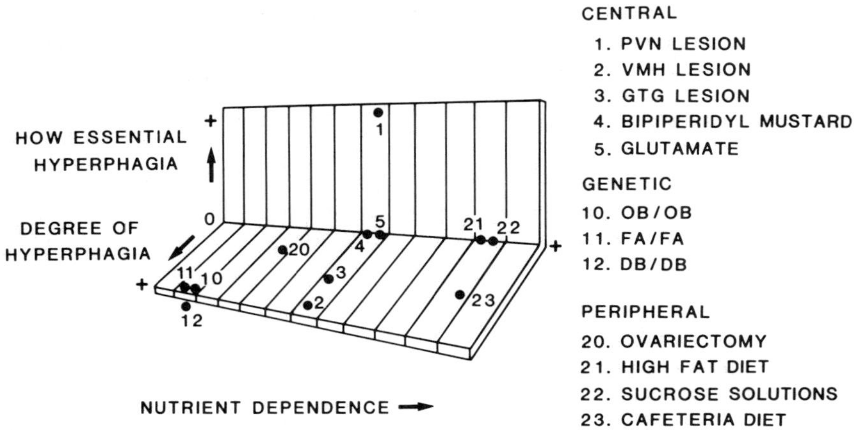


**Fig. 3.** This three-dimensional diagram shows relative nutrient dependence in animal models of hypothalamic (central), genetic, and dietary (peripheral) obesity. Also shown are the presence and degree of hyperphagia in each model and the dependence on hyperphagia for development of obesity. (Copyright 1987, George A. Bray. Reprinted with permission.)

probably in humans as well (Fig. 3). The following animal models reveal that nutrient intake and hyperphagia are separable variables in the obesity equation.

### 1. *Hypothalamic (Central) Obesity*

Animals with lesions in the paraventricular nucleus (PVN) are hyperphagic (Tokunaga *et al.*, 1986; Leibowitz *et al.*, 1981), and hyperphagia appears essential to development of obesity (Weingarten *et al.*, 1985). However, development of obesity in these animals appears to be relatively independent of the nutrient composition of the diet—they become fat on high- or low-carbohydrate diets.

Hypothalamic obesity produced by lesions in the ventromedial hypothalamus (VMH) or by injecting gold thioglucose (GTG) is no more nutrient dependent than obesity produced by PVN lesions (Bray and York, 1979). VMH and GTG also include hyperphagia, but this hyperphagia is not essential for development of these syndromes (Han and Frohman, 1970; Frohman *et al.*, 1969). Further, hypothalamic injuries resulting from injection of bipiperidyl mustard or monosodium glutamate cause obesity on any diet.

### 2. *Genetic Obesity*

Although genetic obesities usually involve hyperphagic mechanisms, hyperphagia is not essential for development of obesity (Bray and York,

1979; Coleman, 1982; Cox and Powley, 1977). Genetically obese animals become fat on high- or low-carbohydrate diets.

*3. Dietary (Peripheral) Obesity*

Of syndromes due to peripheral manipulations, ovariectomy produces a modest hyperphagia that is not essential for development of obesity and increases susceptibility to a high-fat diet (Sclafani, 1984). High-fat diets (Schemmel *et al.*, 1970), access to sucrose solutions (Kanarek and Hirsch, 1977) and cafeteria diets (Rothwell and Stock, 1979) have a high nutrient dependence for development of obesity. Cafeteria-fed rats are the most hyperphagic; the other two show only limited hyperphagia.

## III. THE BRAIN AS CONTROLLER

### A. Anatomy

Several anatomic regions of the brain appear to play important roles in controlling nutrient balance (Luiten *et al.*, 1987). Destruction of the VMH is associated with increased fat stores in most homeothermic species studied (Bray and York, 1979), but destruction of regions in the lateral hypothalamus is associated with reduced fat stores. More recently, the PVN has been shown to be an important site for stimulation of food intake by topical injection of norepinephrine and such neuropeptides as dynorphin and neuropeptide Y (Leibowitz, 1986). The primacy of the PVN in regulating body fat stores is suggested by the fact that chronic infusion of norepinephrine into the VMH induces obesity, whereas chronic infusion into the PVN does not (Shimazu *et al.*, 1986).

### B. Neurotransmitters

Norepinephrine, serotonin, and several peptides may transmit information that regulates food intake and nutrient stores. As noted above, norepinephrine infusions into the VMH can increase fat stores. Serotonin also plays an important role in regulating food intake and nutrient stores (Blundell, 1984). Tryptophan and 5-hydroxytryptophan, two serotonin precursors, both decrease food intake (Wurtman and Wurtman, 1984). Drugs that block serotonin release can increase body weight, and those that stimulate its release or inhibit its reuptake from nerve endings can reduce body weight. Thus norepinephrine and serotonin appear to regulate food intake through structures located in the medial and lateral hypothalamus.

Several peptides also modulate food intake and may influence nutrient storage (Baile *et al.*, 1986; Morley and Levine, 1985; Leibowitz, 1986). Neuropeptide Y, beta-endorphin, dynorphin, and galanin stimulate food intake when injected in the VMN or PVN (Leibowitz, 1986; Morley and Levine, 1981). In contrast, other peptides, including bombesin, cholecystokinin, neurotensin, somatostatin, and corticotropin-releasing factor (CRF), inhibit feeding when injected topically in the VMN region or when infused into the third ventricular system (Baile *et al.*, 1986; Morley and Levine, 1985; Leibowitz, 1986). Evidence also suggests that raising the insulin concentration in cerebrospinal fluid decreases food intake in several species, but the physiological importance of this finding remains unclear (Woods *et al.*, 1979; Brief and Davis, 1984).

## IV. FEEDBACK SIGNALS

The central neurotransmitters that regulate nutrient balance are activated by afferent signals transmitted through the blood or the autonomic nervous system. Carbohydrate balance appears to be regulated on a day-to-day basis in mice (Flatt, 1987). Because carbohydrate stores are concentrated as glycogen in muscle and liver, carbohydrate balance might be modulated by hepatic glycogen stores. Glucoreceptors in the liver send information to the brain through vagal afferent nerves (Niijima, 1984). Vagal afferent nerve fibers have been traced from the liver to the nucleus of the tractus solaritarius (NTS), to the parabrachial nucleus, to the lateral hypothalamus, and to the PVN (Novin *et al.*, 1981). Cholecystokinin, which inhibits food intake in humans and animals (Baile *et al.*, 1986), may be involved in this afferent vagal system because it fails to lower food intake after vagotomy or in the presence of NTS or PVN lesions. These data suggest that the afferent vagal pathway to the PVN may be one way in which changes in glucose balance are transmitted, thus inducing changes in food intake.

Glucose balance may also be modulated by the direct action of glucose on the central nervous system (Le Magnen, 1983). Hauger and associates (1986) have demonstrated that glucose regulates the binding of amphetamine to the sodium pump ($Na^+$–$K^+$ ATPase) in the hypothalamus and that this activity is modulated by glucose intake. Thus, at least two mechanisms may regulate glucose balance.

The potential role of serotonin in regulating protein intake and/or carbohydrate balance is suggested by the relationship between tryptophan, a serotonin precursor, and food intake (Wurtman and Wurtman, 1984). Tryptophan, 5-hydroxytryptophan, and drugs like fenfluramine that increase serotonin concentrations at neuroeffector junctions alter the preference for carbohydrates and modify the preference for protein

(Rowland and Carlton, 1986). Amphetamines, which influence the noradrenergic system, alter the preference for protein (Rowland and Carlton, 1986).

Fat balance presents a more complicated problem. When the percentage of dietary fat increases, body fat stores rise in most animal species (Schemmel *et al.*, 1970). However, within each species, some animals consuming a high-fat diet are considerably more resistant to developing obesity than others.

We found important differences in the responses of rats sensitive or resistant to a high-fat diet. Changes in food intake in response to insulin and anorectic drugs differed significantly (Fisler and Bray, 1985). Changes in insulin concentrations may explain the increase in blood ketones, the product of fatty-acid metabolism by the liver, observed in resistant rats. Ketones are secreted and transported to other tissues, where they provide metabolic fuel. They may also signal the status of fatty-acid oxidation to the liver or brain. We observed that the transport of 3-hydroxybutyrate across the blood–brain barrier is significantly higher in rats resistant to high-fat diets than in sensitive rats (Bray *et al.*, 1987).

In other studies, we observed that microinjections of ketones into the VMH enhance sympathetic activity, as reflected by the increased thermogenic properties of brown adipose tissue (BAT) (Arase *et al.*, 1987) and by the increased sympathetic firing rate of nerves to BAT (Sakaguchi and Bray, 1988). These findings, in harmony with observations of Davis and associates (1981), suggest that the VMH plays a pivotal role in producing resistance to obesity in rats eating a high-fat diet.

The importance of the VMH in the resistant rat is underlined by the fact that VMH lesions convert the resistant rat into one that is sensitive to a high-fat diet (Oku *et al.*, 1984). Resistant rats also show an altered pattern of response to drugs that attenuate food intake (Fisler and Bray, 1985) but not to castration- or sucrose-diet-induced obesity (Schemmel *et al.*, 1982).

Resistant and sensitive rats also exhibit differences in efferent controls. Sympathetic nervous system activity is higher in the resistant animal (Fisler *et al.*, 1984). The response to ketones infused into the cerebroventricular system does not appear to vary with diet. The concentration of ketones available to brain tissue is a function of the rate of transport across the blood–brain barrier. Thus, higher blood–brain-barrier transport of ketones following exposure to a high-fat diet leads to greater quantities of ketones in the brain and to greater activation of the sympathetic nervous system by this mechanism.

## V. EFFERENT CONTROLS

Efferent controls represent the final section of the nutrient control model for obesity.

## A. Motor Activities

One efferent control is the complex sequence of motor activities that lead to seeking, identification, killing, and inges,tion of food. These activities seem to be integrated in the lateral hypothalamus because electrical stimulation of this area leads to ingestive behavior.

## B. Autonomic Nervous System

Efferent controls also include internal regulators of nutrient intake and stores. In animals whose obesity follows hypothalamic lesions, vagal system activity increases (Bray and York, 1979; Bray *et al.*, 1981; Cox and Powley, 1981; Inoue *et al.*, 1983). This provides one explanation for the increase in insulin that characterizes this syndrome. However, reduced sympathetic activity may be more characteristic of obesity and may enhance insulin secretion (Niijima *et al.*, 1984; Yoshimatsu *et al.*, 1984; Nishizawa and Bray, 1978). Sympathetic activity normally increases in response to sucrose (Young and Landsberg, 1977a) or glucose (Sakaguchi and Bray, 1987).

In our animal studies, sympathetic activity appeared to be inversely related to food intake (Sakaguchi *et al.*, 1986). During spontaneous eating, a negative correlation between basal activity of the sympathetic nervous system and food intake is found ($r = -0.91$). Apparent exceptions are observed in fasted animals (Young and Landsberg, 1977b) and in animals eating a cafeteria or supermarket diet (Young *et al.*, 1982). Sympathetic nervous system activity declines in fasted rats (Young and Landsberg, 1977b; Yoshida *et al.*, 1983). However, this reduced sympathetic activity may be consistent with the negative correlation between food intake and sympathetic activity if one considers how much the fasted animal might have eaten if food were available. With our model of a negative correlation between food intake and resting sympathetic activity, the low sympathetic activity observed with fasting would predict an increase in food intake when food first becomes available. Van Itallie and Kissileff (1985) observed precisely this relationship: initial food intake increased as the length of the fast increased.

The increased food intake in the cafeteria-fed rat (Young *et al.*, 1982) and in the sucrose-fed rat (Young and Landsberg, 1977a) may mean that positive feedback signals are overriding the normal reciprocal relationship between food intake and the sympathetic nervous system.

Table I summarizes the effects of various maneuvers on the sympathetic nervous system. Clearly, this system plays an important role in regulating many of the body's basic functions as well as in its adaptation to a variety of signals.

TABLE I

**Factors Affecting Sympathetic Activity[a]**

| | Sympathetic activity | | |
|---|---|---|---|
| Physiologic variable | Low | Normal | High |
| Hypothalamic lesion[a] | VMH | PVN | LH |
| Food intake (quality) | High fat | Mixed diet | High carbohydrate |
| Food intake (quantity) | Fasting | Average | Overeating |
| Genetic obesity | Fatty (*fa/fa*) | — | — |
| | Obese (*ob/ob*) | — | — |
| | Diabetic (*db/db*) | — | — |
| Corticosteroid level | High | — | Low (adrenalectomy) |
| Insulin level | Low | — | High |
| Thyroid hormone level | High | — | Low |
| Temperature | Hot | Neutral | Cold |
| Lactation | Lactating | — | — |

[a]VMH is ventromedial hypothalamus, PVN is paraventricular nucleus, and LH is lateral hypothalamus.

## C. Adrenal Steroids

Adrenalectomy plays an important role in sympathetic activity and its regulation of nutrient control: it reverses or attenuates the development or progression of experimental obesity (Bray, 1982; Bruce *et al.*, 1982; Mook *et al.*, 1972). This striking observation (Bray, 1986; Bray, 1984; Saito and Bray, 1984; Holt and York, 1982; Marchington *et al.*, 1983) requires special consideration because it suggests that glucocorticoids might play a key role in the development of obesity.

Adrenalectomy produces two effects on nutrient balance (Fukushima *et al.*, 1985). First, nutrient intake returns nearly, if not completely, to normal levels after adrenalectomy in genetically obese animals, in those with castration-induced obesity (Mook *et al.*, 1972), and in those with hypothalamic obesity (Bruce *et al.*, 1982). Second, feeding patterns also revert to normal (Saito and Bray, 1984). Leibowitz (1986) has observed that adrenalectomy almost completely abolishes the stimulation of food intake normally induced by norepinephrine injections into the PVN. Treatment with corticosterone rapidly reverses this effect. Loss of sensitivity to norepinephrine may explain why food intake returns to normal after adrenalectomy.

Energy expenditure also increases after adrenalectomy (Holt and York, 1982; Marchington *et al.*, 1983; vander Tuig *et al.*, 1984). We (vander Tuig *et al.*, 1984) and others (York *et al.*, 1985; Holt and York, 1982) have also shown increased sympathetic activity, measured by increased norepinephrine turnover in nerve endings in BAT (vander Tuig *et al.*, 1984) and by increased thermogenic activity—binding of guanosine 5′-diphosphate to mitochondria from BAT (Marchington *et al.*, 1983). Effects of corticosteroids on thermogenic activity can be observed in normal (Fukushima *et al.*, 1985) as well as obese animals (Marchington *et al.*, 1983).

Because removal of glucocorticoids by adrenalectomy affects efferent systems for food intake and sympathetic activity, nutrient control appears to be regulated at yet another site than those involved in genetic, dietary, or hypothalamic obesity. After adrenalectomy, the negative feedback signal produced by corticosterone is absent, and CRF released into hypothalamic portal circulation stimulates increased ACTH output from the pituitary. Increased release of CRF may be the principal stimulus for reduced food intake and increased sympathetic activity. CRF injections into the ventricle of the rat decrease food intake (Levine *et al.*, 1983; Morley *et al.*, 1983) and increase circulating epinephrine and norepinephrine (Brown *et al.*, 1982). Because adrenalectomy attenuates obesity in genetically obese animals, the mechanism by which CRF influences food intake and sympathetic activity appears to work differently from mechanisms associated with neurotransmitter systems involved in hypothalamic, genetic, or dietary obesity (Fig. 4).

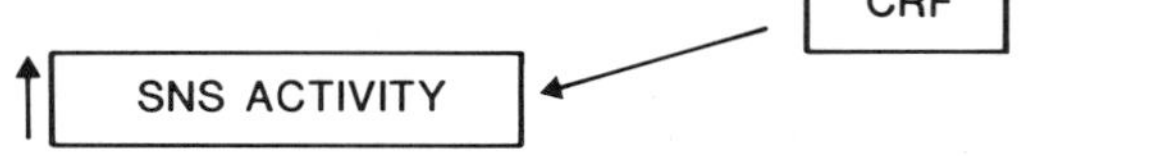


**Fig. 4.** The effects of adrenalectomy on control of sympathetic nervous activity and food intake are shown in this model. The central actor in this system is corticotropin-releasing factor (CRF), which can modulate reciprocal changes in food intake and sympathetic nervous system (SNS) activity. (Copyright 1987, George A. Bray. Reprinted with permission.)

## VI. SUMMARY

Nutrient intake is a regulated system, whose principal feedback elements involve vagal afferent fibers from the liver, stomach, and pancreas. Nutrients from food—including ketones produced by fatty-acid oxidation in the liver—and circulating hormones released during ingestion, digestion, and storage of nutrients may also provide feedback signals to the brain. Positive feedback is also associated with the smell and taste of food. Social occasions and other events that lead to overriding the normal satiety mechanisms can lead to enhanced food intake.

The brain has receptor systems that integrate messages that normally control the feeding system. The lateral and ventromedial hypothalamus act reciprocally to control the parasympathetic and sympathetic nervous system. Following adrenalectomy, the increase in CRF may override the defects of genetic and hypothalamic obesity.

The model described here suggests that new therapeutic approaches to obesity should involve strategies to modulate each nutrient. The concept that nutrient balance is regulated by controlling the balance of individual nutrients supports the following important advice regulating obesity through diet and exercise: Eat a high-carbohydrate, low-fat diet, and exercise to maintain muscles at a moderate degree of training.

## ACKNOWLEDGMENTS

This work is supported in part by Grant AM RO1-AM 32018.

## REFERENCES

Arase, K., York, D. A., Shargill, N. S., and Bray, G. A. (1987). Effect of cerebroventricular infusions of insulin and beta-hydroxybutyrate on food intake and thermogenesis in the rat [Abstract]. *Clin. Res.* **35**, 767A.

Baile, C. A., McLaughlin, C. L., and Della-Fera, M. A. (1986). Role of cholecystokinin and opioid peptides in the control of food intake. *Physiol. Rev.* **66**, 172–234.

Blundell, J. E. (1984). Serotonin and appetite. *Neuropharmacology* **23**, 1537–1552.

Bray, G. A. (1976). "The Obese Patient. Major Problems in Internal Medicine," Vol. 9. W. B. Saunders Company, Philadelphia.

Bray, G. A. (1982). Regulation of energy balance: Studies on genetic, hypothalamic and dietary obesity. *Proc. Nutr. Soc.* **41**, 95–108.

Bray, G. A. (1984). Integration of energy intake and expenditure in animals and man: The autonomic and adrenal hypothesis. *Clin. Endocrinol. Metab.* **13**, 521–546.

Bray, G. A. (1986). Autonomic and endocrine factors in the regulation of energy balance. *Fed. Proc.* **45**, 1404–1410.

Bray, G. A. (1987). Obesity—A disease of nutrient or energy balance? *Nutr. Rev.* **45**, 33–43.

Bray, G. A., and York, D. A. (1979). Hypothalamic and genetic obesity in experimental animals: An autonomic and endocrine hypothesis. *Physiol. Rev.* **59**, 719–809.

Bray, G. A., Inoue, S., and Nishizawa, Y. (1981). Hypothalamic obesity. The autonomic hypothesis and the lateral hypothalamus. *Diabetologia* **20**, 366–377.

Bray, G. A., Teague, R. J., and Lee, C. K. (1987). Brain uptake of ketones in rats with differing susceptibility to dietary obesity. *Metabolism* **36**, 27–30.

Brief, D. J., and Davis, J. D. (1984). Reduction of food intake and body weight by chronic intraventricular insulin infusion. *Brain Res. Bull.* **12**, 571–575.

Brown, M. R., Fisher, L. A., Rivier, J., Spiess, J., Rivier, C., and Vale, W. (1982). Corticotropin-releasing factor: Effects on the sympathetic nervous system and oxygen consumption. *Life Sci.* **30**, 207–210.

Bruce, B. K., King, B. M., Phelps, G. R., and Veitia, M. C. (1982). Effects of adrenalectomy and corticosterone administration on hypothalamic obesity in rats. *Amer. J. Physiol.* **243**, E152–E157.

Carlson, L. D., and Hsieh, A. C. L. (1970). "The Control of Energy Exchange." MacMillan Company, New York.

Coleman, D. L. (1982). Thermogenesis in diabetes-obesity syndromes in mutant mice. *Diabetologia* **22**, 205–211.

Cox, J. E., and Powley, T. L. (1977). Development of obesity in diabetic mice pair-fed with lean siblings. *J. Comp. Physiol. Psychol.* **91**, 347–358.

Cox, J. E., and Powley, T. L. (1981). Prior vagotomy blocks VMH obesity in pair-fed rats. *Amer. J. Physiol.* **240**, E573-E583.

Davis, J. D., Wirtshafter, D., Asin, K. E., and Brief, D. (1981). Sustained intracerebroventricular infusion of brain fuels reduces body weight and food intake in rats. *Science* **212**, 81–83.

Donato, K., and Hegsted, D. M. (1985). Efficiency of utilization of various sources of energy for growth. *Proc. Nat. Acad. Sci. USA* **82**, 4866–4870.

Fisler, J. S., and Bray, G. A. (1985). Dietary obesity: Effects of drugs or food intake in S5B/P1 and Osborne-Mendel rats. *Physiol. Behav.* **34**, 225–231.

Fisler, J. S., Yoshida, T., and Bray, G. A. (1984). Catecholamine turnover in S5B/P1 and Osborne-Mendel rats: response to a high-fat diet. *Amer. J. Physiol.* **247**, R290-R295.

Flatt, P. R. (1987). Dietary fat, carbohydrate balance, and weight maintenance: Effects of exercise. *Amer. J. Clin. Nutr.* **45**, 296–306.

Frohman, L. A., Bernardis, L. L., Schnatz, J. D., and Burek, L. (1969). Plasma insulin and triglyceride levels after hypothalamic lesions in weanling rats. *Amer. J. Physiol.* **216**, 1496–1501.

Fukushima, M., Lupien, J., and Bray, G. A. (1985). Interaction of light and corticosterone on food intake and interscapular brown adipose tissue of rats. *Amer. J. Physiol.* **249**, R753-R757.

Garrow, J. S. (1978). "Energy Balance and Obesity in Man," 2nd ed. Elsevier/North Holland Biomedical Press, Amsterdam.

Han, P. W., and Frohman, L. A. (1970). Hyperinsulinemia in tube-fed hypophysectomized rats bearing hypothalamic lesions. *Amer. J. Physiol.* **219**, 1632–1636.

Hauger, R., Hulihan-Giblin, B., Angel, I., Luu, M. D., Janowsky, A., Skolnick, P., and Paul, S. M. (1986). Glucose regulates ($^3$H)(+)-amphetamine binding and $Na^+K^+$ ATPase activity in the hypothalamus: A proposed mechanism for the glucostatic control of feeding and satiety. *Brain Res. Bull.* **16**, 281–288.

Holt, S., and York, D. A. (1982). The effect of adrenalectomy on GDP binding to brown adipose tissue mitochondria of obese rats. *Biochem. J.* **208**, 819–822.

Inoue, S., Mullen, Y. S., and Bray, G. A. (1983). Hyperinsulinemia in rats with hypothalamic obesity. Effects of autonomic drugs and glucose. *Amer. J. Physiol.* **245**, R372–R378.

Kanarek, R. B., and Hirsch, E. (1977). Dietary-induced overeating in experimental animals. *Fed. Proc.* **36**, 154–158.

Leibowitz, S. F. (1986). Brain monoamines and peptides: Roles in the control of eating behavior. *Fed. Proc.* **45**, 1396–1403.

Leibowitz, S. F., Hammer, N. J., and Chang, K. (1981). Hypothalamic paraventricular nucleus lesions produce overeating and obesity in the rat. *Physiol. Behav.* **27**, 1031–1040.

Le Magnen, J. (1983). Body energy balance and food intake: A neuroendocrine regulatory mechanism. *Physiol Rev.* **63**, 314–386.

Levine, A. S., Rogers, B., Kneip, J., Grace, M., and Morley, J. E. (1983). Effect of centrally administered corticotropin release factor (CRF) on multiple feeding paradigms. *Neuropharmacol.* **22**, 337–339.

Luiten, P. G. M., ter Horst, G. J., and Steffens, A. B. (1987). The hypothalamus, intrinsic connections and outflow pathways to the endocrine system in relation to the control of feeding and metabolism. *Prog. Neurobiol.* **28**, 1–54.

Marchington, D., Rothwell, N. J., Stock, M. J., and York, D. A. (1983). Energy balance, diet-induced thermogenesis and brown adipose tissue in lean and obese (fa/fa) Zucker rats after adrenalectomy. *J. Nutr.* **113**, 1395–1402.

Mook, D. G., Kenney, N. J., Roberts, S., Nussbaum, A. I., and Rodier, W. I. III (1972). Ovarian-adrenal interactions in regulation of body weight by female rats. *J. Comp. Physiol. Psychol.* **81**, 198–211.

Morley, J. E., and Levine, A. S. (1981). Dynorphin (1–13) induces spontaneous feeding in rats. *Life Sci.* **29**, 1901–1903.

Morley, J. E., and Levine, A. S. (1985). The pharmacology of eating behavior. *Rev. Pharmacol. Toxicol.* **25**, 127–146.

Morley, J. E., Levine, A. S., and Rowland, N. E. (1983). Stress-induced eating. *Life Sci.* **32**, 2169–2182.

Niijima, A. (1984). The effect of D-glucose on the firing rate of glucose-sensitive vagal afferents in the liver in comparison with the effect of 2-deoxy-D-glucose. *J. Autonom. Nerv. Syst.* **10**, 255–260.

Niijima, A., Rohner-Jeanrenaud, F., and Jeanrenaud, B. (1984). Role of ventromedial hypothalamus on sympathetic efferents of brown adipose tissue. *Amer. J. Physiol.* **247**, R650–R654.

Nishizawa, Y., and Bray, G. A. (1978). Ventromedial hypothalamic lesions and the mobilization of fatty acids. *J. Clin. Invest.* **61**, 714–721.

Novin, D., Rogers, R. D., and Hermann, G. (1981). Visceral afferent and efferent connections in the brain. *Diabetologia* **20**, 331–336.

Oku, J., Bray, G. A., Fisler, J. S., and Schemmel, R. A. (1984). Ventromedial hypothalamic knife-cut lesions in rats resistant to dietary obesity. *Amer. J. Physiol.* **246**, R943–R948.

Rothwell, N. J., and Stock, M. J. (1979). A role for brown adipose tissue in diet-induced thermogenesis. *Nature* **281**, 31–35.

Rowland, N. E., and Carlton, J. (1986). Neurobiology of an anorectic drug: Fenfluramine. *Prog. Neurobiol.* **27**, 13–62.

Saito, M., and Bray, G. A. (1984). Adrenalectomy and food restriction in the genetically obese (*ob/ob*) mouse. *Amer. J. Physiol.* **246**, R20–R25.

Sakaguchi, T., and Bray, G. A. (1987). The effect of intrahypothalamic injections of glucose on sympathetic efferent firing rate. *Brain Res. Bull.* **18**, 591–595.

Sakaguchi, T., and Bray, G. A. (1988). Microinjection of beta-hydroxybutyrate into the ventromedial or paraventricular nucleus of the hypothalamus stimulates the sympathetic nervous system. *Metabolism.* (In press.)

Sakaguchi, T., Takahashi, M., and Bray, G. A. (1986). The diurnal pattern of food intake is controlled by the suprachiasmatic nucleus (SCN) [Abstract]. *Clin. Res.* **34**, 553A.

Schemmel, R., Mickelson, O., and Gill, J. L. (1970). Dietary obesity in rats. Body weight and body fat accretion in seven strains of rats. *J. Nutr.* **100**, 1041–1048.

Schemmel, R. A., Teague, R. J., and Bray, G. A. (1982). Obesity in Osborne–Mendel and S5B/P1 rats: Effects of sucrose solutions, castration, and treatment with estradiol or insulin. *Amer. J. Physiol.* **243**, R347–R353.

Sclafani, A. (1984). Animal models of obesity: Classification and characterization. *Int. J. Obesity* **8**, 491–508.

Shimazu, T., Noama, M., and Saito, M. (1986). Chronic infusion of norepinephrine into the ventromedial hypothalamus induced obesity in rats. *Brain Res.* **369**, 215–223.

Tokunaga, K., Fukushima, M., Kemnitz, J. W., and Bray, G. A. (1986). Comparison of ventromedial and paraventricular lesions in rats that become obese. *Amer. J. Physiol.* **251**, R1221–R1227.

vander Tuig, J. G., Ohshima, K., Yoshida, T., Romsos, D. R., and Bray, G. A. (1984). Adrenalectomy increases norepinephrine turnover in brown adipose tissue of obese (*ob/ob*) mice. *Life Sci.* **31**, 1423–1432.

Van Itallie, T. B., and Kissileff, H. R. (1985). Physiology of food intake: an inventory control model. *Amer. J. Clin. Nutr.* **42**, 914–923.

Weingarten, J. P., Chang, P., and McDonald, T. J. (1985). Comparison of the metabolic and behavioral disturbances following paraventricular and ventromedial hypothalamic lesions. *Brain Res. Bull.* **14**, 551–559.

Woo, R., Daniels-Kush, R., and Horton, E. S. (1985). Regulation of energy balance. *Ann. Rev. Nutr.* **5**, 411–433.

Woods, S. C., Lotter, E. C., McKay, L. D., and Porte, D., Jr. (1979). Chronic intracerebroventricular infusion of insulin reduces food intake and body weight of baboons. *Nature* **282**, 503–505.

Wurtman, R. J., and Wurtman, J. J. (1984). Nutrients, neurotransmitter synthesis, and the control of food intake. *In* "Eating and Its Disorders" (A. J. Stunkard and E. Stellard, eds.), pp. 77–96. Raven Press, New York.

York, D. A., Marchington, D., Holt, S. J., and Allars, J. (1985). Regulation of sympathetic activity in lean and obese Zucker rats. *Amer. J. Physiol.* **249**, E299–E305.

Yoshida, T., Kemnitz, J. W., and Bray, G. A. (1983). Lateral hypothalamic lesions and norepinephrine turnover in rats. *J. Clin. Invest.* **72**, 919–927.

Yoshimatsu, H., Niijima, A., Oomura, Y., Kazutoshi, Y., and Katafuchi, T. (1984). Effects of hypothalamic lesions on pancreatic autonomic nerve activity in the rat. *Brain Res.* **303**, 147–152.

Young, J. B., and Landsberg, L. (1977a). Stimulation of the sympathetic nervous system during sucrose feeding. *Nature* **269**, 615–617.

Young, J. B., and Landsberg, L. (1977b). Suppression of sympathetic nervous system during fasting. *Science* **196**, 1473–1475.

Young, J. B., Saville, E., Rothwell, N. J., Stock, M. J., and Landsberg, L. (1982). Effect of diet and cold exposure on norepinephrine turnover in brown adipose tissue of the rat. *J. Clin. Invest.* **69**, 1061–1071.

# 10

# Essential Obesity and the Pathogenetic Role of a Low Metabolic Rate

Clifton Bogardus and Eric Ravussin

*Clinical Diabetes and Nutrition Section*
*National Institute of Diabetes and Digestive and Kidney Diseases*
*National Institutes of Health*
*Phoenix, Arizona*

## I. INTRODUCTION

Nutritional disorders underlie many world health problems. In developed countries, obesity is a common disorder associated with considerable morbidity in connection with hypertension, noninsulin-dependent diabetes mellitus and cardiovascular and other diseases. Obesity also decreases longevity (Maison *et al.*, 1987; Simopolous and Van Itallie, 1984). The increasing prevalence of obesity and its associated health problems has increased interest in determining its pathogenesis.

The word obesity, derived from the Latin *ob* (over) and *edere* (to eat), implies that obesity is simply caused by overeating. This is true, of course, because to become obese, a person must eat more calories than needed to maintain lean body weight. However, the overeating hypothesis is insufficient to describe the pathogenesis of human obesity. It fails to explain *why* some people overeat and others do not. It also fails to consider variability in caloric needs as a contributor to imbalance in the human energy equation. Attributing obesity solely to overeating also accuses the overweight person of gluttony. This is convenient because it relieves physicians of their helplessness to treat the disease and fixes the blame on the obese patient.

Although useful for the physician, the gluttony theory of obesity does not fit well with current data regarding the pathogenesis of obesity in humans and experimental animals. Human obesity has long been established as a familial disorder and is now known to have genetic determinants. Stunkard and associates (1986), who studied adopted children and their biological and adoptive parents in Denmark, found the estimated degree of obesity in adopted children more similar to that of their biological than adoptive parents. If gluttony were the only cause of obesity, these data would suggest that gluttony is inherited. This seems quite unlikely. Therefore, excess caloric intake as a cause of obesity should more appropriately be examined in terms of complex pathophysiological mechanisms of appetite regulation and/or feeding behavior rather than in terms of simple lack of self-control.

The gluttony theory also fits poorly with obesity models in rodents. Some species of rats and mice can be bred to become obese. Their obesity is frequently associated with hyperphagia, but pair-feeding experiments have shown that they become obese while eating the same food as their lean littermates (Cleary *et al.*, 1980; Cox and Powley, 1977). Livestock researchers have shown that strains of pigs and cows can be bred to be more calorie efficient and obese eating the same food as leaner strains (Ferrell and Jenkins, 1984; Koong *et al.*, 1983).

These findings provide good reasons to discard the hypothesis that gluttony is the only mechanism leading to human obesity. Humans with genetically determined disorders of appetite regulation and feeding behavior or with genetically determined greater ''caloric efficiency'' are likely to exist. We will review current data relevant to the pathogenesis of human obesity collected among a population of Native Americans, the Pima Indians.

## II. PIMA INDIANS

The Pima Indians are relatively genetically homogeneous (Matson *et al.*, 1968) and geographically isolated; they have lived in the same arid environment in the southwestern United States for nearly 2,000 years. The Pima were farmers who, for centuries, irrigated their fields with water from the Gila River. With the arrival of the white man, who settled in increasing numbers upstream on the Gila River, their water supplies decreased. Water supplies eventually became too scarce to permit their continued reliance on the river and farming for their food. Their diet changed rapidly from naturally grown produce to commercially produced foods.

By the mid 1970s, the Pima were more obese than similarly aged Caucasians (Knowler *et al.*, 1981). Their obesity is associated with the highest reported prevalence and incidence of noninsulin-dependent diabetes mellitus of any population in the world (Knowler *et al.*, 1978).

In 1982, cross-sectional and longitudinal studies were begun among the Pima to determine the metabolic defect(s) that could predict the development of diabetes among nondiabetic Pimas. In conjunction with these studies, we performed studies of their energy expenditure in relation to obesity.

## III. COMPONENTS OF DAILY ENERGY EXPENDITURE

Daily energy expenditure has three major components (Fig. 1): the resting metabolic rate (RMR), the thermic effect of food and the caloric cost of physical activity. In most sedentary adults, RMR accounts for about 60–70% of daily caloric expenditure. The thermic effect of food, usually about 10% of caloric intake, accounts for another 10%. The contribution of physical activity to daily caloric expenditure is much more variable.

In recent years, studies of energy metabolism in lean and obese persons have focused predominantly on the thermic effect of food. This seems to have occurred for two reasons. First, it was assumed that RMR is constant for a given body size and therefore an unlikely cause of variations in daily caloric expenditure among individuals. Second, studies have failed to prove that obese subjects are consistently less active than lean persons.

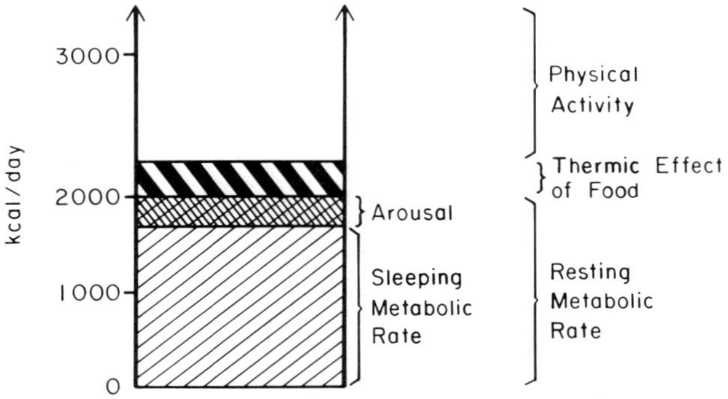


**Fig. 1.** Components of daily energy expenditure in man include the resting metabolic rate (RMR), the thermic effect of food, and physical activity. RMR can be subdivided into "sleeping metabolic rate" and "arousal," the change in metabolic rate associated with being awake but motionless.

Thus, the thermic effect of food appeared to be the only component of daily energy expenditure that could cause variations in predisposition to obesity among individuals.

However, because RMR accounts for a much greater portion of daily energy expenditure than the thermic effect of food, a 10% reduction in RMR would have a much greater impact on daily caloric expenditure than a 10% reduction in the thermic effect of food. Therefore, our initial studies reassessed the variability of RMR among persons of similar body size.

## IV. RESTING METABOLIC RATE

### A. The Variability of the Resting Metabolic Rate

RMR was measured using the ventilated-hood method of indirect calorimetry. Body composition was assessed by underwater weighing, and fat-free body mass was calculated (Bogardus *et al.*, 1986). In our studies, RMR correlated more closely with fat-free body mass than body weight in men and women, but considerable variance in RMR was still apparent at any given fat-free body mass (Fig. 2).

Previous investigators have observed a similar variance in RMR within the normal range (Boothby and Sandiford, 1922). They were more concerned, however, with defining the limits of the normal range to identify such disease states as hypo- or hyperthyroidism. As a result, because of the generally good correlation between body size and RMR, RMR was considered constant for a given body size. This led to use of equations to predict RMR based on height and weight.

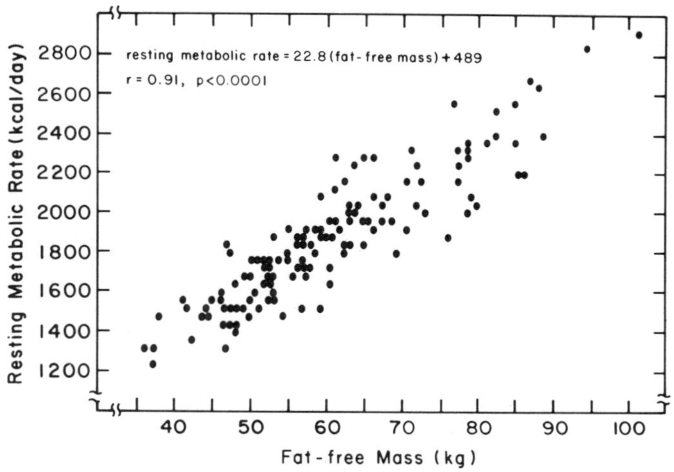


**Fig. 2.** The relationship between resting metabolic rate and fat-free body mass in 130 nondiabetic Pima Indians is plotted above. In our studies, RMR was significantly correlated to the fat-free body mass ($r = 0.91$; $p < 0.0001$). (From Bogardus *et al.*, 1986. Reprinted with permission.)

In our studies (Bogardus *et al.*, 1986), we wanted to know why RMR varies among normal persons. To determine whether the variation in RMR at a given fat-free body mass was attributable to the indirect calorimetric method, we determined its variance by repeated measurements of burning acetone within the hood. To determine whether RMR varies from one time to another in a given individual, we repeatedly measured RMR in several subjects on different days at intervals of 1 week to 21 months. As shown (Fig. 3), the variability of the method or of RMR in a given individual could not account for the variability around the regression line when RMR was regressed on fat-free body mass. Nor was the variance accounted for by differences in age or sex. These data demonstrate that individuals vary in RMR more than can be accounted for by differences in the fat-free body mass.

## B. Familial Aggregation of the Resting Metabolic Rate

As mentioned earlier, obesity aggregates in families. It was of interest, therefore, to determine whether RMR aggregates in families, independent of similarities among siblings in body size, age, and sex. The 130 subjects whose RMR we had measured represented 54 different families. Among them were 37 families with 2 siblings, 12 with 3 siblings, and 5 with 4 siblings. After adjusting for individual differences in body size, age, and sex, RMR was significantly aggregated in families. Familial aggregation

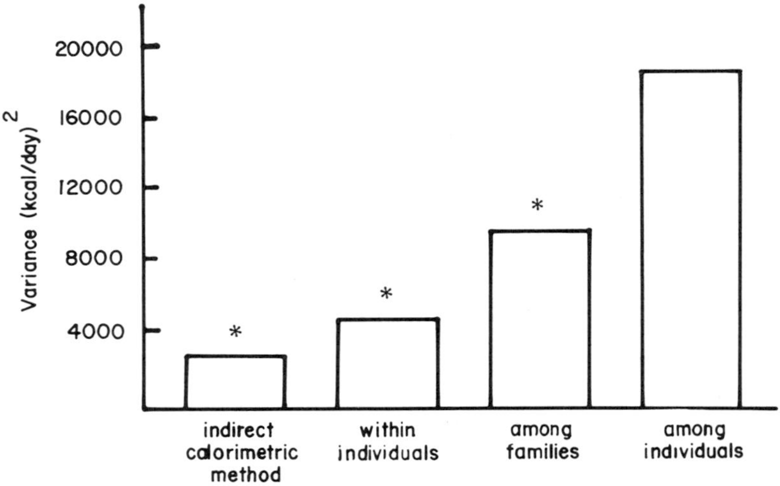


**Fig. 3.** The variance in resting metabolic rate (RMR) among all subjects (''among individuals'') was compared to variances in RMR attributable to the method (''indirect calorimetry method''), to variances in RMR in a given individual (''within individuals''), and to variances in RMR among members of the same family (''among families''). After adjusting for individual differences in body size, age, and sex, the variance in RMR among members of the same family was less than the variance in RMR among all individuals measured ($p < 0.0001$). (Data from Bogardus *et al.*, 1986.)

of RMR is best represented by grouping each individual's RMR, adjusted for fat-free body mass, age, and sex, with adjusted RMRs of siblings (Fig. 4). The mean range of RMR within families differed by as much as 450 kcal/day from that among families.

The intraclass correlation coefficient (Fisher, 1958) for the family effect on the RMR was 0.41 (Bogardus *et al.*, 1986). This suggests that the familial effect accounted for about 41% of the variance in RMR after adjusting for covariates. This intraclass correlation coefficient can be compared to those for other biological variables among adult siblings. In Tecumseh, Michigan, for example, the intraclass correlation coefficients were 0.22–0.35 for total serum cholesterol, 0.17 for body mass index, and 0.14–0.22 for blood pressure (Sing and Orr, 1978; Longini *et al.*, 1984a; Longini *et al.*, 1984b).

The above analyses demonstrated that RMR varies more among individuals than accounted for by individual differences in fat-free body mass, age, and sex and that adjusted RMR is a familial trait, as might be expected if it contributes to obesity in humans. But these were only cross-sectional data; longitudinal studies were required to demonstrate that a low RMR is associated with increased risk of developing obesity.

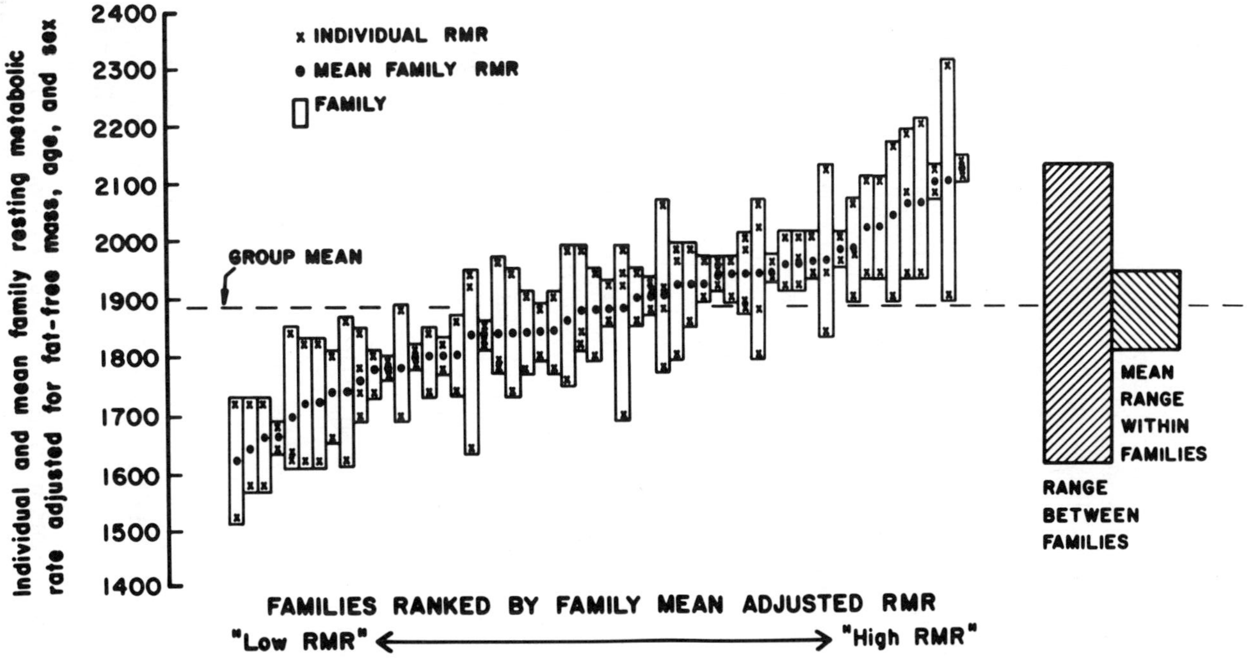


**Fig. 4.** Measured mean family (−) and individual (+) resting metabolic rates (RMRs) were adjusted for the covariates of fat-free mass, age, and sex. Adjusted RMR was calculated as residual from the regression model with covariates only, plus the mean RMR for the whole sample. Families ([ ]) are ranked according to adjusted RMR. The range of mean family adjusted RMR (''between families'') and the range of mean RMR among members of the same family (''within families'') are depicted by the hatched bars on the right. (From Bogardus *et al.*, 1986. Reprinted with permission.)

### C. A Low Resting Metabolic Rate as a Predictor of Weight Gain

Follow-up data on body weight and composition were available on 126 Pimas whose RMR had previously been measured (Ravussin *et al.*, 1987). Subjects were divided into gainers ($n$ = 15) and nongainers ($n$ = 111), using 10 kg as an arbitrary definition of significant weight gain. At initial examination, gainers were of similar age, height, weight, and degree of obesity as nongainers. However, the RMR (mean ± SD) of gainers (1,694 ± 103 kcal/day) was lower than that of nongainers (1,764 ± 109 kcal/day) ($p < 0.03$).

The mean duration of follow-up in gainers was shorter (21 ± 7 months) than in nongainers (38 ± 6 months). To adjust for differences in duration of follow-up between groups and to estimate the level of risk of weight gain associated with a low RMR, data were analyzed using a Cox regression analysis (Harrel, 1983). This analysis showed that a low RMR was associated with a significantly increased risk of weight gain of 10 kg or more (Ravussin *et al.*, 1987). After four years of follow-up, the risk was approximately 7 times greater in those with the lowest RMR compared with those with the highest RMR. Using other arbitrary definitions of significant weight gain, such as a gain of >5 or >7.5 kg, Cox regression analyses also showed a significantly greater risk of weight gain in those with the lowest RMR.

Cross-sectional and longitudinal RMR data collected among the Pima Indians suggest that RMR varies more among individuals than can be explained by differences in their fat-free body mass, age, and sex; RMR, adjusted for these covariates, is a familial trait; and a low RMR is associated with significantly higher risk of weight gain. These data suggest that a low RMR may contribute to familial aggregation of human obesity.

## V. 24-HOUR ENERGY EXPENDITURE

### A. The Human Respiratory Chamber in Phoenix

To measure 24-hour energy expenditure (24EE), including RMR, the thermic effect of food, and the caloric cost of physical activity, a human respiratory chamber was constructed at the Clinical Diabetes and Nutrition Section of the National Institute of Diabetes and Digestive and Kidney Diseases in Phoenix (Fig. 5A; Fig. 5B) (Ravussin *et al.*, 1986). The chamber is an open-circuit, indirect calorimeter modeled after the chamber constructed in the laboratory of Prof. E. Jequier in Lausanne, Switzerland. To approximate normal living conditions, the small room contains a convertible sofa, desk, chair, television, coffee table, sink, and toilet. Two radar devices, mounted on opposite walls of the chamber, are calibrated to measure any physical activity beyond respiration.

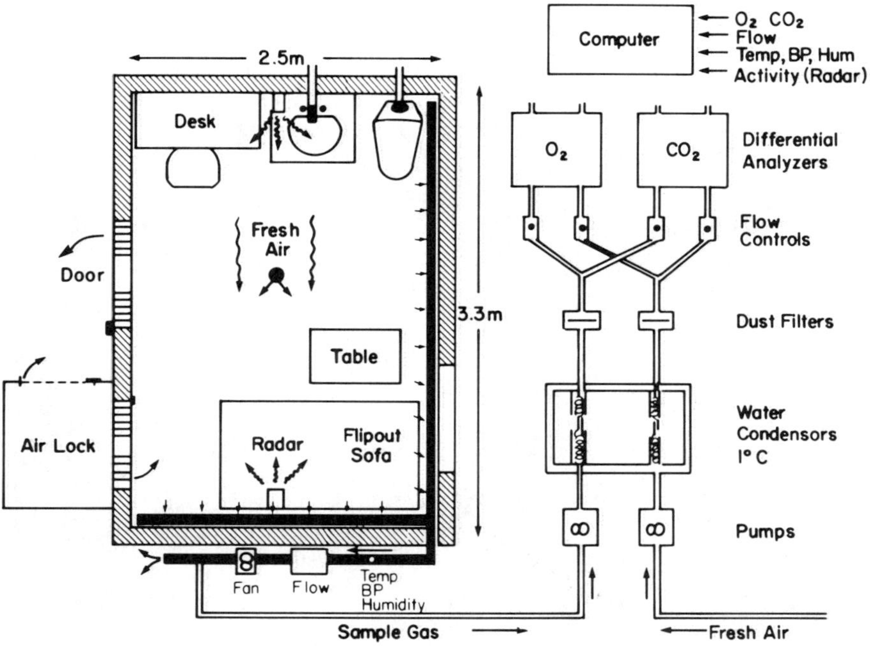


**Fig. 5A.** This schematic drawing of the Phoenix respiratory chamber system shows an open-system indirect calorimeter through which air is drawn by a fan. Flow, temperature, barometric pressure, and humidity of this air, similar in physical characteristics to that of the chamber, are measured. A sample is then dried and measured for $O_2$ and $CO_2$ concentrations by differential analyzers.

Data collected in the chamber were corrected for differences in fat-free body mass, age, and sex. Then, much like those for RMR data, our initial analyses focused on variations in 24EE and on effects of the measurement method and of variations within a given individual on variations in 24EE.

## B. Variability and Familial Aggregation of the Rate of 24-Hour Energy Expenditure

Fat-free body mass was the major determinant of 24EE, but, as shown in Fig. 6, considerable variation in 24EE occurs at any given fat-free body mass. The variance in 24EE could not be attributed to the indirect calorimetric method itself or to variations within each individual, as shown by repeated measures of burning propane in the chamber and of 24EE in several individuals (Fig. 7). A significant portion of the variance in 24EE, adjusted for the three covariates, was accounted for by individual differences in spontaneous physical activity within the chamber as measured by radar (Ravussin *et al.*, 1986).

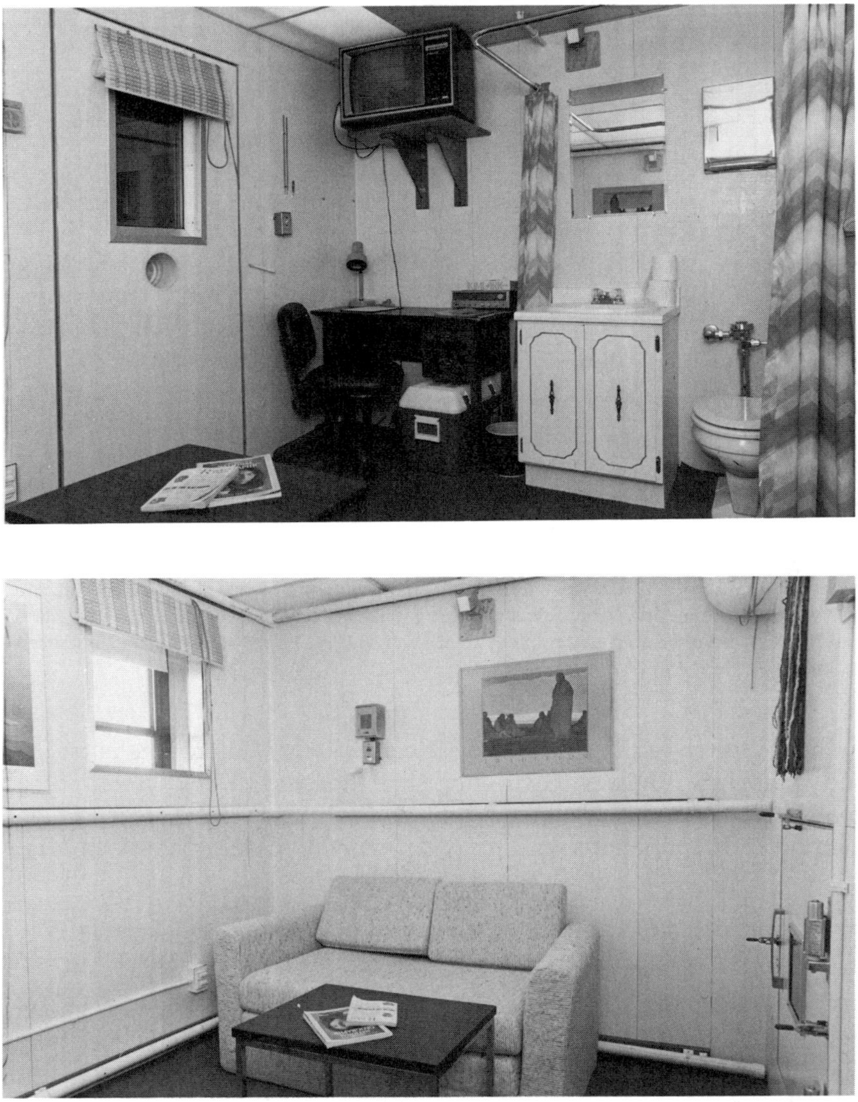

**Fig. 5B.** Interior views of the Phoenix respiratory chamber.

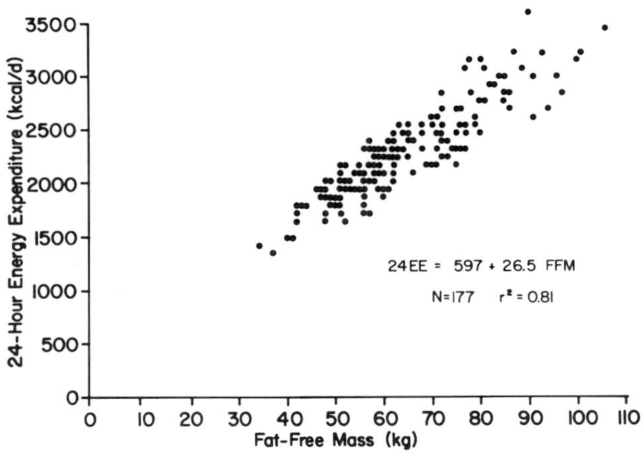


**Fig. 6.** The relationship between 24-hour energy expenditure (24EE) and fat-free body mass are plotted above. Despite considerable variation at any given fat-free body mass, this covariate was the major determinant of 24EE ($r$ = 0.81; $p < 0.0001$). (From Ravussin *et al.*, 1986. Reprinted with permission.)

Data from the chamber were also analyzed to determine whether 24EE, adjusted for four covariates—fat-free body mass, fat mass, age, and sex—aggregated in families as did RMR. 24EE data were available on 94 siblings from 36 families—22 with 2 siblings, 9 with 3 siblings, 2 with 4 siblings, and 3 with 5 siblings. Analysis showed that 24EE, adjusted for the covariates, varied significantly less within families than among all of the individuals measured ($p < 0.02$). Thus, adjusted 24EE aggregates in families. The intraclass correlation coefficient for family effect on adjusted 24EE was 0.28. (Intraclass correlation coefficients for other biological variables were presented above.) Therefore, data on 24EE and RMR are quite similar. The 24EE varied more among individuals than can be explained by body composition, age, and sex and aggregated in families.

## C. A Low 24-Hour Metabolic Rate as a Predictor of Weight Gain

Longitudinal studies were performed to determine whether a low 24EE is associated with a greater risk of weight gain. Follow-up body weights were available on 95 subjects who had previously been studied for 24 hours in the respiratory chamber. The rate of 24EE, adjusted for fat-free body mass, fat mass, age, and sex, correlated negatively with the amount of weight change ($r$ = 0.33; $p < 0.001$) and with the rate of weight change ($r$ = 0.39; $p < 0.001$). The rate of weight change was calculated as the difference in body weight between initial examination and subsequent peak weight at follow-up, divided by the time between these measurements.

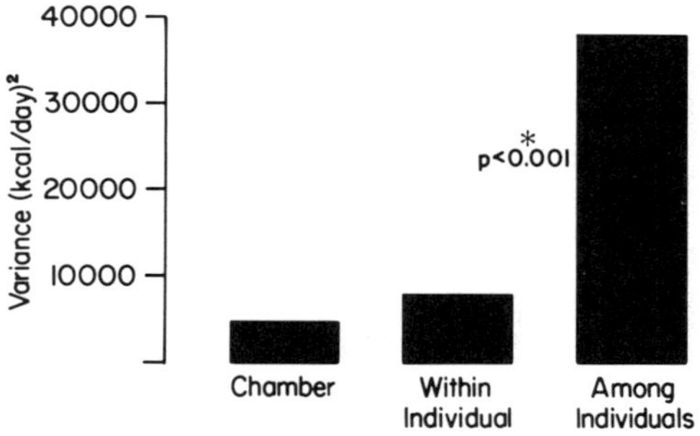


**Fig 7.** The variance in 24-hour energy expenditure (24EE) among all subjects (''among individuals'') was compared to variances in 24EE attributable to the method (''chamber'') and to the variances in 24EE in a given individual (''within individuals''). After adjusting for individual differences in body size, age, and sex, variances in 24EE attributable to the method or to variances within a given individual were significantly lower than variances among individuals. (From Ravussin *et al.*, 1986. Reprinted with permission.)

Data were also analyzed using a Cox regression analysis (Harrel, 1983). Individuals with a low 24EE were at significantly greater risk of weight gain ($p < 0.03$). After 24 months of follow-up, the risk of gaining 7.5 kg was 8 times higher for those with the lowest 24EE compared with those with the highest 24EE.

These data are similar to those for RMR. Both RMR and 24EE data suggest that metabolic rate is an individual characteristic, independent of body size, age, and sex, and that a low metabolic rate is associated with an increased risk of weight gain. Although a low metabolic rate clearly predicts weight gain, it is clearly not the only contributor to the pathogenesis of obesity. Excess caloric intake and decreased physical activity also contribute, but the relative contribution of each remains to be determined.

## VI. OBESITY AS A REGULATORY MECHANISM

RMR was measured at each follow-up examination in Pimas for whom baseline RMR had been determined. As described above, the initial mean adjusted RMR of the 15 who gained more than 10 kg was significantly less than the mean RMR of nongainers. However, on follow-up examination, the differences in mean adjusted RMR of gainers (1,813 $\pm$ 134 kcal/day) versus nongainers (1,795 $\pm$ 151 kcal/day) were not significant (Ravussin *et al.*, 1987).

Thus, weight gain among gainers was associated with a ''normalization'' of RMR. Also, assuming no significant decrease in physical activity, their energy cost of physical activity must also have increased as a result of greater body weight. Possible changes in the thermic effect of food were not measured at follow-up. Nonetheless, the increases in adjusted RMR and in energy cost of physical activity after initial weight gain could be viewed as regulatory mechanisms to resist further weight gain and to "normalize" daily energy expenditure.

## VII. COMPARISON OF PIMA AND CAUCASIAN DATA

Although it seems clear that a low metabolic rate predisposes to obesity in Pima Indians, it is reasonable to question the applicability of this finding to other populations. Unfortunately, no longitudinal data on Caucasians are available for direct comparison with Pima data. However, cross-sectional data are quite comparable between the two populations.

Earlier investigators studying Caucasians observed a ±10% variation in RMR at any given body height, weight, and sex among "normal" subjects (Fisher, 1958). In other studies of Caucasian groups, several have observed considerable variability in RMR among individuals of the same size (Warwick *et al.*, 1978; Booyens and McCance, 1957; Edholm *et al.*, 1955). More recently, Fontaine and associates (1985) determined that the RMR, adjusted for differences in body size, was more similar between monozygotic than dizygotic twins. These data show that genetic determinants of RMR are independent of genetic determinants of body size. Data on familial aggregation of RMR among Pima Indians are similar. The Caucasian data also suggest that familial aggregation of RMR and 24EE among the Pima may result from genetic rather than environmental influences.

Although no strictly comparable prospective study has related metabolic rate to weight gain among Caucasians, Caucasian studies do suggest that the outcome would be similar to studies among the Pima Indians. The rate of weight loss among obese Caucasian women has been found to be lower in women with a lower metabolic rate (Garrow *et al.*, 1978). Other investigators have found that the RMR or weight-maintenance energy requirements of obese women were lower than expected for their reduced body weight following caloric restriction (Finer *et al.*, 1986; Leibel and Hirsch, 1984). These observations could be explained by an adaptive response to prolonged caloric restriction, but they could also result from a low RMR among women predisposed to obesity.

The Caucasian and Pima energy expenditure data appear quite similar with regard to both familial aggregation and variation among groups of individuals. Because data comparable to the Pima longitudinal data do not exist, we believe that a prospective Caucasian study, relating metabolic rate to subsequent weight gain, is not only warranted on the basis of the Pima data but is also sorely needed.

## VIII. DIRECTIONS FOR FUTURE RESEARCH

Prospective studies of the determinants of weight gain among Caucasians are needed. Among Pima Indians, longer follow-up studies will address the long-term consequences of initial lower or higher metabolic rates. Studies are also underway to determine the mechanism(s) responsible for variances in RMR and 24EE at any given body size. Ongoing and future studies should allow for determining: the relationship between metabolic rate and thyroid hormone status among clinically euthyroid individuals; sympathetic nervous system activity; sodium-potassium ATPase activity in different tissues, including skeletal muscle; protein turnover rates; and metabolic rates of different tissues.

More consideration should also be given to effective ways to increase 24EE and to decrease energy intake in order to prevent weight gain in individuals predisposed to obesity. High-risk persons might be identified on the basis of a family history of obesity or an increased risk associated with a particular heritage, as in the Pima. Approaches to increasing energy expenditure should include the behavioral (to motivate increased physical activity and reduced food intake) as well as the pharmacological (to develop safe aids to increase energy expenditure and/or to decrease energy intake). Given the considerable morbidity and mortality associated with obesity, it is surprising that more pharmacological strategies for weight loss have not been tried. Inertia in this area may reflect the conventional gluttony theory of obesity discussed earlier. This unfortunate theory categorizes obese patients as blameful, recalcitrant, and wholly guilty for their health problem.

Although we know behavioral factors influence serum cholesterol and blood pressure, we also accept the role genetic factors play in determining the observed variation in these biological variables. Similarly, although overeating plays a role in causing human obesity, current data suggest we should now also accept that genetic influences on metabolic rate and on obesity are at least as great as those on total serum cholesterol and blood pressure.

Persons with hypertension of a presumed genetic basis are frequently referred to as having "essential hypertension." In this context, "essential" means the cause of the hypertension is unknown and also implies that the increased blood pressure is inherent and not the result of external, environmental causes. We readily accept this construct of the uncontrollable nature of "essential hypertension," even though the condition is known to be aggravated by excess salt intake, overeating, etc. The similarity to human obesity is apparent. Some people are obese as a result of intrinsic metabolic forces beyond their control. One force that we have identified is a reduced rate of energy expenditure. In many persons, superimposed environmental mechanisms may also contribute to obesity. This should not negate the fact that in some, and perhaps in many, is an underlying condition best described as "essential obesity."

Treatment of obesity, therefore, should be approached as objectively and thoroughly as that of essential hypertension. When behavioral strategies fail, the physician should be able to turn to a combined approach using behavioral and pharmacological therapies. More research is needed to develop a first generation of safe, effective ''anti-obesity'' agents.

## IX. CONCLUSIONS

Obesity is a familial, and to a significant extent, a genetic disorder caused by an excess of caloric intake over expenditure. Accurate methods to assess the impact of disorders of feeding behavior and appetite regulation on the imbalance in this energy equation are currently unavailable. Studies of energy expenditure among the Pima Indians have shown that:

1. Rates of energy expenditure vary more among individuals than can be accounted for by differences in body size, age, or sex.
2. Rates of energy expenditure aggregate in families, independent of these covariates.
3. A low rate of energy expenditure is associated with an increased risk of weight gain.

These data suggest that a low metabolic rate contributes to the familial aggregation of obesity. It seems evident that as sure as there is ''essential hypertension,'' there is ''essential obesity.'' Research is urgently needed to develop new pharmacological agents to treat this disorder that is associated with significant morbidity and mortality.

## REFERENCES

Bogardus, C., Lillioja, S., Ravussin, E., Abbott, W., Zawadzki, J., Young, A., Knowler, W. C., Jacobowitz, R., and Moll, P. P. (1986). Resting metabolic rate is a familial trait. *N. Engl. J. Med.* **315**, 96–100.

Boothby, W.M., and Sandiford, I. (1922). Summary of the basal metabolism data on 8,614 subjects with special reference to the normal standards for the estimation of the basal metabolic rate. *J. Biol. Chem.* **54**, 783–803.

Booyens, J., and McCance, R. A. (1957). Individual variations in expenditure of energy. *Lancet* **1**, 225–229.

Cleary, P. M., Vasselli, J. R., and Greenwood, R. C. (1980). Development of obesity in Zucker obese (*fa/fa*) rat in absence of hyperphagia. *Amer. J. Physiol.* **238**, E284–E292.

Cox, J. E., and Powley, T. L. (1977). Development of obesity in diabetic mice pair-fed with lean siblings. *J. Comp. Physiol.* **91**, 347–358.

Edholm, O. G., Fletcher, J. G., Widdowson, E. M., and McCance, R. A. (1955). The energy expenditure and food intake of individual men. *Brit. J. Nutr.* **9**, 286–300.

Ferrell, C. L., and Jenkins, T. G. (1984). Energy utilization by mature, nonpregnant, nonlactating cows of different types. *J. Amer. Sci.* **58**, 234–243.

Finer, N., Swan, P. C., and Mitchell, F. T. (1986). Metabolic rate after massive weight loss in human obesity. *Clin. Sci.* **70**, 395–398.

Fisher, R. A. (1958). "Statistical Methods for Research Workers," 13th ed., pp. 211–247. Hafner, New York.

Fontaine, E., Savard, R., Tremblay, A., Despies, J. P., Pochlman, E., and Boochard, C. (1985). Resting metabolic rate in monozygotic and dizygotic twins. *Acta Genet. Med. Gemellol (Roma)* **34**, 41–47.

Garrow, J. S., Durant, M. L., Mann, S., Stalley, S. F., and Warwick, P. M. (1978). Factors determining weight loss in obese patients in a metabolic ward. *Int. J. Obes.* **2**, 441–447.

Harrel, F. E. (1983). The PHGIM procedure. *In*: "SUGI (Supplemental Library Users' Guide)" (S. P. Joiner, ed.), pp. 267–294. SAS Institute Inc., Cary, North Carolina.

Knowler, W. C., Bennett, P. H., Hamman, R. F., and Miller, M. (1978). Diabetes incidence and prevalence in Pima Indians: a 19-fold greater incidence than in Rochester, Minnesota. *Amer. J. Epidemiol.* **108**, 497–505.

Knowler, W. C., Pettitt, D. J., Savage, P. J., and Bennett, P. H. (1981). Diabetes incidence in Pima Indians: contributions of obesity and parental diabetes. *Amer. J. Epidemiol.* **113**, 114–156.

Koong, L. J., Nienaber, J. A., and Hershman, H. J. (1983). Effect of plane of nutrition on organ size and fasting heat production in genetically lean and obese pigs. *J. Nutr.* **113**, 1626–1631.

Leibel, R. L., and Hirsch, J. (1984). Diminished energy requirements in reduced-obese patients. *Metabolism* **33**, 164–170.

Longini, I. M., Higgins, M. W., Hinton, P. C., Moll, P. P., and Keller, J. B. (1984a). Environmental and genetic sources of familial aggregation of blood pressure in Tecumseh, Michigan. *Amer. J. Epidemiol.* **120**, 131–144.

Longini, I. M., Higgins, M. W., Hinton, P. C., Moll, P. P., and Keller, J. B. (1984b). Genetic and environmental sources of familial aggregation of body mass in Tecumseh, Michigan. *Hum. Biol.* **56**, 733–757.

Maison, J. E., Stamp, M. J., Sr., Hennekens, C. H., and Willett, W. C. (1987). Body weight and longevity. *JAMA-J. Am. Med. Assn.* **257**(3), 353–358.

Matson, G. A., Burch, T. A., and Polesky, H. F. (1968). Distribution of hereditary factors in the blood of Indians of the Gila River, Arizona. *Amer. J. Physiol. Anthropol.* **29**, 311–338.

Ravussin, E., Lillioja, S., Anderson, T. E., Christin, L., and Bogardus, C. (1986). Determinants of 24-hour energy expenditure in man: Methods and results using a respiratory chamber. *J. Clin. Invest.* **78**, 1568–1578.

Ravussin, E., Lillioja, S., Knowler, W. C., Christin, L., Freymond, D., Abbott, W., Boyce, V., Howard, B., and Bogardus, C. (1987). Reduced rate of energy expenditure as a risk factor for body weight gain. *N. Engl. J. Med.* **318**, 467–472.

Simopolous, A. P., and Van Itallie, T. B. (1984). Body weight, health and longevity. *Ann. Intern. Med.* **100**, 285–295.

Sing, C. F., and Orr, J. D. (1978). Analysis of genetic and environmental sources of variation in serum cholesterol in Tecumseh, Michigan. IV. Separation of polygene from common environment effects. *Amer. J. Human Genetics* **30**, 491–504.

Stunkard, A. J., Sorenson, T. I. A., Harris, C., Teasdale, T. W., Chakraborty, R., Schull, W., and Schulsinger, F. (1986). An adoptive study of human obesity. *N. Engl. J. Med.* **314**, 193–198.

Warwick, P., Toft, R., and Garrow, J. S. (1978). Individual differences in energy expenditure [Abstract]. *Int. J. Obes.* **2**, 396.

# 11

# Nutritional Consequences of the Aminoacidurias

Russell W. Chesney

*Department of Pediatrics*
*University of California, Davis*
*School of Medicine*
*Davis, California*



## I. INTRODUCTION

The renal tubular reabsorption of amino acids is very efficient. Indeed, most amino acids are 98% reabsorbed, and only 1–2% of the filtered load appears in the urine (Foreman and Segal, 1985).

The main site of active, uphill transport of amino acids is the $S_1$ segment of the renal proximal convoluted tubule. Amino acids appear to be transported across plasma membranes of the tubular epithelium by multiple pathways, including diffusion and sodium-independent and sodium-dependent carriers

(Stevens *et al.*, 1984). Active transport of many amino acids occurs on the luminal or brush-border surface, and energy for uphill uptake is symport (cotransport) with the sodium ion (Barfuss and Schafer, 1981), which goes down its concentration gradient as it enters the cell. The complex of sodium and amino acid has a net positive charge that favors its entry into the cell. This favorable electrochemical gradient is perpetuated by the adenosine triphosphate (ATP)-dependent extrusion of sodium at the basolateral membrane (Foreman and Segal, 1985). Amino acids within the cell can be further metabolized, incorporated into protein, or transported across the basolateral membrane into the interstitium of the kidney. Net arteriovenous differences between renal artery and vein are small for most amino acids. Thus, most amino acids appear to be returned to the blood after glomerular filtration and transepithelial transport (Mitch and Chesney, 1983).

Separate transport processes have been described for at least four groups of amino acids: *dibasic* (lysine, arginine, ornithine, and cystine), *acidic* or dicarboxylic (aspartic and glutamic acids), *neutral* (alanine, serine, threonine, valine, isoleucine, phenylalanine, glutamine, histidine, asparagine, tyrosine, tryptophan, and citrulline), and *beta* (taurine, beta-alanine, and beta-amino isobutyrate) (Scriver *et al.*, 1976). Transport is competitive among amino acids within each group, but not among amino acids in different groups.

About 2–3% of total urinary nitrogen is comprised of amino acids, and of the 70 g of amino acids filtered, about 1 g is excreted (Mitch and Chesney, 1983). Thus, under normal circumstances, little amino nitrogen is lost, and nutritional consequences of urine nitrogen excretion are minimal. If an excess of amino acid is excreted into the urine, aminoaciduria occurs. This pathologic process can involve a single amino acid, a group transported by a related process, or essentially all amino acids (''generalized'' aminoaciduria). The precise mechanisms by which aminoaciduria occurs are unknown, but the following factors may contribute to its development:

1. Whenever the filtered load of an amino acid exceeds its transport capacity by the tubular epithelium, an ''overload'' aminoaciduria occurs. This overload characterizes most inborn errors of amino acid metabolism that result in a high level of unmetabolized amino acid in the plasma.
2. A defective transport protein may result in high urinary excretion the affected amino acid, leading to aminoaciduria and depletion of the affected amino acid.
3. Low absorption of a given amino acid results in relatively increased tubular concentration and depressed competitive transport of other amino acids that use the same transport system.
4. If the luminal or basolateral membrane is ''leaky,'' back diffusion of transported amino acid may occur and overwhelm the reabsorptive process.

The nutritional consequences of aminoaciduria are significant because amino acids lost in the urine are unavailable for protein synthesis and metabolism.

## II. INHERITED AMINOACIDURIAS

The inherited aminoacidurias represent a group of disorders in which a single amino acid or a group of amino acids is lost (Foreman and Segal, 1985; Scriver *et al.*, 1976). Recognized human aminoacidurias include: *classical cystinuria*, with loss of cystine as well as ornithine, arginine, and lysine; *Hartnup disease*, with loss of the neutral monoamino-monocarboxylic acid group; *hypermethioninuria; histidinuria; iminoglycinuria*, with loss of glycine, proline, and hydroxyproline; *glycinuria;* and *dicarboxylic aminoaciduria*, with loss of glutamic and aspartic acids. Hartnup disease, hypermethioninuria, and cystinuria have the most significant nutritional consequences (Foreman and Segal, 1985; Scriver *et al.*, 1976).

### A. Hartnup Disease

Named for the *propositus* family, Hartnup disease is a disorder of intestinal malabsorption and massive aminoaciduria of the neutral monoamino-monocarboxylic amino acids. It results in an intermittent red, scaly rash in sun-exposed sites, cerebellar ataxia, and dementia—in effect, the features of pellagra (Jepson, 1983). This pellagra-like state is caused, in part, by nicotinamide deficiency. Bacterial decomposition of the malabsorbed amino acids results in production of indoles and indicans, which are absorbed by the gut and excreted in the urine. In particular, the intestinal malabsorption of *L*-tryptophan results in low nicotinamide because its availability for metabolic conversion to nicotinamide via the kynurenine pathway is low. Poorly nourished patients with low nicotinamide intake appear to be the most extensively affected. This disorder rarely occurs in North Americans, who ingest 20 or more mg of nicotinamide per day, the amount required to prevent deficiency.

### B. Hypermethioninuria

Methionine malabsorption is also called ''oasthouse syndrome'' because the patient's urine smells like an oasthouse or somewhat like celery (Foreman and Segal, 1985). Urinary concentrations of methionine, phenylalanine, tyrosine and alpha-hydroxybutyric acid are above normal, and fecal methionine and alpha-hydroxybutyrate are also elevated.

Oral methionine administration results in diarrhea, tachypnea, methioninuria, and the urinary excretion of alpha-hydroxybutyric acid, a product of colonic bacterial decomposition of methionine. A low-methionine diet causes alpha-hydroxybutyric acid to fall, reverses neurological symptoms such as convulsions and somnolence, and results in an improved electroencephalogram. Hence, clinical symptoms in this disorder may result from intestinal malabsorption of methionine or from its conversion to a ketoacid, which may itself be toxic (Smith and Strang, 1958).

## C. Cystinuria

Cystinuria represents an important cause of renal stones in humans because of the relative insolubility of cystine, a disulfide amino acid (Segal and Thier, 1983). The presence of dibasic aminoaciduria in conjunction with cystine hyperexcretion has been shown to be related to a defect in the low-$K_m$, high-affinity shared transport system that functions in both intestinal and kidney brush-border membranes. Cystinuric patients without dibasic aminoaciduria may have a defect in the high-$K_m$, nonshared cystine transport system. Likewise, dibasic aminoaciduria patients without cystinuria may have a defect in the high-$K_m$, nonshared dibasic transport system (Segal and Thier, 1983).

Cystine hyperexcretion results in stone formation, staghorn calculi, urinary stasis, infection, and, in some cases, kidney loss. Therefore, therapy should be directed toward reducing urinary cystine excretion. Treatments have included high fluid intake, alkalinization of the urine, and administration of D-penicillamine or other sulfhydryl agents that undergo *in vivo* disulfide exchange with cystine. Administration of compounds such as D-penicillamine or 2-mercaptopropionyl glycine (alpha-MPG) results in excretion of penicillamine-cysteine- or alpha-MPG-cysteine-mixed disulfides. Production of more soluble compounds results in a marked decline in urinary cystine excretion (Pak *et al.*, 1986).

Dietary restriction of cystine and methionine have been tried without notable success. However, urinary cystine excretion was significantly reduced in cystinuric patients switched from a diet high in animal protein to a vegetarian regimen (Rodman *et al.*, 1984). In one study, urinary cystine fell from 6.13 to 4.89 m*M*/day when cystinuric patients ingested a low-protein, vegetarian diet.

A report that L-glutamine supplementation can markedly reduce urinary cystine was met with skepticism (Skovky *et al.*, 1980). However, a newer investigation of the potential anticystinuric effects of oral glutamine dosing in cystinuria demonstrated that glutamine reduces cystine excretion only in patients on a high-sodium diet (Jaeger *et al.*, 1986). When dietary sodium was restricted below 150 micromoles/day, glutamine had no anticystinuric influence. However, low sodium intake did reduce the excretion of cystine and dibasic amino acids. The mechanism by which glutamine exerts its anticystinuric effect when sodium intake is high is unclear. Glutamine may affect the permeability of the paracellular shunt pathway, which would be evident in a hypervolemic, or sodium-loaded, state (Jaeger *et al.*, 1986). By inference, L-glutamine therapy would be unlikely to be useful in patients ingesting a normal diet, but dietary sodium restriction could be beneficial. The role of lower sodium intake in the earlier observation that a vegetarian diet reduces cystine excretion (Rodman *et al.*, 1984) is unclear.

## III. AMINOACIDURIA OF VITAMIN D DEFICIENCY

Vitamin D deficiency results in hypocalcemia, hypophosphatemia, tetany, rickets, and bowing of the limbs (DeLuca, 1979), as well as poor dentition, fractures, pneumonia, infections, systemic metabolic acidosis, and the Fanconi syndrome—a renal proximal tubulopathy including bicarbonaturia, glucosuria, phosphaturia, and aminoaciduria (Scriver, 1974). Many features of vitamin D deficiency—including bicarbonaturia, phosphauria, and erosion of bone—are caused by secondary hyperparathyroidism. However, deficiency of vitamin D may have critical effects at its nontraditional target sites—bone, muscle, pancreas, lymphocytes, stem cells and parathyroid gland—where receptors for 1,25-$(OH)_2D_3$ are demonstrable (Pike, 1985).

Tubulopathy and aminoaciduria have been ascribed to elevated parathyroid hormone (PTH) levels, which are thought to modulate renal function by changing renal blood flow and/or glomerular filtration rate (GFR) or by generating 3′:5′-cyclic phosphate (cAMP), which phosphorylates proximal tubule membrane proteins (Fraser *et al.*, 1967). However, few patients with primary hyperparathyroidism have generalized aminoaciduria, and there is no correlation between aminoaciduria and PTH levels in nutritional rickets (DeRubertis and Craven, 1976). The possibility that vitamin D deficiency, *per se*, has a direct, PTH-independent effect on amino acid reabsorption merits further study.

Most animal studies of vitamin D deficiency and the mechanisms of aminoaciduria have been limited in scope (Vainsel *et al.*, 1974) or have used vitamin D-replete animals and relied on inferences to the deficient state. Our study in vitamin D-deficient rats evaluated whether variations in dietary calcium (Ca) and/or phosphorus (P) would influence renal handling of these divalent ions and of amino acids of all transport classes (unpublished observations).

Studies were performed in Sprague Dawley rats born of mothers fed a diet containing minimal vitamin D (0.2 IU/g chow). At weaning, rats were fed one of six diets: control (Con), very low calcium (VLC), very low calcium plus 3 days of 1,25-$(OH)_2D_3$ (VLC+1,25-$(OH)_2D_3$), low calcium (LC), high calcium (HC), or low phosphorus (LP) (Table I). Rats were housed in a room with tungsten lighting and no windows. Most rats were killed at 55 days of age, but VLC and LP rats were killed at 48 days because they tended to die of tetany and/or pneumonia shortly thereafter.

On the day before they were killed, rats were placed in cages for 14 to 17 hours, and blood and urine were collected. Calcium and phosphorus were measured by autoanalyzer. After deproteinization of plasma, renal cortex, and urine, amino acids were determined on an amino acid analyzer. Immunoreactive PTH was measured by a rat-specific anti-PTH antibody (Chanard *et al.*, 1977) and vitamin D metabolites by a calf thymus assay (Reinhardt *et al.*, 1984). Brush-border membrane vesicles (BBMV) were prepared by the $CaCl_2$ precipitation method (Chesney *et al.*, 1985a), and the uptake of [$^3$H]taurine and [$^3$H]proline was measured by Millipore filtration.

Vitamin D concentrations in all five deficient groups were markedly lower than in controls (Table I). Serum calcium was 40–50% lower than normal in VLC, VLC+1,25-$(OH)_2D_3$, and LC rats; 18% below normal in HC rats; and normal in LP and control rats (Table I). All rats had high or normal phosphorus levels except LP rats, whose serum phosphorus was low (Table I).

Serum PTH was above normal in all vitamin D-deficient groups except LP, and the HC group was closest to normal (Fig. 1). Plasma PTH correlated with plasma calcium, $PO_4$, and urinary cAMP. The urinary calcium to creatinine ratio was quite high (0.72 ± 0.11) in LP rats, but $<0.05$ in all other groups. High urinary phosphorus excretion in VLC rats was corrected by 1,25-$(OH)_2D_3$ therapy, and tubular phosphorus reabsorption was $>99\%$ in HC and LP rats (data not shown). A high level of urinary cAMP was noted in all experimental groups except LP (Fig. 2) and was highly correlated ($r = 0.544$, $p < 0.001$) with plasma PTH values (unpublished observations).

Few changes in plasma and renal cortex levels of the eleven measured amino acids were detected (Table II). In some but not all rats fed the experimental diets, mean plasma levels of aspartic acid and glutamic acid were below normal, and levels of threonine, glutamine, and citrulline were above normal. In marked contrast, extremely high urinary excretion of all 11 amino acids was observed in all rats fed vitamin D-deficient diets, irrespective of the dietary calcium or phosphorus content, the PTH level or the urinary cAMP level (Table II). The intervention of 3 days of intraperitoneal 1,25-$(OH)_2D_3$ administration, which raised plasma calcium and reduced urinary $PO_4$ excretion, had little effect on observed aminoaciduria. Furthermore, no correlation was found between urinary

**TABLE I**

**Influence of Calcium and Phosphorus Intake on Vitamin D Concentration In Vitamin D-Deficient Rats[a]**

| Group | Dietary content | | | Serum concentrations | | | |
|---|---|---|---|---|---|---|---|
| | Calcium[b] | Phosphorus[b] | Vitamin D | Calcium[c] | Phosphorus[c] | 25-OH-$D_3$[d] | 1,25-$(OH)_2D_3$[e] |
| Control (Con) | 1.10 | 0.74 | 4.4 IU $D_2$/g | 9.7 ± 0.2 | 9.8 ± 0.2 | 52 ± 8 | 32 ± 4 |
| Very low calcium (VLC) | 0.02 | 0.30 | — | 4.3 ± 0.3 | 11.3 ± 0.3 | 4 ± 1 | 2 ± 1 |
| Very low calcium (VLC + 1,25-$(OH)_2D_3$) | 0.02 | 0.30 | 500 pg[f] | 5.7 ± 0.3 | 10.8 ± 0.4 | 9 ± 1 | 98 ± 21 |
| Low calcium (LC) | 0.47 | 0.30 | — | 4.1 ± 0.3 | 11.2 ± 0.3 | 6 ± 1 | 1 ± 1 |
| High calcium (HC) | 2.50 | 0.30 | — | 8.0 ± 0.4 | 5.0 ± 0.3 | 7 ± 1 | 4 ± 2 |
| Low phosphorus (LP) | 1.20 | 0.10 | — | 9.4 ± 0.3 | 6.4 ± 0.6 | 7 ± 1 | 2 ± 1 |

[a]Data from unpublished observations.
[b]Amounts stated as percentages of total diet.
[c]Amounts stated as mg/dl ± SEM.
[d]Amounts stated as ng/ml ± SEM.
[e]Amounts stated as pg/nl ± SEM.
[f]Daily amount of 1,25-$(OH)_2D_3$ fed for 3 days prior to being killed.

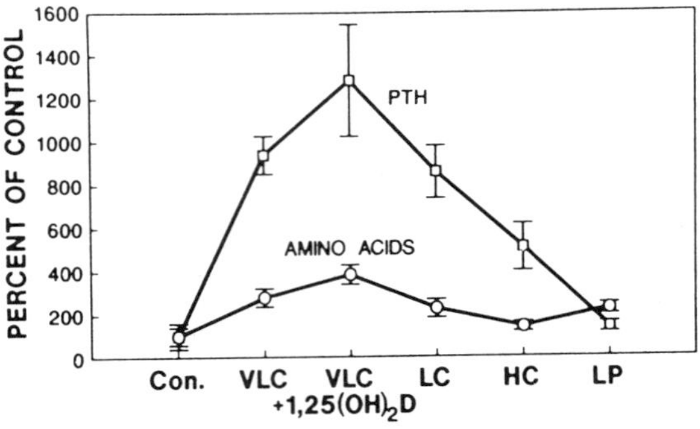


**Fig. 1.** Plasma parathyroid hormone (PTH) and urinary amino acid excretion were measured in vitamin-D deficient rats placed on one of 6 diets at weaning: control (Con), very low calcium plus 3 days of 1,25-$(OH)_2D_3$](VLC + 1,25-$(OH)_2D_3$)], very low calcium (VLC), low calcium (LC), high calcium (HC), or low phosphorus (LP). Plasma PTH values and urinary amino acids are expressed as a percent of control (Con), where control = 100%. Each point is the mean of 9–12 values. (Data from unpublished observations.)

cAMP or plasma PTH and excretion of taurine or proline, test amino acids that were more carefully monitored than the other nine.

To further emphasize the independence of PTH secretion in aminoaciduria, we examined the influence of dibutyryl-cyclic AMP (dbcAMP) on taurine uptake by rat brush-border membrane vesicles (BBMV). Because PTH binds to its receptor at the peritubular membrane before cAMP is generated, we hypothesized that cAMP or a more soluble and stable

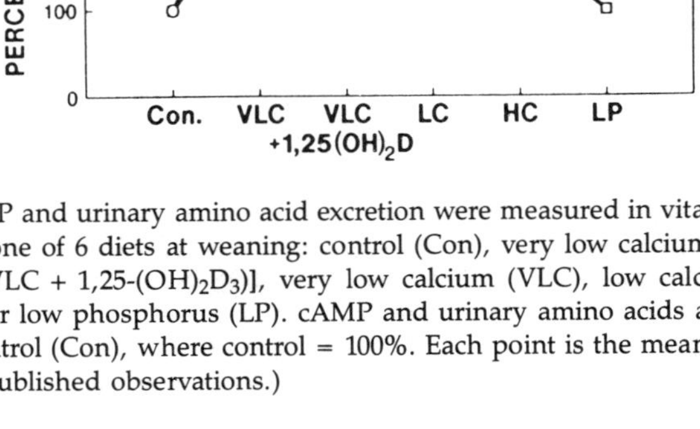


**Fig. 2.** cAMP and urinary amino acid excretion were measured in vitamin-D deficient rats placed on one of 6 diets at weaning: control (Con), very low calcium plus 3 days of 1,25-$(OH)_2D_3$[(VLC + 1,25-$(OH)_2D_3$)], very low calcium (VLC), low calcium (LC), high calcium (HC), or low phosphorus (LP). cAMP and urinary amino acids are expressed as a percent of control (Con), where control = 100%. Each point is the mean of 9–12 values. (Data from unpublished observations.)

**TABLE II**

**Profile of Amino Acid Excretion in Vitamin D Deficiency**[a]

| Diet | Taurine | Aspartic acid | Threonine | Serine | Glutamine | Methionine | Proline | Glutamic acid | Citrulline | Glycine | Alanine |
|---|---|---|---|---|---|---|---|---|---|---|---|
| Normal ($n$ = 7) | 5.92 ± 1.16 | 0.012 ± 0.004 | 0.16 ± 0.020 | 0.16 ± 0.020 | 1.37 ± 0.020 | 0.29 ± 0.05 | 0.037 ± 0.009 | 0.07 ± 0.009 | 0.004 ± 0.001 | 0.32 ± 0.004 | 0.14 ± 0.020 |
| VLC ($n$ = 6) | 18.73 ± 1.66 $p < 0.001$ | 0.046 ± 0.012 $p < 0.020$ | 0.50 ± 0.080 $p < 0.01$ | 0.340 ± 0.070 $p < 0.02$ | 1.95 ± 0.29 NS | 0.68 ± 0.12 $p < 0.02$ | 0.370 ± 0.080 $p < 0.01$ | 0.46 ± 0.070 $p < 0.001$ | 0.46 ± 0.070 $p < 0.001$ | 0.75 ± 0.090 $p < 0.01$ | 0.44 ± 0.040 $p < 0.001$ |
| VLC + $1,25(OH)_2D_3$ ($n$ = 6) | 26.44 ± 4.26 | 0.093 ± 0.010 | 0.49 ± 0.070 | 0.570 ± 0.110 | 2.93 ± 0.36 | 1.03 ± 0.08 | 0.380 ± 0.090 | 0.24 ± 0.030 | 0.038 ± 0.009 | 1.17 ± 0.170 | 0.48 ± 0.050 |
| LC ($n$ = 6) | 14.52 ± 2.71 $p < 0.02$ | 0.053 ± 0.015 $p < 0.01$ | 0.35 ± 0.090 $p < 0.05$ | 0.260 ± 0.070 NS | 1.64 ± 0.42 NS | 0.63 ± 0.08 $p < 0.01$ | 0.480 ± 0.090 $p < 0.001$ | 0.63 ± 0.140 $p < 0.01$ | 0.028 ± 0.006 $p < 0.001$ | 1.16 ± 0.220 $p < 0.01$ | 0.48 ± 0.090 $p < 0.01$ |
| HC ($n$ = 7) | 9.58 ± 1.15 $p < 0.05$ | 0.320 ± 0.006 $p < 0.02$ | 0.18 ± 0.020 NS | 0.096 ± 0.014 $p < 0.05$ | 0.58 ± 0.06 $p < 0.01$ | 0.21 ± 0.04 NS | 0.180 ± 0.010 $p < 0.01$ | 0.25 ± 0.020 $p < 0.001$ | 0.006 ± 0.003 NS | 0.50 ± 0.060 $p < 0.02$ | 0.19 ± 0.014 NS |
| VLP ($n$ = 8) | 13.74 ± 1.84 $p < 0.01$ | 0.066 ± 0.020 $p < 0.05$ | 0.42 ± 0.034 $p < 0.001$ | 0.320 ± 0.069 $p < 0.05$ | 1.88 ± 0.020 NS | 0.58 ± 0.06 $p < 0.01$ | 0.440 ± 0.070 $p < 0.001$ | 0.43 ± 0.060 $p < 0.001$ | 0.017 ± 0.004 $p < 0.01$ | 1.09 ± 0.140 $p < 0.001$ | 0.34 ± 0.030 $p < 0.001$ |

[a]Test animals were fed one of six diets: normal, very low calcium (VLC), very low calcium plus 3 days of $1,25\text{-}(OH)_2D_3$ (VLC + $1,25\text{-}(OH)_2D_3$), low calcium (LC), high calcium (HC), or very low phosphorus (VLP). Values are stated as micromoles/mg creatinine. All results represent mean ± SEM. (Data from unpublished observations.)

chemical analog like dbcAMP, could influence the brush-border membrane accumulation of amino acids if PTH were a modulating mechanism in amino acid reabsorption. Most amino acids are accumulated at a greater rate in the presence of sodium; this difference in sodium-dependent and sodium-independent uptake is termed the ''overshoot.'' The peak of the uptake curve over time is called the ''peak overshoot.'' PTH has been shown to influence phosphorus reabsorption in the proximal tubule, and reduced phosphorus uptake is related to cAMP-dependent protein phosphorylation in canine BBMV (Hammerman *et al.*, 1983). Direct exposure of intact vesicles to dbcAMP did not alter initial (15 sec), later (60 sec), or peak (360 sec) sodium-dependent overshoot rates of taurine uptake at $10^{-3}$ to $10^{-8}$ *M*. However, at $10^{-2}$ *M*, a nonphysiologic, hyperosmolar level, uptake was minimally but significantly reduced. Neither prolonged preincubation in dbcAMP nor exposure to the nucleotide at temperatures between 4°–40° C affected taurine uptake (unpublished observations).

Hypotonic lysis, which opens the vesicles and permits dbcAMP access to sites on the inner face of the membrane, was used next. Vesicles were resealed by raising the osmolality of the incubation solution. Even in the presence of additional ATP and potassium fluoride, dbcAMP did not influence taurine uptake.

We next studied the accumulation of proline and taurine in BBMV prepared from normal and vitamin D-deficient rats. In both cases, uptake of these alpha- and beta-amino acids was significantly lower at the peak of the sodium-dependent overshoot in vesicles from animals fed each vitamin D-deficient diet than in brush-border vesicles from animals fed normal diets (Table III). Addition of dietary 1,25-$(OH)_2D_3$ in VLC+1,25-$(OH)_2D_3$ rats corrected the defect in peak uptake of proline but not of taurine.

Differences in amino acid uptake by BBMV were studied over a broad range of values, and the $K_m$ of uptake was ascertained. Vitamin D deficiency had no influence on the $K_m$ of uptake for either proline or taurine. However, $V_{max}$ data for taurine accumulation showed a reduced rate of

**TABLE III**

**Peak Overshoot Value of Proline and Taurine Uptake**[a]

| Amino acid | Control | VLC | VLC + 1,25 | LC | HC | LP |
|---|---|---|---|---|---|---|
| Proline | 181 ± 44 | 110 ± 31 | 182 ± 67 | 133 ± 33 | 133 ± 33 | 134 ± 33 |
| Taurine | 50 ± 6 | 37 ± 6 | 28 ± 8 | 39 ± 7 | 38 ± 7 | 39 ± 4 |

[a]Results stated as pmoles/mg protein/30 sec. (Data from unpublished observations.)

uptake at 60 sec (the linear portion of the curve) in all vitamin D-deficient groups; this was corrected by supplementation with 1,25-$(OH)_2D_3$. No similar change was found for proline. Finally, no correlation was found between peak overshoot rate of uptake and plasma calcium, phosphorus, PTH, or urinary cAMP for either amino acid. However, if the overshoot was low, more taurine appeared in the urine.

Our examination of vitamin D deficiency in the albino rat utilized wide variations in dietary calcium and phosphorus, and all experimental groups achieved vitamin D deficiency as defined by plasma levels of the metabolites 25-$(OH)D_3$ and 1,25-$(OH)_2D_3$. Calcium and phosphorus intake appeared to have direct effects on plasma concentrations of calcium and phosphorus and on circulating immunoreactive PTH, as would be anticipated. Dietary mineral intake also influenced urinary calcium, phosphorus, and cAMP excretion. For example, the LP diet led to a low PTH value, normal serum calcium, hypercalciuria, hypophosphatemia, and no urinary phosphorus excretion, as described elsewhere (Brantbar *et al.*, 1979). However, despite these changes in mineral homeostasis and in circulating PTH, vitamin D deficiency was associated with generalized aminoaciduria. The mechanism underlying this aminoaciduria is unclear, but it appears to be totally PTH-independent.

In these experiments, we also examined cAMP, an end product of PTH activity, and found no evidence for cAMP-induced inhibition of sodium-dependent taurine uptake. This finding was more firmly established by the lack of external and internal cAMP and by the failure of potassium fluoride or excess ATP, known stimulators of adenylate cyclase activity, to alter taurine accumulation into vesicles. This provides further evidence that PTH modulation of tubule function does not have a role in generalized aminoaciduria.

The defect in renal transport of all major classes of amino acids is manifest at the brush-border surface. These findings suggest that the aminoaciduria of vitamin D deficiency is an apical surface event. Although the usual kinetic parameters—$K_m$ and $V_{max}$—were not consistently affected, a consistently and significantly lower peak of sodium-dependent overshoot was present. The mechanism of this defect is unclear but is dissimilar to the aminoaciduria of immaturity (Chesney *et al.*, 1986a) or of dietary amino acid excess (Chesney *et al.*, 1985a), in which the initial rate of sodium-dependent taurine uptake is affected. Intracellular calcium and/or phosphorus may influence amino acid transport (Hruska *et al.*, 1984), but a liposomic effect of 1,25-$(OH)_2D_32$ cannot be excluded. Evidence exists that 1,25-$(OH)_2D_3$ induces a change in the phospholipid composition of intestinal brush-border membranes that coincides with changes in calcium transport across the membrane (Matsumoto *et al.*, 1981). Whether vitamin D deficiency induces similar changes in renal brush-border membranes in the rat is unclear and needs to be evaluated.

To conclude, these data suggest that vitamin D deficiency, *per se*, results in aminoaciduria, independent of PTH or of any interaction of cAMP with the brush-border surface. The aminoaciduria we found is expressed at the brush-border surface, and it represents a low overshoot rather than a change in initial $V_{max}$. These results require further investigation to better understand the membrane event underlying this change.

## IV. AMINOACIDURIA OF IMMATURITY

Neonates of all mammalian species have a generalized aminoaciduria, which most likely reflects an immaturity of proximal tubule function in the postnatal period (Brodehl and Gellissen, 1968). Nevertheless, this aminoaciduria is illogical in that it represents the loss of nutrients in the face of growth demands. Postnatal development of renal amino acid transport involves an enhancement of amino acid reabsorption in the presence of an enormous two- to threefold increase in GFR and an increased filtered amino acid load (Arant, 1978). The percentage of reabsorption of all classes of filtered amino acids increases over the first weeks to months of life. The generalized aminoaciduria of immaturity then abates (Baerlocher *et al.*, 1971a), unless an inherited disorder of amino acid transport, such as cystinuria, is present (Lashley and Scriver, 1979). Indeed, it can be difficult to distinguish homozygotes from heterozygotes for cystinuria in the first few months of life (Scriver *et al.*, 1985). The pathophysiological mechanisms causing neonatal aminoaciduria and the factors responsible for the maturation of absorption of organic solutes are of interest to the developmental physiologist and the nutritionist.

Three potential mechanisms underlie this maturation process:

1. The transport site, shared or single, may be inserted into the plasma membrane of a renal epithelial cell as a postnatal event. This event could result in a change in the observed $K_m$ or affinity of the carrier for its substrate (Baerlocher *et al.*, 1971b).

2. An age-related increase in the number of transport sites per unit area of cell membrane could occur postnatally. This net increase in sites would not alter affinity ($K_m$) but rather would be detected as an increase in rate of transport ($V_{max}$). This postnatal enhancement of transport rate is relevant in many systems, including the higher accumulation of taurine by slices or isolated tubules of immature rat kidney (Chesney *et al.*, 1985c).

3. A reduced efflux of a specific amino acid across the basolateral membrane of the cell into the interstitium could increase intracellular pools to such an extent that back-diffusion of amino acid into urine could occur. This mechanism has also been shown to be relevant (Segal, 1982).

We have explored the mechanisms of aminoaciduria using dietary manipulation to influence amino acid transport systems. The renal tubular epithelium conserves ions and organic solutes during periods of low dietary intake and allows increased excretion with dietary excess. Taurine was used as a probe of the renal adaptive response to altered intake.

In rodents fed low amounts of sulfur amino acids (methionine, cysteine, and taurine), renal tubular reabsorption, collagenase-isolated tubule accumulation, and solute BBMV uptake of taurine was extremely high (Friedman *et al.*, 1983; Chesney *et al.*, 1983; Chesney *et al.*, 1985a). A diet containing normal methionine (0.7%) and high taurine (3%) produced a sixfold increase in taurine excretion and low taurine uptake by both tubules and vesicles. These opposing adaptive responses in adult animals occur because of a change in the initial $V_{max}$ of sodium-dependent taurine transport and not because of a change in the $K_m$ of the substrate for the transport site (Friedman *et al.*, 1983; Chesney *et al.*, 1983; Chesney *et al.*, 1985a).

Our group also examined factors important to amino acid transport processes, whose full expression develops with maturation (Chesney and Jax, 1979a; Chesney and Jax, 1979b; Chesney *et al.*, 1984; Chesney *et al.*, 1985c; Friedman *et al.*, 1981). At 28 days, young weanling rats fed a low-sulfur taurine diet (LTD) or high-sulfur taurine diet (HTD) have the same patterns of uptake and transport kinetics as adult animals, but their urinary taurine excretion is five times greater, in keeping with their relative immaturity (Chesney *et al.*, 1985a; Chesney and Jax, 1979a; Chesney and Jax, 1979b; Chesney *et al.*, 1984). Although this adaptive response is completely expressed at the apical surface in weanling rats, the manner in which this adaptive response is expressed in nursing animals is unclear.

Our BBMV studies employed rat pups born of mothers fed the LTD, HTD, or normal-sulfur taurine diet (NTD). The full compositions of the diets are described elsewhere (Chesney *et al.*, 1986b). The taurine content of milk from nursing dams was low after feeding the LTD and high after feeding the HTD (Chesney *et al.*, 1986b). At days 7, 14, and 21, both urine and plasma samples were collected from pups for analysis of taurine and creatinine (Chesney *et al.*, 1983). Kidney cortex was used to prepare BBMV (Chesney *et al.*, 1983), which were isolated using a modification of the method of Booth and Kenny (1974). Marker enzyme measurements were made for each BBMV preparation to evaluate its purity. An 8- to 11-fold increase in gamma glutamyl transferase activity was achieved between the final BBMV preparation and the initial cortex homogenate preparation (Friedman *et al.*, 1983; Chesney *et al.*, 1983; Chesney *et al.*, 1985a). Taurine was determined by high-pressure liquid chromatography (Chesney *et al.*, 1986b). Accumulation of [$^3$H]taurine was measured by the rapid Millipore filtration method of Chesney and associates (1973). To evaluate the kinetic properties of transport, uptake was determined over a wide range of concentrations (10–5,000 $\mu M$) at 15 sec, which was in the linear portion of the uptake curve.

To assure that the sodium–taurine accumulation represented entry into vesicles, we used sucrose, a nonpermeant solute, to study the effect of increasing external osmolarity on taurine accumulation at equilibrium (45 sec). In membranes prepared from animals aged 7, 14, 28 and 58 (adult) days, uptake was inversely related to external osmolarity, indicating that it occurs in an intravesicular space. Binding, which appeared to represent 5–7% of uptake at 300 mOsm, was not changed by diet.

These results summarize findings in four studies of immature rats (Chesney *et al.*, 1984; Chesney *et al.*, 1986b; Chesney *et al.*, 1986a; Chesney *et al.*, 1987). At all ages, immature nursing rats born to mothers consuming the NTD excreted more taurine in urine than adult rats (Table IV). Nursing rats whose mothers consumed the LTD conserved taurine, whereas those whose mothers ingested the HTD hyperexcreted taurine. Thus, rat pups expressed the renal adaptive response to altered sulfur taurine intake by lactating dams at the renal tubular epithelial surface (Chesney *et al.*, 1986b).

The time-dependent uptake of taurine (10 micromolar) was similar at all ages, reaching a peak at 3–6 min, but the height of the sodium-dependent overshoot was greatest in the oldest animals. A progression

**TABLE IV**

**Urine Taurine Excretion in Nursing and Adult Rats[a]**

| Age | LTD | NTD | HTD | LTD vs. NTD | NTD vs. HTD |
|---|---|---|---|---|---|
| 7 days ($n$ = 12) | 6.12 ± 0.47 | 207.89 ± 8.11 | 407.63 ± 39.01 | $p < 0.001$ | $p < 0.01$ |
| 14 days ($n$ = 12) | 3.45 ± 0.27 | 195.79 ± 45.32 | 462.83 ± 51.11 | $p < 0.001$ | $p < 0.02$ |
| 21 days ($n$ = 9) | 12.60 ± 3.37 | 309.00 ± 39.19 | 473.52 ± 65.30 | $p < 0.001$ | $p < 0.05$ |
| Adult ($n$ = 1) | 13.05 ± 1.91 | 100.00 ± 11.20 | 821.68 ± 144.25 | $p < 0.001$ | $p < 0.001$ |

[a]Results are stated as a percentage of the value in an adult rat fed NTD. Each value represents the mean ± SEM of the number of pooled urine samples indicated: 7-day = 11–15 pups; 14-day = 7–9 pups; 21-day = 4–6 pups; adult = 1 rat. (From Chesney *et al.*, 1986a. Reprinted with permission.)

of uptake was found: 7 day <14 day <21 day <28 day = adult (Chesney *et al.*, 1986a). Taurine uptake in relation to diet is shown in Fig. 3. Sodium-taurine symport was highest in membranes from 14-day-old pups, 21-day-old pups, and adults exposed to LTD. However, no diet-induced changes were found in preparations from 7-day-old animals. Exposure to the HTD reduced taurine accumulation in BBMV at all ages greater than 7 days. By contrast, no effect of diet or age was seen when uptake was examined at a high taurine concentration (5 m*M*) (Fig. 4).

Dietary change increased the $V_{max}$ of sodium-taurine symport in BBMV at 14, 21, and 58 days but not at 7 days (Chesney *et al.*, 1986a). The $V_{max}$ of uptake was lower in BBMV from animals exposed to the HTD but again only after 7 days of age. The $V_{max}$ of sodium-taurine symport was 25–50% above normal in nursing pups of mothers fed the LTD and 16–50% below normal in those of mothers fed the HTD ($p < 0.05$ to $< 0.02$). By Lineweaver-Burk kinetic analysis, the $K_m$ varied from $35 \pm 8$ $\mu M$ to $68 \pm 8$ $\mu$M, which was not statistically different among the three diets at each of four ages.

These results lead to the speculation that the physiological taurinuria of immature rats may result from a low rate of uptake at the apical surface of the proximal tubule, the second mechanism proposed above. However,

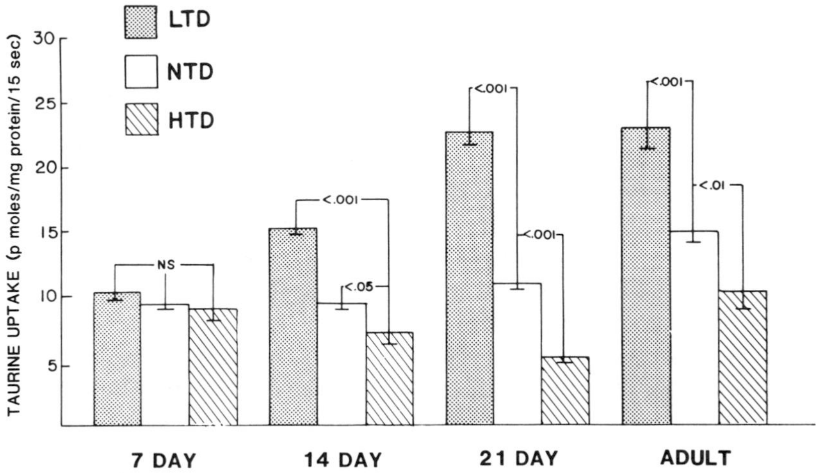


**Fig. 3.** Taurine uptake was studied in brush-border membrane vesicles of young weanling rats born of mothers fed a low-sulfur taurine diet (LTD), a high-sulfur taurine diet (HTD) or normal-sulfur taurine diet (NTD). The initial (15 sec) rate of taurine (10 micromolar) accumulation was measured in relation to diet and age. Each point represents a mean ± SEM of 4–5 determinations performed in triplicate. (From Chesney *et al.*, 1986a. Reprinted with permission.)

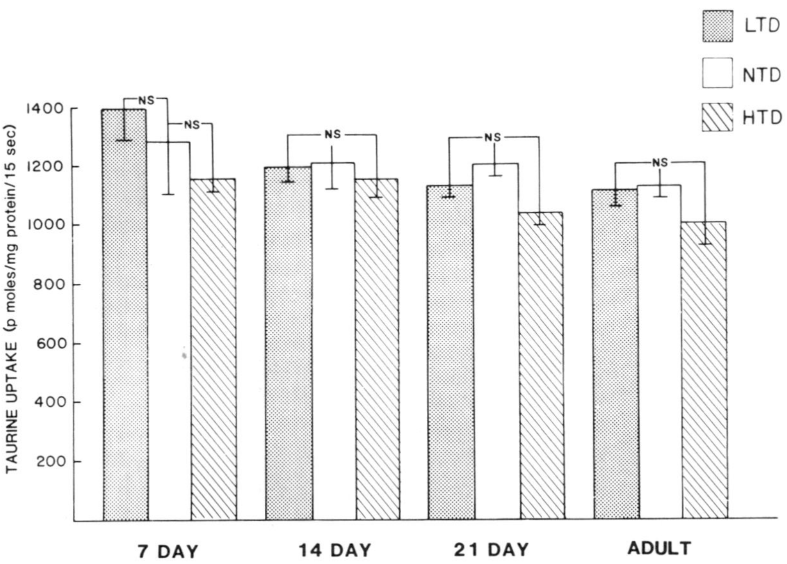


**Fig. 4.** Taurine uptake was studied in brush-border membrane vesicles of young weanling rats born of mothers fed a low-sulfur taurine diet (LTD), a high-sulfur taurine diet (HTD) or normal-sulfur taurine diet (NTD). The influence of age and diet on the initial (15 sec) rate of taurine (5 m*M*) accumulation was measured. (From Chesney *et al.*, 1986a. Reprinted with permission.)

at some time between one and two weeks of age, the adaptive response to dietary changes in sulfur taurine begins to be expressed at the brush-border surface.

These and previous studies (Chesney *et al.*, 1986a; Friedman *et al.*, 1983; Chesney *et al.*, 1983; Chesney *et al.*, 1985a) show that the renal adaptive response is membrane-related. Therefore, the LTD or HTD might alter the microviscosity and phospholipid composition of brush-border membranes (Chesney *et al.*, 1987). Changes in the physical characteristics or lipid composition of biological membranes can affect the movement of ions and solutes across these membranes (Jain, 1980). Alterations in fluidity and membrane phospholipid composition may also influence the activity or accessibility of membrane-bound enzymes and transport systems. Further, lipid–protein interactions may modify the function of proteins inserted into the membrane.

Fluorescence polarization has been employed to study plasma membrane fluidity (Molitoris and Simon, 1985). We incubated BBMV isolated in our earlier studies with 1-6-diphenyl-1,3,5-hexatriene (DPH), a fluorescent probe, and measured membrane fluidity at intervals in temperature between 4°–56° F. Membrane fluorescence was determined in an Elscient

Model MV-1a microviscosimeter, and the Perrin equation was used to interpret the data (Gourley *et al.*, 1983a). The best fit was assessed with a F-test from a computer program based on the theory of Hudson, as modified by Gourley and associates (1983b).

Membrane phospholipid content was determined after lipid extraction and analysis of phospholipids by established methods (Bligh and Dyer, 1954; Perleman *et al.*, 1982). Phospholipids were separated by two-dimensional thin-layer chromatography employing an internal standard of [$^{14}$C]dipalmitoyl phosphatidyl choline to establish recoveries.

The best fit for DPH membrane fluorescence in terms of absolute temperature was a two-limb, single-breakpoint curve (Table V) (Chesney *et al.*, 1987). Data showed:

1. The transition or ''break'' temperature between the upper and lower slopes was 23 ± 3° C for nearly all ages and diets.
2. The polarization fluorescence ($p$) value varied between 0.305 and 0.337.
3. The slopes of the upper and lower segments were similar and unrelated to diet or age.
4. Neither diet nor age altered the transition temperature or the $p$ value, but fluidity increased with age regardless of diet (Chesney *et al.*, 1987).

**TABLE V**

**Membrane Fluidity Measurements in Brush-Border Membrane Vesicles From Rats of Ages 7, 14, and 21 Days and Adult**[a]

| Age | Diet[b] | Break temperature[c] | Polarization fluorescence[d] | Upper slope | Lower slope |
|---|---|---|---|---|---|
| 7 days | LTD | 21.3 ± 2.2 | 0.320 ± 0.009 | 341.3 | 211.3 |
| | NTD | 24.7 ± 4.2 | 0.305 ± 0.025 | 313.5 | 181.8 |
| | HTD | 27.7 ± 1.8 | 0.323 ± 0.005 | 316.8 | 189.6 |
| 14 days | LTD | 23.2 ± 1.5 | 0.320 ± 0.010 | 334.4 | 198.2 |
| | NTD | 23.3 ± 3.3 | 0.312 ± 0.026 | 329.1 | 187.5 |
| | HTD | 24.9 ± 1.5 | 0.323 ± 0.015 | 350.3 | 207.4 |
| 21 days | LTD | 24.0 ± 1.2 | 0.327 ± 0.015 | 328.9 | 192.1 |
| | NTD | 23.0 ± 3.6 | 0.312 ± 0.034 | 311.7 | 175.1 |
| | HTD | 23.9 ± 3.5 | 0.326 ± 0.032 | 326.1 | 209.2 |
| Adult | LTD | 25.3 ± 3.3 | 0.334 ± 0.012 | 353.0 | 204.8 |
| | NTD | 20.0 ± 3.8 | 0.334 ± 0.016 | 334.1 | 170.3 |
| | HTD | 23.6 ± 1.6 | 0.337 ± 0.021 | 341.7 | 196.8 |

[a]From Chesney *et al.*, 1987. Reprinted with permission.

[b]Diets contained low taurine (LTD), normal taurine (NTD) or high taurine (HTD).

[c]Break temperature, stated in degrees centigrade, is the mean ± SD of 4 determinations.

[d]Polarization fluorescence is the mean ± SD of 4 determinations.

5. The lipid microenvironment was not significantly influenced by age or diet.

In BBMV of rats of all ages, the most abundant phospholipids were phosphatidyl choline, phosphatidyl serine, and phosphatidyl ethanolamine, but adults had lower levels of phosphatidyl choline and higher levels of phosphatidyl serine than young rats. Therefore, phospholipid composition of BBMV is a function of age rather than diet (Chesney *et al.*, 1987). These results permit the tentative conclusion that the high level of sodium-taurine symport found with the LTD and the low level of symport found with the HTD do not relate to physical changes in BBMV. Further, the change in phospholipid composition that occurs with maturation may play a role in the adaptive process.

As previously noted, taurine accumulation into BBMV from 7-day-old pups was significantly lower than that from older animals, and no dietary influence was found. These findings support the hypothesis that the aminoaciduria of immaturity may result, in part, from low brush-border surface uptake. Segal's group (Meadow *et al.*, 1983) has also found low vesicle accumulation of proline in nursing pups. Nonetheless, *in vivo*, a noteworthy discrepancy exists between urinary taurine excretion patterns and BBMV uptake: urinary taurine excretion is high in pups nursed by HTD mothers and low in those nursed by LTD mothers (Chesney *et al.*, 1986b; Chesney *et al.*, 1986a), but BBMV uptake is similar in both. Changes in sodium entry into membranes or other ionic factors may be responsible for the age-related low amino acid uptake, for the failure of BBMV to express the adaptive response, and for the discrepancy between membrane-related events and urinary excretion (Chesney *et al.*, 1985b). Low sodium-glucose cotransport by immature rabbit renal vesicles has also been shown. This finding relates to greater sodium permeability in these membranes, which appear to be more "leaky" (Beck, 1985). Low sodium entry would reduce initial taurine uptake. Diametrically opposite findings indicate that uptake of $^{22}$Na into rat jejunal BBMV is more brisk. Thus, low sodium–glucose uptake may be caused by rapid dissipation of the inwardly directed sodium-gradient, which is the driving force for sodium-coupled symport (Grishan and Wilson, 1985). In our preliminary studies comparing sodium uptake in membranes from immature and older animals, findings related to sodium–taurine uptake and sodium/hydrogen exchange suggest that rapid dissipation of $^{22}$Na may be the operative mechanism (Zelikovic *et al.*, 1987).

From a nutritional standpoint, the renal adaptive response may be pivotal in conserving and concentrating taurine in tissues. Prominent among these is the brain, where taurine serves as a neuromodulator and an osmoregulator (Chesney, 1985). Taurine is probably an osmolar substance that maintains cell volume. Brain concentrations of taurine are stable, even in the presence of diet-induced changes in plasma and renal taurine levels, which are high in HTD-fed and low in LTD-fed animals (Chesney *et al.*, 1986b).

In summary, higher BBMV uptake of taurine occurred with increasing age, and the renal adaptive response was expressed in BBMV sometime between 7–14 days after birth (Chesney *et al.*, 1986a). This response was affected by dietary taurine levels in both directions—upregulation and downregulation—and was caused by a change in the initial sodium–taurine cotransport rate. No changes in the lipid microenvironment of the membrane were detectable by membrane fluidity studies (Chesney *et al.*, 1987). Although vesicles from 7-day-old pups did not show the adaptive response and accumulated little taurine, the entry of sodium, which energizes uptake, may be altered at this age, thereby preventing full expression of the adaptive response (Zelikovic *et al.*, 1987).

Finally, our study indicates that the adaptive response occurred early in the development of transport, and this may be important in maintaining stable brain levels of taurine during a period of rapid growth. However, the relationship between the kidney, where adaptation is expressed, and the brain, where taurine homeostasis is maintained, is not well defined.

## V. AMINOACIDURIA OF INCREASED AMINO ACID INTAKE

As noted previously, ingestion of a high amino acid load or a high-protein diet results in an "overflow" aminoaciduria (Scriver *et al.*, 1976). Again, the taurine dietary model can be used to explore this pattern of aminoaciduria. In rats fed a high (3%) taurine diet (HTD), plasma taurine content was $606 \pm 155$ m*M*, versus $367 \pm 50$ m*M* for normal (NTD) controls ($n = 8$, $p < 0.02$) (Chesney *et al.*, 1985a). Urinary taurine excretion in HTD rats was $63.4 \pm 3.2$ micromoles/mg creatinine, versus $8.7 \pm 1.2$ micromoles/mg creatinine for NTD rats ($p < 0.001$). Taurine concentration in the renal cortex of HTD rats was $7.1 \pm 0.9$ $\mu M$/g net weight, versus $4.2 \pm 0.8$ for NTD rats ($p < 0.05$). Hence, high taurine intake was associated with hypertaurinemia, hypertaurinuria, and high taurine content in the renal cortex. As noted previously, the HTD also caused a lower initial rate of taurine uptake—$33.16 \pm 3.76$ pmole/mg protein/60 sec, versus $48.6 \pm 1.31$ for NTD ($p < 0.001$).

When these rats were fasted and/or fed 3% beta-alanine in their drinking water, renal cortex taurine content fell, and plasma taurine values changed slightly but not significantly (Chesney *et al.*, 1985a). Although urinary taurine excretion was only modestly reduced following fasting or beta-alanine exposure, renal cortex taurine content fell to 62% of the control value. Both of these maneuvers increased BBMV accumulation of taurine (Fig. 5).

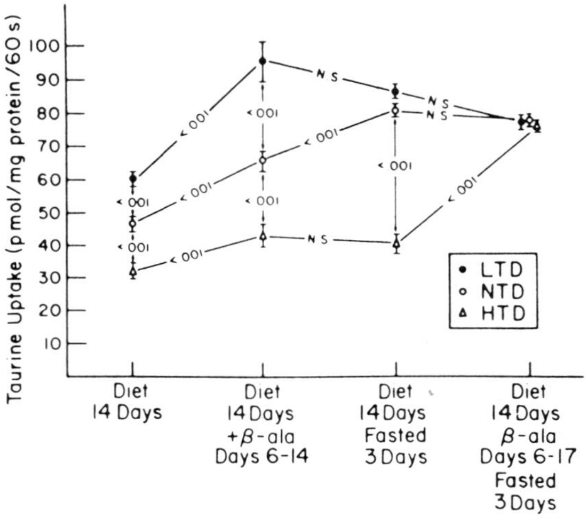


**Fig. 5.** Taurine uptake was studied in brush-border membrane vesicles (BBMV) of young weanling rats born of mothers fed a low-sulfur taurine diet (LTD), a high-sulfur taurine diet (HTD) or normal-sulfur taurine diet (NTD). During the study, rats on these diets were also fasted and/or fed 3% beta-alanine (b-ala) in their drinking water. Taurine uptake by BBMV over 60 sec, using 25 $\mu M$ taurine, was determined for each diet. Each point represents the mean ± SEM of 4–6 determinations, performed in triplicate (From Chesney *et al.*, 1985a. Reprinted with permission.)

Hence, events that deplete renal cortex taurine result in greater accumulation of this amino acid by BBMV, despite only minor changes in plasma taurine values.

These data suggest that trans-stimulation of amino acid uptake occurs. Thus, a reduction in intracellular taurine content serves as a signal for increased sodium–taurine cotransport across the brush-border surface (Chesney *et al.*, 1985a). Further, in the presence of an excess of dietary taurine, tissue and plasma taurine levels rise, thereby negating the signal for trans-stimulation. As a result, sodium–taurine cotransport system activity and taurine uptake are low.

Our laboratory has preliminary evidence that the adaptive response reflects incorporation of preformed transporter into the BBMV. In membranes prepared from rats fed 3% taurine, transport activity falls then rises after an overnight fast. When rats were injected with colchicine, a known inhibitor of intracellular microtubules, this rise was blocked, and these rats did not express the adaptive response. This finding implies that inhibition of microtubule function, and therefore of cotransporter insertion, blocks this brush-border membrane function (unpublished observation).

Although we know that the $T_m$ or maximal tubule transport rate is high, the mechanisms of diet-induced aminoaciduria are imperfectly understood. However, our studies in hypertaurinemic and taurine-supplemented rats provide physiologic clues to the mechanisms involved in diet-induced aminoaciduria. As previously noted, renal cortex pool size governs the activity of the transporter for taurine—with low dietary intake, the sodium-taurine cotransport rate increases; with dietary surfeit, the cotransport rate falls. With cotransport falls, less taurine is reabsorbed, and more is excreted into the urine (Chesney *et al.*, 1985a). These studies show that aminoaciduria caused by high dietary amino acid intake probably reflects a membrane-related event, with the signal being the transmembrane amino acid ratio.

The nutritional implication of such a system is that in periods of dietary surfeit, the transporter could be could downregulated, possibly by being shifted back into the microtubule system within the cytoplasm, and more amino acid would be excreted. Further, this mechanism could maintain tissue pool size of a specific amino acid.

## ACKNOWLEDGMENTS

Supported in part by NIH grants DK 37233 and P30 AM 35747.

## REFERENCES

Arant, B. S., Jr. (1978). Glomerulotubular balance following saline loading in developing canine kidney. *Amer. J. Physiol.* **235**, F417–F425.

Baerlocher, K. E., Scriver, C. R., and Mohyuddin, F. (1971a). The ontogeny of amino acid transport in the kidney. I. Effect on distribution ratios and intracellular metabolism of proline and glycine. *Biochim. Biophys. Acta* **249**, 353–363.

Baerlocher, K. E., Scriver, C. R., and Mohyuddin, F. (1971b). The ontogeny of amino acid transport in rat kidney. II. Kinetics of uptake and effect of anoxia. *Biochim. Biophys. Acta* **249**, 364–372.

Barfuss, D. W., and Schafer, J. A. (1981). Differences in active and passive glucose transport along the proximal nephron. *Amer. J. Physiol.* **240**, 597–608.

Beck, J. C. (1985). Glucose and sodium transport in brush border membrane vesicles from fetal rabbit kidney. *Ann. N.Y. Acad. Sci.* **246**, 456–458.

Bligh, E. G., and Dyer, W. J. (1954). A rapid method of total lipid extraction and purification. *Can. J. Biochem. Physiol.* **37**, 911–917.

Booth, A. G., and Kenny, A. J. (1974). A rapid method for the preparation of microvilli from rabbit kidney. *Biochem. J.* **142**, 575–581.

Brantbar, N., Walling, M. W., and Coburn, J. (1979). Interactions between vitamin D deficiency and phosphorus depletion in the rat. *J. Clin. Invest.* **63**, 335–341, 1979.

Brodehl, J., and Gellissen, K. (1968). Endogenous renal transport of free amino acids in infancy and childhood. *Pediatrics* **42**, 395–404.

Chanard, J., Black, R., Pulkerson, M., Lewis, J., Klahr, S., and Slatopolsky, E. (1977). The effect of colchicine and vinblastine on parathyroid hormone in the rat. *Endocrinology* **101**, 1792–1800.

Chesney, R. W. (1985). Taurine: Biological role and clinical perspective. *Adv. Pediatr.* **32**, 1–42.

Chesney, R. W., and Jax, D. K. (1979a). Developmental aspects of renal beta-amino acid transport. I. Ontogeny of taurine reabsorption and accumulation in rat renal cortex. *Pediatr. Res.* **13**, 854–860.

Chesney, R. W., and Jax, D. K. (1979b). Developmental aspects of renal beta-amino acid transport. II. Ontogeny of uptake and efflux processes and effect of anoxia. *Pediatr. Res.* **13**, 861–867.

Chesney, R. W., Sacktor, B., and Rosen, R. R. (1973). The binding of D-glucose to the isolated rabbit renal brush border. *J. Biol. Chem.* **248**, 2182–2191.

Chesney, R. W., Gusowski, N., and Friedman, A. L. (1983). Renal adaptation to altered dietary sulfur amino acid intake occurs at the luminal brush border membrane. *Kidney Int.* **24**, 588–594.

Chesney, R. W., Gusowski, N., and Theissen, M. (1984). Developmental aspects of renal beta-amino acid transport. IV. Brush border membrane response to altered intake of sulfur amino acids. *Pediatr. Res.* **18**, 611–618.

Chesney, R. W., Gusowski, N., and Dabbagh, S. (1985a). Renal cortex taurine content regulates renal adaptive response to altered dietary intake of sulfur amino acids. *J. Clin. Invest.* **76**, 2213–2221.

Chesney, R. W., Gusowski, N., Dabbagh, S., Theissen, N. M., Padilla, M., and Drehl, A. (1985b). Factors affecting the transport of beta-amino acids in rat renal brush-border membrane vesicles: The role of external chloride. *Biochim. Biophys. Acta* **812**, 702–712.

Chesney, R. W., Gusowski, N., Friedman, A. L., Dabbagh, S., and Diehl, A. (1985c). Divergent membrane maturation in rat kidney: Exposure by dietary taurine manipulation. *Int. J. Pediatr. Nephrol.* **6**, 93–100.

Chesney, R. W., Gusowski, N. Zelikovic, I, and Padilla, M. (1986a). Developmental aspects of renal beta-amino acid transport. V: Brush border membrane transport in nursing animals—Effects of age and diet. *Pediatr. Res.* **20**, 890–894.

Chesney, R. W., Lippencott, S., Gusowski, N., Padilla, M., and Zelikovic, I. (1986b). Studies on renal adaptation to altered dietary amino acid intake: Tissue taurine responses in nursing and adult rats. *J. Nutr.* **116**, 1965–1976.

Chesney, R. W., Gusowski, N., and Zelikovic, I. (1987). Developmental aspects of renal beta-amino acid transport. VI: The role of membrane fluidity and phospholipid composition in the renal adaptive response in nursing animals. *Pediatr. Res.* **22**, 163–167.

DeLuca, H. F. (1979). The vitamin D system in the regulation of calcium and phosphorus metabolism. *Nutr. Rev.* **37**, 161–193.

DeRubertis, F. R., and Craven, P. A. (1976). Hormonal modulation of cyclic adenosine 3μ,5μ)monophosphate dependent protein kinase activity in rat renal cortex. *J. Clin. Invest.* **57**, 1442–1450.

Foreman, J. W., and Segal, S. (1985). Aminoacidurias. *In* "Renal Tubular Disorders: Pathophysiology, Diagnosis and Management (H. C. Gonick and V. M. Buckalew, Jr., eds.), pp. 131–158. Marcel Decker, New York.

Fraser, D., Kooh, S.W., and Scriver, C. R. (1967). Hyperparathyroidism as the cause of hyperaminoaciduria and phosphaturia in human vitamin D deficiency. *Pediatr. Res.* **1**, 425–435.

Friedman, A. L., Jax, D. K., and Chesney, R. W. (1981). Developmental aspects of renal beta-amino acid transport. III. Characteristics of transport in isolated renal tubules. *Pediatr. Res.* **15**, 10–13.

Friedman, A. L., Albright, P. W., Gusowski, N., Padilla, M., and Chesney, R. W. (1983). Renal adaptation to alteration in dietary amino acid intake. *Amer. J. Physiol.* **245**, F159–F166.

Gourley, G. R., Korsmo, H. A., and Olsen, W. A. (1983a). Intestinal mucosa in diabetic rats: Studies of microvillus membrane composition and microviscosity. *Metabolism* **30**, 1053–1058.

Gourley, G. R., Mogilevsky, W., and Odell, G. B. (1983b). Hepatic microsomal composition studies in the Gunn rat. *Biochim. Biophys. Acta* **750**, 419–423.

Grishan, F. K., and Wilson, F. A. (1985). Developmental maturation of D-glucose transport by rat jejunal brush-border membrane vesicles. *Amer. J. Physiol.* **248**, G87–G92.

Hammerman, M. R., Hansen, V. A., and Morrissey, J. J. (1983). Cyclic AMP-dependent protein phosphorylation and dephosphorylation alter phosphate transport in canine renal brush border vesicles. *Biochim. Biophys. Acta* **755**, 10–16.

Hruska, K. A., Mulls, S., and Westbrook, S. (1984). Regulation of proximal tubular cell cystolic calcium ($Ca^{++}$) by parathyroid hormone (PTH) [Abstract]. *Clin. Res.* **32**, 801A.

Jaeger, P., Portmann, L., Saunders, A., Rosenberg, L. E., and Thier, S. O. (1986). Anticystinuric effect of glutamine and dietary sodium restriction. *N. Engl. J. Med.* **315**, 1120–1123.

Jain, M. K. (1980). Phase properties of bilayers. *In* "Introduction to Biological Membranes" (M. K. Jain and R. C. Wagner, eds.), pp. 53–175. Wiley, New York.

Jepson, J. B. (1983). Hartnup disease. *In* "The Metabolic Basis of Inherited Disease" (J. B. Stanbury, J. B. Wyngaarden, D. S. Fredrickson, J. L. Goldstein, and M. S. Brown, eds.), 5th ed., pp. 1804–1805. McGraw-Hill, New York.

Lashley, L., and Scriver, C. R. (1979). Ontogeny of amino acid reabsorption in human kidney: Evidence from the homozygous infant with familial renal immunoglycinuria for multiple proline and glycine systems. *Pediatr. Res.* **13**, 65–70.

Matsumoto, T., Fontaine, O., and Rasmussen, H. (1981). Effect of 1,25-dihydroxyvitamin $D_3$ on phospholipid metabolism in chick duodenal mucosal cell. *J. Biol. Chem.* **256**, 3353–3360.

Meadow, M. E., Roth, K. S., Foreman, J. W., Bover, K. C., and Segal, S. (1983). Renal brush-border membrane vesicles from newborn rat by free flow electrophoresis and their proline uptake. *Biochem. J.* **214**, 209–214.

Mitch, W. E., and Chesney, R. W. (1983). Amino acid metabolism of the kidney. *Mineral Electrolyte Metab.* **9**, 190–202.

Molitoris, B. A., and Simon, F. R. (1985). Renal cortical brush-border and basolateral membranes: Cholesterol and phospholipid composition and relative turnover. *J. Membrane Biol.* **83**, 207–215.

Pak, C. Y. C., Fuller, C., Sakhall, K., Zerwekh, J. E., and Adams, B. V. (1986). Management of cystine nephrolithiasis with alpha-mercaptopropionyl glycine. *J. Urol.* **136**, 1003–1008.

Perleman, R. H., Engle, M. J., Kemnitz, J. W., Kotas, R. V., and Farrell, P. M. (1982). Biochemical and physiological development of fetal rhesus lung. *J. Appl. Physiol.* **53**, 230–235.

Pike, J. W. (1985). Intracellular receptors mediate the biologic action of 1,25-dihydroxy vitamin $D_3$. *Nutr. Rev.* **43**, 161–168.

Reinhardt, T. A., Horst, R. L., Orf, J. W., and Hollis, B. W. (1984). A microassay for 1,25-dihydroxy-vitamin D not requiring high performance liquid chromatography: Application to clinical studies. *J. Clin. Endocrinol. Metab.* **58**, 91–98.

Rodman, J. S., Blackburn, P., Williams, J. J., Brown, A., Pospischil, M. A., and Peterson, C. M. (1984). The effect of dietary protein on cystine excretion in patients with cystinuria. *Clin. Nephrol.* **22**, 273–278.

Scriver, C. R. (1974). Rickets and the pathogenesis of impaired tubular transport of phosphate and other solutes. *Amer. J. Med.* **57**, 43–54.

Scriver, C. R., Chesney, R. W., and McInnes, R. R. (1976). Genetic aspects of renal tubular transport: Diversity and topology of carriers. *Kidney Int.* **9**, 149–171.

Scriver, C. R., Clow, C. L., Reade, T. M., Goodyer, P., Auray-Blais, C., Giguere, R., and Lemieux, B. (1985). Ontogeny modifies manifestations of cystinuria genes: Implications for counseling. *J. Pediatr.* **106**, 411–416.

Segal, S. (1982). Regulatory aspects of transport during development. *In* "The Kidney During Development" (A. Spitzer, ed.), pp. 363–372. Masson, New York.

Segal, S., and Thier, S. O. (1983). Cystinuria. *In* "The Metabolic Basis of Inherited Disease" (J. B. Stanbury, J. B. Wyngaarden, D. S. Fredrickson, J. L. Goldstein, and M. S. Brown, eds.), 5th ed., pp. 1774–1791. McGraw-Hill, New York.

Skovky, F., Rosenberg, L. E., and Thier, S. O. (1980). No effect of L-glutamine on cystinuria. *N. Engl. J. Med.* **302**, 236–237.

Smith, A. J., and Strang, L. B. (1958). An inborn error of metabolism with the urinary excretion of alpha-hydroxybutyric acid and phenylpyuric acid. *Arch. Dis. Child.* **33**, 109–113.

Stevens, B. P., Kaunitz, J. D., and Wright, E. M. (1984). Intestinal transport of amino acids and sugars: Advances using membrane vesicles. *Ann. Rev. Physiol.* **46**, 417–433.

Vainsel, M., Manderlier, T. H., Corvilain, J., and Vis, H. L. (1974). Study of secondary hyperparathyroidism in vitamin D rickets: II. Aspects of amino acid metabolism. *Biomedicine* **20**, 404–409.

Zelikovic, I., Stejskal, E., Lohstroh, P., and Chesney, R. W. (1987). $Na^+/H^+$ exchange is enhanced in neonatal rat renal brush border membrane vesicles (BBMV) [Abstract]. *The Physiologist* **30**, 148.

# 12

# Amino Acid Abnormalities in Renal Failure

Jonas Bergström

*Department of Renal Medicine*
*Karolinska Institute*
*Huddinge University Hospital*
*Stockholm, Sweden*



## I. INTRODUCTION

Protein malnutrition is common in chronic renal failure in nondialyzed, hemodialyzed, and peritoneal dialyzed patients. Signs of this malnutrition include: weight loss, decreases in muscle and lean body mass, low plasma proteins, low alkali-soluble cell proteins in muscle, and impaired cellular immune response (Guarnieri *et al.*, 1983). In patients treated with intermittent hemodialysis, protein malnutrition is strongly associated with increased morbidity and mortality (Acchiardo *et al.*, 1983).

Many factors contribute to protein malnutrition in renal failure. These include low protein and energy intake, physical inactivity, metabolic acidosis; resistance to the anabolic action of insulin and other hormones; and high levels of parathyroid, glucagon, and other catabolic hormones. Protein malnutrition in renal failure contributes to symptoms of anorexia, nausea, and depression and to the further complications of anemia, myopathy, neuropathy, and bone disease. Patients with chronic renal failure may exhibit several signs of impaired amino acid metabolism, some of them nonspecific signs of protein malnutrition and others resulting from loss of renal mass, reduced excretory function, endocrine abnormalities, and uremic toxicity.

The plasma aminogram in chronic renal failure is, in many respects, similar to that found in protein malnutrition. Levels of most essential amino acids are low (except for methionine, which is usually normal), and levels of several nonessential amino acids are high. This plasma aminogram is consistent with other evidence of protein malnutrition in patients with renal failure. Other characteristics of the aminogram for uremia include: relatively high concentrations of cystine, citrulline, methylated histidines, hydroxylysine, and hydroxyproline; relatively low levels of tyrosine, serine, and tryptophan; and a low tyrosine/phenylalanine ratio (Kopple, 1983).

Hyperinsulinemia in uremic subjects appears to be an adaptive response to peripheral tissue insensitivity to insulin required for glucose metabolism. In contrast, tissue sensitivity to insulin for amino acid metabolism seems to be normal (DeFronzo *et al.*, 1983; Alvestrand *et al.*, 1987). Hence, hyperinsulinemia may contribute to low plasma concentrations of essential amino acids in patients with renal failure.

Effective protein synthesis does not occur in the presence of low amino acid concentrations at sites of protein synthesis. Evidence suggests that protein synthesis rates relate more closely to amino acid concentrations in the intracellular or muscle pool than to concentrations in the extracellular or plasma pool. Intracellular free amino acids in muscle are of special interest because muscle contains the largest pool of protein and free amino acids. An increase or decrease in the concentration of a single free amino acid in muscle may more accurately reflect an excess or deficiency than its concentration in plasma. However, protein and free amino acid pools are in dynamic equilibrium, and amino acids liberated during protein breakdown are extensively reused. Thus, the rate of protein synthesis and degradation in adults is about 5 g/kg/day—four to six times higher than recommended protein intake (Young and Pellett, 1987).

The intracellular concentration of most amino acids in muscle is higher than the concentration in plasma. This concentration gradient, or ratio of a given amino acid's intracellular to extracellular concentration, is especially high for taurine and glutamine, but is only slightly greater than one for the branched-chain amino acids phenylalanine and tyrosine (Bergström *et al.*, 1978). In untreated patients with chronic renal failure, the intracellular free amino acid profile in muscle exhibits several features typical of uremia (Bergstrom *et al.*, 1978; Alvestrand *et al.*, 1982).

Table I summarizes a number of studies of amino acid concentrations muscle in chronic renal failure. These studies were carried out in untreated patients, in patients undergoing dialysis treatments, and in patients treated with a low-protein diet (15–20 g/day), supplemented with two to three times the minimum requirements of essential amino acids (Rose's formula) (Rose *et al.*, 1955) plus added amounts of one or more specific amino acids. Table I shows the effects of two such diets, one supplemented with essential amino acids and histidine (EAAH) and the other with a new amino acid formula (NAAF) including more valine than leucine and adding histidine and tyrosine (Alvestrand *et al.*, 1982).

Both oral and parenteral amino acid solutions were tested. The evidence suggests that treatment with the EAAH diet, the NAAF diet (Alvestrand *et al.*, 1982) or chronic hemodialysis (Alvestrand *et al.*, 1983b; Lindholm *et al.*, 1986) normalizes some but not all intracellular amino acid deficiencies (Table I). This normalization may result from improved nutrition. However, the distribution of branched-chain amino acids became even more abnormal in patients treated with intermittent peritoneal dialysis for 24 hours twice weekly than in patients treated with other forms of therapy (Bergström *et al.*, 1978) (Table I).

Broyer's group reported normal branched-chain amino acid concentrations in muscle of children with severe renal failure (Delaporte *et al.*, 1978). However, in moderate renal failure, low concentrations of all three branched-chain amino acids were observed in muscle, with valine most markedly below normal (Broyer *et al.*, 1980).

The etiologies of amino acid disturbances in uremia are incompletely understood. The posttranscriptionally modified amino acids, 1- and 3-methyl histidine, hydroxyproline, and hydroxylysine, are not reused in protein synthesis and are excreted by the kidneys. Their accumulation is similar to that of creatinine when the glomerular filtration rate decreases (Kopple, 1983).

Because the kidneys are also important in metabolizing certain amino acids, loss of renal function may cause or contribute to low plasma levels of serine and tyrosine and high plasma levels of citrulline. Uremic toxins may affect metabolism by their influence on key enzymes involved in the transport and metabolism of specific amino acids.

**TABLE I**

**Concentrations of Selected Amino Acids in Muscle of Patients with Chronic Uremia[a]**

| Amino acid | Untreated | EAAH diet[b] | NAAF diet[c] | Chronic hemodialysis | Continuous ambulatory peritoneal dialysis (CAPD) | Intermittent peritoneal dialysis[d] |
|---|---|---|---|---|---|---|
| Essential amino acids | | | | | | |
| Histidine[e] | Low/borderline | Normal | Normal | Normal | Normal | Normal |
| Isoleucine | Normal | Normal | Normal | Normal | Normal | High |
| Leucine | Normal | Normal | Normal | Normal | Normal | High |
| Lysine | Low | Normal | Normal | Normal | High | High |
| Methionine | Normal | Normal | Normal | Normal | High | — |
| Phenylalanine | Normal | Normal | Normal | Normal | Normal | Normal |
| Threonine | Low | Normal | Normal | Normal | Normal | Low |
| Tyrosine[e] | Normal | Low | Borderline low | Normal | Low | Low |
| Valine | Low | Low | Normal | Low | Borderline Low | Low |
| Nonessential amino acids | | | | | | |
| Alanine | Normal | Normal | Normal | Normal | Normal | High |
| Arginine | Low/normal | Normal | Normal | Normal | Normal | Normal |
| Asparagine | Normal | Normal | Normal | Normal | High | Normal |
| Aspartic acid | Normal | Normal | High | Normal | High | — |
| Citrulline | Normal | Normal | Normal | Normal | Normal | High |
| Glutamate | Normal | Normal | Normal | Normal | High | High |
| Glutamine | Normal | Normal | Normal | Normal | Normal | High |
| Glycine | Normal | Normal | Normal | Normal | Normal | Normal |
| Ornithine | Normal | Normal | Normal | Normal | Normal | High |
| Serine | Normal | Borderline low | Borderline low | Low | Borderline low | Normal |

[a]Data from Bergström *et al.*, 1978; Alvestrand *et al.*, 1982; Alvestrand *et al.*, 1983b; Lindholm *et al.*, 1986.

[b]This low-protein diet consisted of 15–20 g protein/day, supplemented with two to three times the minimum requirements of essential amino acids in humans (Rose's formula) (Rose *et al.*, 1955) plus histidine (EAAH).

[c]This new amino acid formula (NAAF) consisted of 15–20 g protein/day, supplemented with two to three times the minimum requirements of essential amino acids in humans (Rose's formula) (Rose *et al.*, 1955) with high valine plus histidine and tyrosine (Alvestrand *et al.*, 1982).

[d]Patients were treated for 24 hours twice weekly.

[e]This amino acid is considered essential in uremia.

## II. SPECIFIC AMINO ACID ABNORMALITIES

### A. Branched-Chain Amino Acid Metabolism

Branched-chain amino acid metabolism in renal failure has been reviewed extensively (Bergström and Alvestrand, 1984). Of the branched-chain amino acids in plasma, valine is most consistently low; it is also the plasma amino acid most closely interrelated with other nutritional variables used to assess protein–energy malnutrition (Young *et al.*, 1982). Administration of oral pyridoxine (vitamin $B_6$) supplements to chronic dialysis patients for two weeks normalized low plasma valine and leucine levels (Kleiner *et al.*, 1980). Plasma levels of all three ketoanalogs of the branched-chain amino acids were low in adults with chronic renal failure (Schauder *et al.*, 1979), and plasma levels of 2-ketoisocaproic acid (KICA) were low in uremic children (Jones *et al.*, 1983).

Changes in branched-chain amino acid concentrations in erythrocytes of chronically uremic patients were similar to those in plasma. Cerebrospinal fluid concentrations of valine and leucine are also lower in uremic patients than in controls (Pye *et al.*, 1979).

Pharmacokinetic studies of amino acid elimination after intravenous injection of amino acid mixtures in nondialyzed chronically uremic patients showed low plasma clearance of valine (Takala, 1983) or of all three branched-chain amino acids (Druml *et al.*, 1983). Metabolic clearance rates for isoleucine and leucine were low in chronic hemodialysis patients (Chami *et al.*, 1976; Chami *et al.*, 1978). Pyridoxine supplements, which normalized low plasma valine and leucine concentrations, did not influence their plasma clearance rate (Kleiner *et al.*, 1980). After bolus injection of an amino acid mixture, the metabolic clearance rate of valine was lower in hemodialysis patients than in controls (Druml *et al.*, 1983). In experiments with [$^{14}$C]valine, free valine pools and valine turnover appeared to be lower in postabsorptive, nondialyzed patients than in controls (Jones and Kopple, 1978; Kopple *et al.*, 1981).

Observations on splanchnic uptake of branched-chain amino acids in the fasting state are inconsistent. Alvestrand *et al.* (1987) found a high splanchnic uptake of valine in chronically uremic patients, which may contribute to decreases in free valine pools in plasma and muscle. In contrast, others described normal splanchnic uptake of valine in chronically uremic patients (Tizianello *et al.*, 1980b; Tizianello *et al.*, 1983). However, the less severe renal failure in Tizianello's patients may explain this discrepancy. Low cerebral uptake of branched-chain amino acids correlated with low plasma levels in chronic renal failure (Deferrari *et al.*, 1981; Tizianello *et al.*, 1983), but renal metabolism of branched-chain amino acids did not differ from that of controls (Tizianello *et al.*, 1980a; Tizianello *et al.*, 1983).

The pathogenesis of branched-chain amino acid abnormalities in chronic renal failure is unclear. Low plasma levels of all three branched-chain amino acids have been found, along with selective intracellular depletion of valine in the presence of normal (Alvestrand *et al.*, 1978) or high (Fürst *et al.*, 1980a) muscle levels of isoleucine and leucine. Selective depletion of free valine in uremia would require preferential catabolism of this amino acid. The same transaminase is generally thought to be involved in degradation of all branched-chain amino acids (Ichihara and Koyama, 1966), and a single dehydrogenase complex is believed to control the rate-limiting decarboxylation of branched-chain ketoacids (Odessey and Goldberg, 1972). However, the demonstration in humans of metabolic defects involving only one or two branched-chain amino acids (Budd *et al.*, 1967) suggests that decarboxylation of branched-chain ketoacids may occur by more than one enzymatic mechanism (Connelly *et al.*, 1968). The affinity of individual branched-chain ketoacids for one or more enzymes of the dehydrogenase complex may be changed by a change in pH (Randle, 1981) or by the presence of high concentrations of one or more of the metabolites that accumulate in the uremic state.

The fractional splanchnic uptake for valine, but not for leucine or isoleucine was markedly enhanced in the basal preabsorptive state in uremic patients. The same was true in euglycemic clamp studies of hyperinsulinemia (Alvestrans *et al.*, 1987). These data suggest that degradation in the liver may contribute to depletion of valine pools. However, the postprandial splanchnic uptake of valine from an oral amino acid mixture was no higher in uremic than normal subjects (DeFerrari *et al.*, 1987), but isoleucine uptake by the splanchnic bed was low as were uptakes of threonine, histidine, and phenylalanine.

Because long-term treatment with the EAAH diet did not normalize low valine concentrations in plasma and muscle (Table I), low valine intake in itself is probably not a major factor in depletion of valine pools. In untreated uremia and in patients treated with an EAAH diet, the abnormal branched-chain amino acid pattern resembles that induced by nutritional antagonism among these amino acids in rats fed a low-protein diet containing an excess of leucine (Shinnic and Harper, 1977). Thus, the relative proportions of dietary branched-chain amino acids appear to be significant.

Hyperinsulinemia elicits similar decreases in plasma branched-chain amino acids in uremic and normal subjects, indicating that insulin resistance in uremia does not influence transport and metabolism of branched-chain amino acids (DeFronzo *et al.*, 1983). Thus, hyperinsulinemia may contribute to low plasma branched-chain amino acid levels in chronic renal failure.

The sensitivity to insulin of branched-chain amino acid metabolism in muscle is also normal in uremia (Alvestrand *et al.*, 1987). Other findings indicate that the metabolism of valine differs from that of other branched-chain amino acids in uremia. For example, an oral glucose load produced a decline in all branched-chain amino acids in healthy subjects, whereas only alpha-ketoisovaleric acid (the ketoacid of valine) declined in uremic patients (Schauder *et al.*, 1981).

The intracellular-extracellular gradients of leucine and isoleucine rose in uremia, while the valine gradient remained normal (Alvestrand *et al.*, 1978; Fürst *et al.*, 1980a). These changes suggest that membrane transport or permeability of leucine and isoleucine may be altered, either as a direct effect of uremia or as a secondary effect of disturbed amino acid metabolism or endocrine abnormalities (Manchester, 1970).

## B. Phenylalanine and Tyrosine Metabolism

The tyrosine/phenylalanine ratio tends to be low in uremic plasma and muscle (Bergström *et al.*, 1978; Alvestrand *et al.*, 1982). Phenylalanine loading tests and studies with [$^{14}$C]phenylalanine in chronic renal failure indicate that metabolic clearance is low, oxidation is impaired, and phenylalanine conversion to tyrosine is slower than normal (Pickford *et al.*, 1973; Young and Parsons, 1973; Letteri and Scipione, 1974; Jones *et al.*, 1978). Serum from uremic patients inhibited phenylalanine hydrolase activity in normal rat liver by about 15% (Young and Parsons, 1973). The inhibitor is diffusible *in vitro* and appears to have a molecular weight of approximately 800 daltons (Stonier *et al.*, 1984). Studies of liver homogenates from chronically uremic and control rats showed a direct relation between protein intake and liver phenylalanine hydroxylase activity. In uremic rats, normal activity was found for this hydrolase and for tyrosine amino transferase, the first enzymatic step in the degradation of tyrosine (Wang *et al.*, 1975). Studies in normal humans also suggest that phenylalanine hydroxylation decreased during restricted protein intake (Jones *et al.*, 1978). Against an important role of the liver in reducing conversion of phenylalanine to tyrosine are observations that the splanchnic exchange of tyrosine and phenylalanine is normal in patients with chronic renal failure (Tizianello *et al.*, 1980b; Alvestrand *et al.*, 1987). However, tyrosine release from leg muscle was lower in uremic patients than in controls (Alvestrand *et al.*, 1987).

The diseased kidney may play a role in the reduced conversion of phenylalanine to tyrosine. The kidney produces tyrosine from phenylalanine in normal dogs and humans, and this activity decreased in renal deficiency (Fukuda and Kopple, 1980; Tizianello *et al.*, 1980b). Phenylalanine hydroxylase activity in uremic rat kidney was lower than that in controls (Wang *et al.*, 1975). We found that patients with renal failure on a low-protein plus essential amino acids diet minus tyrosine developed marked tyrosine depletion in muscle (Alvestrand *et al.*, 1982). This finding suggests that tyrosine may be indispensible in uremia and that uremic patients should receive tyrosine supplements.

### C. Tryptophan Metabolism

Tryptophan is unique among plasma amino acids in that 75% of circulating tryptophan is normally bound to serum albumin (Gulyassy *et al.*, 1972; de Torrente *et al.*, 1974). Total tryptophan concentration in plasma generally decreases in renal failure. However, this is largely an effect of reduced albumin binding, which results from displacement of binding sites on the albumin molecule by metabolites retained because of reduced renal function (de Torrente *et al.*, 1974). Free tryptophan concentrations in plasma have been found to be normal (Černáček *et al.*, 1980) or higher than normal (de Torrente *et al.*, 1974) in hemodialysis patients, whereas patients on an EAAH diet showed low free tryptophan concentrations (Černáček *et al.*, 1980). Tryptophan, like phenylalanine and tyrosine, is a precursor of neurotransmitters. It competes for transport into the central nervous system (CNS) with these amino acids and with valine, leucine, and isoleucine (Fernström and Wurtman, 1972). Because plasma levels of these five amino acids may change in uremia, this could affect their transport and metabolism in the CNS, resulting in an imbalance in neurotransmitter synthesis that could cause or contribute to encephalopathy (Biasioli *et al.*, 1986). Tryptophan requirements have not been extensively studied in uremia, and daily requirements remain to be defined.

### D. Histidine Metabolism

In our nitrogen-balance studies, chronically uremic patients on a histidine-free diet were given an intravenous or oral mixture of essential amino acids with added histidine. This treatment improved nitrogen balance more than could be accounted for by the nitrogen content of the added histidine (Bergström *et al.*, 1970; Bergström *et al.*, 1972). Addition of histidine to a histidine-free diet in two patients with chronic uremia also increased incorporation of [$^{14}$C]leucine into hemoglobin (Giordano *et al.*, 1972). In another study of histidine metabolism in chronic renal failure, [$^{15}$N]urea was given to two uremic patients and [$^{15}$N]ammonia to one normal subject and one nonuremic, catabolic subject. Normal and catabolic subjects incorporated the label into plasma and muscle protein, but uremic patients did not (Fürst, 1972). These data suggest that transamination and synthesis of the ketoacid analog of histidine (imidiazolepyruvic acid) do not occur normally in uremia. Histidine appears to be essential for uremic and normal humans, but daily requirements are not well established (Kopple and Swendseid, 1975; Kopple and Swendseid, 1978).

In dogs, rats, and humans, the normal kidney releases histidine, but amounts in humans are insignificant (Tizianello *et al.*, 1980a). Even less is released in chronic renal failure (Fukuda and Kopple, 1980). One explanation may be that carnosine (beta-alanylhistidine), a dipeptide with high intracellular concentration in skeletal muscle, is hydrolyzed by renal carnosinase (Fukuda and Kopple, 1979), and this reaction may be depressed in renal failure.

Rats with experimental chronic renal failure showed evidence of altered histidine metabolism. Muscle histidine levels were low, brain histidine and histamine were elevated, and plasma histidine was normal (Schmid *et al.*, 1978). In patients with chronic renal failure, we observed normal plasma histidine levels and low intracellular histidine concentrations in muscle (Table I) (Bergström *et al.*, 1978). We also found lower carnosine in uremic muscle than in controls (Bergström *et al.*, 1978; Alvestrand *et al.*, 1980; Fürst *et al.*, 1980b). In studies using [$^{14}$C]labeled histidine, no difference in histidine metabolism was found among normal and chronically uremic subjects (Jones *et al.*, 1982).

These data indicate that histidine should be considered an essential amino acid in both normal and uremic persons. It should be provided with other essential amino acids in diets containing low protein plus essential amino acids. The limited evidence that histidine cannot be synthesized by transamination from its 2-ketoacid analog precludes use of the analog as a substitute for the complete amino acid in the diet of uremic patients.

### E. Glycine and Serine Metabolism

The normal kidney converts glycine to serine and is a major endogenous source of serine (Pitts and MacLeod, 1972). Renal production of serine was low in patients with chronic renal failure (Tizianello *et al.*, 1980a). In uremic dogs, the low serine/glycine ratio was directly related to creatinine clearance (Fukuda and Kopple, 1980). These data suggest that the low plasma serine concentrations consistently found in chronic renal failure result from decreased production by the kidney.

In our studies of untreated patients with chronic uremia, intracellular serine concentrations in muscle were normal (Table I). However, intracellular serine concentrations were low in patients on hemodialysis (Table I) or on a low-protein diet supplemented with essential amino acids and ketoacids but without serine (Alvestrand *et al.*, 1983b; unpublished observations). Because serine is the only nonessential amino acid known to stimulate protein synthesis *in vitro* (Galbraith and Buse, 1981), these findings suggest that serine is indispensable for some patients with chronic renal failure.

### F. Metabolism of Urea Cycle Amino Acids

Many have found elevated plasma citrulline concentrations in patients with renal failure (Kopple, 1983). However, muscle concentrations of citrulline were similar in our studies in normal and chronically uremic subjects (Table I) (Alvestrand *et al.*, 1982). Significantly low intracellular arginine concentrations in muscle were found in our studies in one group of untreated patients with severe chronic renal failure but not in another (Table I) (Alvestrand *et al.*, 1982). After treatment with a modified low-protein plus essential amino acids diet, arginine concentrations were marginally low. We also found low plasma ornithine levels in chronically uremic patients without a corresponding decrease in intracellular ornithine in muscle (Table I) (Alvestrand *et al.*, 1982); the mechanism is not known.

It has been demonstrated that the kidney takes up citrulline and produces arginine in the rat (Featherston *et al.*, 1973) and in humans (Tizianello *et al.*, 1980a). Low arginine synthetase activity was observed in the kidney of uremic rats *in vitro* (Chan *et al.*, 1974). In patients with chronic renal failure, renal uptake of citrulline and release of arginine were low (Tizianello *et al.*, 1980a); similar observations were made in uremic dogs (Fukuda and Kopple, 1980). The suggestion that low extraction by the kidneys may cause hypercitrullinemia in renal failure has been questioned (Walser, 1980).

### G. Metabolism of Sulfuric Amino Acids

In chronic renal failure, plasma cystine concentrations are high, whereas methionine and taurine concentrations in plasma and muscle are usually normal. High plasma concentrations of free cystine, homocystine, cysteine–homocysteine disulfide, methionine, and taurine and of protein-bound cystine and homocystine were found in maintenance dialysis patients (Smolin *et al.*, 1987). Patients with acute renal failure receiving an intravenous amino acid mixture showed higher plasma levels and elimination half-life of methionine than normal subjects, but had normal clearance, suggesting that methionine turnover increases in uremia (Druml *et al.*, 1986). Normal metabolic clearance and increased turnover of methionine were also observed in chronic dialysis patients (Chami *et al.*, 1978).

In studies of acute renal failure in rats, plasma and liver concentrations of taurine increased 12–48 hours after nephrectomy (Michalk *et al.*, 1983). Skeletal muscle and brain taurine were normal in nephrectomized rats, but heart muscle taurine decreased. In rats with chronic renal failure (five-sixths nephrectomy), taurine concentrations were normal in plasma, skeletal muscle, and liver but high in heart muscle and brain.

Plasma taurine is usually normal in nondialyzed patients with chronic renal failure and high in male hemodialysis patients. In contrast, muscle intracellular taurine was low in patients treated with a low-protein plus essential amino acid diet and also in patients treated with maintenance hemodialysis and continuous ambulatory peritoneal dialysis (CAPD) (Alvestrand *et al.*, 1982; Lindholm *et al.*, 1986).

The cause of muscle intracellular taurine depletion in patients with chronic uremia is far from clear. Taurine concentrations in skeletal muscle, liver, and heart vary with dietary taurine intake in rats, whereas brain concentrations remain relatively constant irrespective of diet (Chesney *et al.*, 1986). The finding that the precursor amino acids cystine and methionine are normal or elevated in the presence of muscle taurine depletion suggests a metabolic block in taurine synthesis. We recently observed that plasma cysteine sulfinic acid is elevated in patients with chronic renal failure and low muscle taurine; this suggests a decrease in the activity of cysteine sulfinic acid decarboxylase, a key enzyme in taurine synthesis (Bergström *et al.*, 1987). Taurine degradation normally takes place slowly through bacterial action in the intestine. Whether the abnormal colonization of the upper gastrointestinal tract that occurs in uremia (Simenhoff *et al.*, 1978) plays a role by increasing taurine degradation has not been explored.

## III. TREATMENT WITH ESSENTIAL AMINO ACIDS

To compensate for deficiencies caused by specific amino acid abnormalities in muscle and to normalize free amino acid deficiencies, we changed our formulas for amino acid supplements for patients with uremia. Based on our early observations that histidine seemed to be indispensible in uremia, histidine was included in our first amino acid mixture (EAAH diet) for parenteral and oral nutrition of patients being treated with a low-protein plus essential amino acids diet (Bergström *et al.*, 1970; Bergström *et al.*, 1972; Fürst, 1972).

We also modified the proportion of branched-chain amino acids in our oral amino acid preparation by including more valine than leucine and adding tyrosine (NAAF diet). This change was based on our observation that chronically uremic patients on the EAAH diet still exhibited low intracellular valine concentrations in muscle, and also markedly decreased intracellular tyrosine concentrations (Table I). With the NAAF diet, we normalized the plasma aminogram and intracellular valine levels and increased intracellular tyrosine concentrations (Table I) (Alvestrand *et al.*, 1983b; unpublished observations). We also observed a slightly positive nitrogen balance in chronically uremic patients, suggesting that these patients were in nitrogen equilibrium (Alvestrand *et al.*, 1983a).

## IV. KETOACID ANALOGS

The 2-ketoanalogs of valine, leucine, isoleucine, and phenylalanine and the 2-hydroxyanalog of methionine have been used—instead of the corresponding essential amino acids—to supplement low-protein diets (Mitch and Walser, 1977). Transamination reactions transform these nitrogen-free analogs into the corresponding essential amino acids. Animal experiments have shown that all essential amino acids except lysine and threonine can be synthesized in the body (Walser *et al.*, 1973b). It has also been demonstrated that the alpha-ketoanalogs can be substituted for all essential amino acids except lysine and threonine in both healthy and uremic subjects (Richards *et al.*, 1972; Walser *et al.*, 1973a).

Theoretically, substituting ketoanalogs for the corresponding amino acids could provide essential carbon skeletons without nitrogen, thereby decreasing the nitrogen burden in severe renal failure. The ketoacid analog of leucine, alpha-ketoisocaproic acid (KICA), was shown to inhibit protein degradation in skeletal muscle, whereas leucine stimulated protein synthesis (Mitch and Clark, 1984).

The ketoanalogs of valine, isoleucine, leucine, and phenylalanine and the hydroxyanalog of methionine are generally provided as calcium salts, together with the essential amino acids lysine, threonine, histidine, tryptophan and tyrosine (Mitch and Walser, 1977). Ketoanalogs have also been given as salts of the dibasic amino acids ornithine or lysine rather than as calcium salts (Mitch *et al.*, 1982). Such ketoacid salts provide more amino groups on a molar basis than the corresponding essential amino acids because ornithine is a dibasic amino acid. Commercially available products contain ketoanalogs as calcium salts, either in molar proportions of essential amino acids (Rose's formula) (Rose *et al.*, 1955) without tyrosine (Zimmermann *et al.*, 1979) or, to compensate for less than 100% utilization of ketoanalogs as amino acids, in two to three times higher proportions of essential amino acids, with added tyrosine (modified Walser formula) (Rippich *et al.*, 1977).

Conversion of the ketoanalogs ketovaline and ketoleucine to amino acids occurred with about 50% efficacy in the rat (Laouari *et al.*, 1986). In normal and uremic human subjects, conversion of ketovaline and ketoleucine occurred with about 25–50% efficacy (Halliday *et al.*, 1981). However, with a very low-protein diet, ketoleucine conversion occurred with about 68–78% efficacy (Epstein *et al.*, 1980).

In our own studies, supplementing a low-protein plus essential amino acids diet with a ketoacid-analog mixture (modified Walser formula) failed to normalize intracellular amino acids after more than three months of treatment and resulted in a slightly negative nitrogen balance (Alvestrand *et al.*, 1983b). It is not known whether modifying the relative proportions of these ketoanalogs would provide any advantages over existing preparations.

## V. FUTURE TRENDS

Most studies have demonstrated that uremic patients have specific disturbances in amino acid metabolism and special amino acid requirements that cannot be met with a diet that provides optimal nutrition for nonuremic subjects. By providing essential amino acids in altered proportions to patients with chronic renal failure, we showed for the first time that some specific amino acid abnormalities could be corrected and that nitrogen utilization could be improved. However, many problems remain to be solved—especially the determination of requirements for specific amino acids—before optimal nutritional treatment of chronic renal failure can be achieved. These problems are even more important with regard to use of nitrogen-free ketoanalogs.

Based on our results of muscle free amino acid determinations in uremic patients (Table I) we hypothesize that tyrosine may need to be supplied in larger amounts to patients on low protein diets plus essential amino acids and that CAPD patients may also need extra tyrosine. Serine supplementation may also need to be considered in conservatively treated patients and in hemodialysis patients requiring amino acid supplementation.

The clinical importance of low muscle levels of taurine in conservatively treated or dialysis patients is unknown. However, taurine plays an important biological role in calcium transport and binding to membranes, in control of heart muscle contractions, and in the function of the retina (Hayes and Sturman, 1981). Therefore, it may be worthwhile to explore whether supplemental taurine might alleviate the fatigue, myopathy, central nervous system disturbances, and other pathological phenomena frequently encountered in uremic patients.

## ACKNOWLEDGMENTS

This work was supported by grants from the Swedish Medical Research Council, Grant No. 1002, and KabiVitrum AB. I am grateful to Dr. Anders Alvestrand for his help in preparing the manuscript and to Ms. Ann Hellström for outstanding secretarial service.

## REFERENCES

Acchiardo, S. R., Moore, L. W., and Latour, P. A. (1983). Malnutrition as the main factor in morbidity and mortality of hemodialysis patients. *Kidney Int.* **24** (Suppl. 16), S199–S203.

Alvestrand, A. (1983). "Amino Acid and Glucose Metabolism in Patients With Chronic Renal Failure: A Clinical and Experimental Study" (thesis). Karolinska Institute, Stockholm.

Alvestrand, A., Bergström, J., Fürst, P., Germanis, G., and Widstam, U. (1978). The effect of essential amino acid supplementation on muscle and plasma free amino acids in chronic uremia. *Kidney Int.* **14**, 323–329.

Alvestrand, A., Bergström, J., and Fürst, P. (1980). Carnosine metabolism in uremia. *In* "Histidine II. Laboratory and Clinical Aspects. Therapeutic Use of Histidine and Zinc. Proceedings of the 2nd International Workshop on Histidine" (G. Partsch and S. Batsford, eds.), pp. 26–31. Georg Thieme Verlag, Stuttgart.

Alvestrand, A., Fürst, P., and Bergström, J. (1982). Plasma and muscle free amino acids in uremia: influence of nutrition with amino acids. *Clin. Nephrol.* **18**, 297–305.

Alvestrand, A., Ahlberg, M., Fürst, P., and Bergström, J. (1983a). Clinical results of long-term treatment with a low protein diet and new amino acid preparation in patients with chronic uremia. *Clin. Nephrol.* **19**, 67–73.

Alvestrand, A., Fürst, P., and Bergström, J. (1983b). Intracellular amino acids in uremia. *Kidney Int.* **24** (Suppl. 16), S9–S16.

Alvestrand, A., DeFronzo, R. A., Smith, D., and Wahren, J. (1987). Influence of hyperinsulinemia on intracellular amino acid levels and amino acid exchange across splanchnic and leg tissues in uremia. *Clin. Sci.* (In press.)

Bergström, J., and Alvestrand, A. (1984). Therapy with branched-chain amino acids and keto acids in chronic uremia. *In* "Branched-Chain Amino Acids and Keto Acids in Health and Disease" (S. A. Adibi, W. Fekl, and U. Langenbeck, eds.), pp. 391–422. S. Karger, Basel.

Bergström, J., Fürst, P., Josephson, B., and Norée, L. O. (1970). Improvement of nitrogen balance in a uremic patient by the addition of histidine to essential amino acid solutions given intravenously. *Life Sci.* **9**, 787–794.

Bergström, J., Bucht, H., Fürst, P., Hultman, E., Josephson, B., and Norée, L. O. (1972). Intravenous nutrition with amino acid solutions in patients with chronic uremia. *Acta Med. Scand.* **191**, 359–367.

Bergström, J., Fürst, P., Norée, L. O., and Vinnars, E. (1978). Intracellular free amino acids in muscle tissue of patients with chronic uremia: Effect of peritoneal dialysis and infusion of essential amino acids. *Clin. Sci. Mol. Med.* **54**, 51–60.

Bergström, J., Qureshi, G. A., and Rashed Qureshi, A. (1987). Inhibition of cysteine sulphinic acid decarboxylase (CSD) as a cause of taurine (TAU) depletion in uremia [Abstract]. *Nephrol. Dial. Transplant.* (In press.)

Biasioli, S., D'Andrea, G., Feriani, M., Charamonte, S., Fabris, A., Ronco, C., and La Greca, G. (1986). Uremic encephalopathy; an updating. *Clin. Nephrol.* **25**, 57–63.

Broyer, M., Jean, G., Dartois, A. M., and Kleinknecht, C. (1980). Plasma and muscle free amino acids in children at the early stages of renal failure. *Amer. J. Clin. Nutr.* **33**, 1396–1401.

Budd, M. A., Tanaka, K., Holmes, L. B., Efron, M. L., Crawford, J. D., and Isselbacher, K. J. (1967). Isovaleric acidemia: Clinical features of a new genetic defect of leucine metabolism. *N. Engl. J. Med.* **277**, 321–327.

Černáček, P., Becvarova, H., Gerova, Z., Valek, A., and Spustova, V. (1980). Plasma tryptophan level in chronic renal failure. *Clin. Nephrol.* **14**, 246–249.

Chami, J., Reidenberg, M. M., Wellner, D., David, D. S., Rubin, A. L., and Stenzel, K. H. (1976). Essential amino acid metabolism in maintenance dialysis patients. *Trans. Amer. Soc. Artif. Internal Organs* **22**, 168–173.

Chami, J., Reidenberg, M. M., Wellner, D., David, D. S., Rubin, A. L., and Stenzel, K. H. (1978). Pharmacokinetics of essential amino acids in chronic dialysis patients. *Amer. J. Clin. Nutr.* **31**, 1652–1659.

Chan, W., Wang, M., Kopple, J. D., and Swendseid, M. E. (1974). Citrulline levels and urea cycle enzymes in uremic rats. *J. Nutr.* **104**, 678–683.

Chesney, R. W., Lippincott, S., Gusowski, N., Padilla, M., and Zelikovic, I. (1986). Studies on renal adaptation to altered dietary amino acid intake: Tissue taurine responses in nursing and adult rats. *J. Nutr.* **116**, 1965–1976.

Connelly, J. L., Danner, D. J., and Bowden, J. A. (1968). Branched chain alpha-ketoacid metabolism: I. Isolation, purification, and partial characterization of bovine liver alpha-keto-isocaproic: Alpha-keto-beta-methylvaleric acid dehydrogenase. *J. Biol. Chem.* **243**, 1198–1203.

Deferrari, G., Garibotto, G., Robaudo, C., Ghiggeri, G. M., and Tizianello, A. (1981). Brain metabolism of amino acids and ammonia in patients with chronic renal insufficiency. *Kidney Int.* **20**, 505–510.

Deferrari, G., Garibotto, G., Robaudo, C., Saffioti, S., Paoletti, E., Passerone, G. C., and Tizianello, A. (1987). Abnormalities in amino acid metabolism in patients with chronic renal failure. *In* "New Perspectives in Diagnosis and Treatment of Kidney Disease, Contributions to Nephrology" (G. D'Amico and G. Colasanti, eds.), Vol. 55, pp. 11–19. S. Karger, Basel.

DeFronzo, R. A., Smith, D., and Alvestrand, A. (1983). Insulin action in uremia. *Kidney Int.* **24** (Suppl. 16), S102–S114.

Delaporte, C., Jean, G., and Broyer, M. (1978). Free plasma and muscle amino acids in uremic children. *Amer. J. Clin. Nutr.* **31**, 1647–1651.

de Torrente, A., Glazer, G. B., and Gulyassy, P. (1974). Reduced *in vitro* binding of tryptophan by plasma in uremia. *Kidney Int.* **6**, 222–229.

Druml, W., Bürger, U., and Kleinberger, G. (1983). Renal failure: Metabolism and supply of amino acids. *In* "New Aspects of Clinical Nutrition. Proceedings of the 4th Congress of the European Society for Parenteral and Enteral Nutrition" (G. Kleinberger, ed.), pp. 412–421. S. Karger, Basel.

Druml, W., Bürger, U., Kleinberger, G., Lenz, K., and Laggner, A. (1986). Elimination of amino acids in renal failure. *Nephron* **42**, 62–67.

Epstein, C. M., Chawla, R. K., Wadsworth, A., and Rudman, D. (1980). Decarboxylation of alpha-ketoisovaleric acid after oral administration in man. *Amer. J. Clin. Nutr.* **33**, 1968–1974.

Featherston, W. R., Rogers, Q. R., and Freedland, R. A. (1973). Relative importance of kidney and liver in synthesis of arginine by the rat. *Biochem. J.* **224**, 127–129.

Fernström, J. D., and Wurtman, R. J. (1972). Brain serotonin content: Physiological regulation by plasma neutral amino acids. *Science* **178**, 414–417.

Fukuda, S., and Kopple, J. D. (1979). Evidence that dog kidney is an endogenous source of histidine. *Amer. J. Physiol.* **237**, E1–E5.

Fukuda, S., and Kopple, J. D. (1980). Uptake and release of amino acids by the kidney of dogs made chronically uremic with uranyl nitrate. *Min. Elect. Metab.* **3**, 248–260.

Fürst, P. (1972). $^{15}N$-studies in severe renal failure. II. Evidence for the essentiality of histidine. *Scand. J. Clin. Lab. Invest.* **30**, 307–312.

Fürst, P., Alvestrand, A., and Bergström, J. (1980a). Effects of nutrition and catabolic stress on intracellular amino acid pools in uremia. *Amer. J. Clin. Nutr.* **33**, 1387–1395.

Fürst, P., Bergström, J., Holmstrom, B., Liljedahl, S. O., Neuhäuser, M., and Vinnars, E. (1980b). *N*-Methylhistidine (3-methylhistidine) in trauma. *In* "Histidine II. Laboratory and Clinical Aspects. Therapeutic Use of Histidine and Zinc. Proceedings of the 2nd International Workshop on Histidine" (G. Partsch and S. Batsford, eds.), pp. 34–43. Georg Thieme Verlag, Stuttgart.

Galbraith, R. A., and Buse, M. G. (1981). Effects of serine on protein synthesis and insulin receptors. *Amer. J. Physiol.* **241**, C167–C171.

Giordano, C., DeSanto, N. G., Rinaldi, S., De Pascale, C., and Pluvio, M. (1972). Histidine and glycine essential amino acids in uremia. *In* "Uremia: An International Conference on Pathogenesis, Diagnosis, and Therapy" (R. Kluthe, G. Berlyne, and B. Burton, eds.), pp. 138–143. Georg Thieme Verlag, Stuttgart.

Guarnieri, G., Toigo, G., Situlin, R., Faccini, L., Coli, U., Landini, S., Bazzato, G., Dardi, F., and Campanacci, L. (1983). Muscle biopsy studies in chronically uremic patients: Evidence for malnutrition. *Kidney Int.* **24** (Suppl. 16), S187–S193.

Gulyassy, P. F., Peters, J. H., and Schoenfeld, P. (1972). Transport and protein binding of tryptophan in uremia. *In* "Uremia: An International Conference on Pathogenesis, Diagnosis, and Therapy" (R. Kluthe, G. Berlyne, and B. Burton, eds.), pp. 163–170. Georg Thieme Verlag, Stuttgart.

Halliday, D., Madigan, M., Chalmers, R. A., Purkiss, P., Ell, S., Bergström, J., Fürst, P., Neuhäuser, M., and Richards, P. (1981). The degree of conversion of alpha-keto acids to valine and phenylalanine in health and uraemia. *Q. J. Med.* **50**, 53–62.

Hayes, K. C., and Sturman, J. A. (1981). Taurine in metabolism. *Ann. Rev. Nutr.* **1**, 401–425.

Ichihara, A., and Koyama, E. (1966). Transaminase of branched chain amino acids. I. Branched chain amino acids—alpha-ketoglutarate transaminase. *J. Biochem. (Tokyo)* **59**, 160–169.

Jones, M. R., and Kopple, J. D. (1978). Valine metabolism in normal and chronically uremic man. *Amer. J. Clin. Nutr.* **31**, 1660–1664.

Jones, M. R., Kopple, J. D., and Swendseid, M. E. (1978). Phenylalanine metabolism in uremic and normal man. *Kidney Int.* **14**, 169–179.

Jones, M. R., Kopple, J. D., and Swendseid, M. E. (1982). $^{14}CO_2$ expiration after $^{14}C$-histidine administration in normal and uremic men ingesting two levels of histidine. *Amer. J. Clin. Nutr.* **35**, 15–23.

Jones, R., Dalton, N., Turner, C., Start, K., Haycock, G., and Chantler, C. (1983). Oral essential amino acid and keto acid supplements in children with chronic renal failure. *Kidney Int.* **24**, 95–103.

Kleiner, M. J., Tate, S. S., Sullivan, J. F., and Chami, J. (1980). Vitamin $B_6$ deficiency in maintenance dialysis patients: Effects of repletion. *Amer. J. Clin. Nutr.* **33**, 1612–1619.

Kopple, J. D. (1983). Amino acid metabolism in chronic renal failure. *In* "Amino Acids. Metabolism and Medical Applications" (G. L. Blackburn, J. P. Grant, and V. R. Young, eds.), pp. 451–471. John Wright PSG Inc., Boston.

Kopple, J. D., and Swendseid, M. E. (1975). Evidence that histidine is an essential amino acid in normal and chronically uremic man. *J. Clin. Invest.* **55**, 881–891.

Kopple, J. D., and Swendseid, M. E. (1978). Effect of histidine intake on plasma and urine. Histidine levels, nitrogen balance and *N*-methylhistidine excretion in normal and chronically uremic men. *J. Nutr.* **111**, 931–942.

Kopple, J. D., Flugel, R., and Jones, M. R. (1981). Branched chain amino acids in chronic renal failure. *In* "Metabolism and Clinical Implications of Branched Chain Amino and Ketoacids. Developments in Biochemistry" (M. Walser and J. R. Williamson, eds.), Vol. 18, pp. 555–567. Elsevier/North Holland, New York.

Laouari, D., Kamoun, P. P., Rocchiccioli, F., Dodu, C., Kleinknecht, C., and Broyer, M. (1986). Efficiency of substitution of 2-ketoisocaproic acid and 2-ketoisovaleric acid in the diet of normal and uremic growing rats. *Amer. J. Clin. Nutr.* **44**, 832–846.

Letteri, J. M., and Scipione, R. A. (1974). Phenylalanine metabolism in chronic renal failure. *Nephron* **13**, 365–371.

Lindholm, B., Alvestrand, A., and Bergström, J. (1986). Muscle free amino acids in patients treated with CAPD. *In* "Frontiers in Peritoneal Dialysis" (J. F. Maher and J. F. Winchester, eds.), pp. 400–404. Field, Rich and Associates, Inc., New York.

Manchester, K. L. (1970). Sites of hormonal regulation of protein metabolism. *In* "Mammalian Protein Metabolism" (H. N. Munro, ed.), Vol. 4, pp. 229–298. Academic Press, New York.

Michalk, D. V., Essich, H. J., Böhles, H. J., and Schärer, K. (1983). Taurine metabolism in experimental renal failure. *Kidney Int.* **24** (Suppl. 15), S16–S21.

Mitch, W. E., and Clark, A. S. (1984). Specificity of the effect of leucine and its metabolites on protein degradation in skeletal muscle. *Biochem. J.* **222**, 579–586.

Mitch, W. E., and Walser, M. (1977). Nitrogen balance of uremic patients receiving branched-chain keto acids and the hydroxy-analogue of methionine as substitutes for the respective amino acids. *Clin. Nephrol.* **8**, 341–344.

Mitch, W. E., Abras, E., and Walser, M. (1982). Long-term effects of a new keto acid-amino acid supplement in patients with chronic renal failure. *Kidney Int.* **22**, 48–53.

Odessey, R., and Goldberg, A. L. (1972). Oxidation of leucine by rat skeletal muscle. *Amer. J. Physiol.* **22**, 1376–1383.

Pickford, J. C., McGale, E. H. F., and Aber, G. M. (1973). Studies on the metabolism of phenylalanine and tyrosine in patients with renal disease. *Clin. Chim. Acta* **48**, 77–83.

Pitts, R. F., and MacLeod, M. B. (1972). Synthesis of serine by the dog kidney *in vivo*. *Amer. J. Physiol.* **222**, 394–398.

Pye, I. F., McGale, E. H. F., Stonier, C., Hutchinson, E. C., and Aber, G. M. (1979). Studies of cerebrospinal fluid and plasma amino acids in patients with steady-state chronic renal failure. *Clin. Chim. Acta* **92**, 65–72.

Randle, P. J. (1981). Discussion. *In* "Metabolism and Clinical Implications of Branched Chain Amino and Ketoacids. Developments in Biochemistry" (M. Walser and J. R. Williamson, eds.), Vol. 18, p. 619. Elsevier/North Holland, New York.

Richards, P., Brown, C. L., Houghton, B. J., and Lowe, S. M. (1972). Synthesis of tryptophan from 3-indolepyruvic acid by a healthy woman. *J. Nutr.* **102**, 1547–1550.

Rippich, T., Katz, N., Mix, A., and Kluthe, R. (1977). Applikation von Ketoanalogen essentialler Aminosauren bei chronischer Niereninsuffizienz. Erste Erfahrungen. *Z. Ernähr. Wiss.* (Suppl. 19), 43–54.

Rose, W. C., Wixom, R. L., Lockhardt, H. B., and Lambert, G. F. (1955). The amino acid requirements of man. XV. The valine requirement: Summary and final observations. *J. Biol. Chem.* **217**, 987–995.

Schauder, P., Matthaei, D., Scheler, F., Mench-Hoinowski, A., and Langenbeck, U. (1979).

Blood levels of branched-chain alpha-keto acids in uremia: Therapeutic implications. *Klin. Wochenschr.* **57**, 825–830.

Schauder, P., Matthaei, D., Henning, H. V., Scheler, F., and Langenbeck, U. (1981). Blood levels of branched-chain-alpha-keto acids in uremia: Effect of an oral glucose tolerance test. *Klin. Wochenschr.* **59**, 845–849.

Schmid, G., Przuntek, H., Fricke, L., Heidland, A., and Hempel, K. (1978). Increased histidine and histamine content in the brain of chronic uremic rats. Cause of enhanced cerebral cyclic adenosine monophosphate in uremia? *Amer. J. Clin. Nutr.* **31**, 1665–1668.

Shinnic, F. L., and Harper, E. A. (1977). Effects of branched-chain amino acid antagonism in the rat on tissue amino acid and keto acid concentrations. *J. Nutr.* **107**, 887–895.

Simenhoff, M. L., Saukkonen, J. J., Burke, J. F., Wesson, L. G., Schaedler, R. W., and Gordon, S. J. (1978). Bacterial populations of the small intestine in uremia. *Nephron* **22**, 63–66.

Smolin, L. A., Laidlaw, S. A., and Kopple, J. D. (1987). Altered plasma free and protein-bound sulfur amino acids levels in patients undergoing maintenance hemodialysis. *Amer. J. Clin. Nutr.* **45**, 737–743.

Stonier, C., McGale, E. H., and Aber, G. M. (1984). Studies of phenylalanine hydroxylase activity in patients with chronic renal failure: The effect of haemodialysis. *Clin. Chim. Acta* **143**, 115–122.

Takala, J. (1983). Total plasma clearance of intravenous essential amino acids: evidence of abnormal metabolism of amino acids in chronic renal failure. *JPEN* **7**, 146–150.

Tizianello, A., Deferrari, G., Garibotto, G., Gurreri, G., and Robaudo, C. (1980a). Renal metabolism of amino acids and ammonia in subjects with normal renal function and in patients with chronic renal insufficiency. *J. Clin. Invest.* **65**, 1162–1173.

Tizianello, A., Deferrari, G., Garibotto, G., and Robaudo, C. (1980b). Amino acid metabolism and the liver in renal failure. *Amer. J. Clin. Nutr.* **33**, 1354–1362.

Tizianello, A., Deferrari, G., Garibotto, G., Robaudo, C., Lutman, M., Paserone, G., and Bruzzone, M. (1983). Branched-chain amino acid metabolism in chronic renal failure. *Kidney Int.* **24**, 17–22.

Walser, M. (1980). Determinants of ureagenesis, with particular reference to renal failure. *Kidney Int.* **17**, 709–721.

Walser, M., Coulter, A. W., Dighe, S., and Crantz, F. R. (1973a). The effect of keto-analogues of essential amino acids in severe chronic uremia. *J. Clin. Invest.* **52**, 678–690.

Walser, M., Lund, P., Ruderman, N. B., and Coulter, A. W. (1973b). Synthesis of essential amino acids from their alpha-keto analogues by perfused rat liver and muscle. *J. Clin. Invest.* **52**, 2865–2877.

Wang, M., Vyhmeister, I., Swendseid, M. E., and Kopple, J. D. (1975). Phenylalanine hydroxylase and tyrosine aminotransferase activities in chronically uremic rats. *J. Nutr.* **105**, 122–127.

Young, G. A., and Parsons, F. M. (1973). Impairment of phenylalanine hydroxylation in chronic renal insufficiency. *Clin. Sci. Mol. Med.* **45**, 89–97.

Young, G. A., Swanepoel, C. R., Croft, M. R., Hobson, S. M., and Parsons, F. M. (1982). Anthropometry and plasma valine, amino acids, and protein in the nutritional assessment of hemodialysis patients. *Kidney Int.* **21**, 492–499.

Young, V. R., and Pellett, L. (1987). Protein intake and requirements with reference to diet and health. *Amer. J. Clin. Nutr.* **45**, 1323–1343.

Zimmermann, E. W., Meisinger, E., Weinel, B., and Strauch, M. (1979). Essential amino acid/keto analogue supplementation: an alternative to unrestricted protein intake in uremia. *Clin. Nephrol.* **11**, 71–78.

# 13

# Alcohol and Malnutrition in the Pathogenesis of Alcoholic Liver Disease

Esteban Mezey

*Alcohol Research Center*
*Department of Medicine*
*The Johns Hopkins University School of Medicine*
*Baltimore, Maryland*



## I. INTRODUCTION

In the pathogenesis of alcoholic liver disease, the incidence of alcoholic hepatitis and cirrhosis correlates with the amount and duration of alcohol consumption (Lelbach, 1972). Cirrhosis has developed in baboons fed an adequate diet containing 50% of calories as ethanol (Lieber *et al.*, 1975). However, only one-third or less of heavy drinkers (Mezey, 1982) or baboons fed alcohol (Lieber *et al.*, 1975) develop cirrhosis. For these reasons, other factors—including genetic predisposition, immune response, hormones, environment, and nutrition—may be important in the pathogenesis of alcoholic liver disease.

The following observations suggest an influence of nutritional deficiencies in the cause and progression of alcoholic liver disease:

1. Nutritional deficiencies frequently occur in alcoholic patients.
2. An association has been found between the degree of malnutrition and the severity of liver disease.
3. Fibrosis and cirrhosis have developed in some animals fed alcohol combined with a lipotrope-deficient diet.
4. A high prevalence of fatty liver and cirrhosis exists in malnourished populations.
5. The histopathology of alcoholic hepatitis bears a striking resemblance to that of liver diseases attributed to metabolic abnormalities such as liver injury arising after jejunoileal bypass, and in diabetes mellitus.
6. Nutritional therapy has lowered morbidity and mortality in patients with alcoholic hepatitis.

## II. RELATIONSHIP BETWEEN NUTRITIONAL STATUS AND SEVERITY OF LIVER DISEASE

Nutritional deficiencies are well-documented in alcoholic liver disease, but their role in the development of liver disease remains controversial. In the Veterans Administration (VA) Cooperative Study on alcoholic hepatitis, an association was found between the degree of protein-calorie malnutrition and the severity of illness and mortality (Mendenhall *et al.*, 1986). This finding underscores the importance of nutritional status in alcoholic liver disease.

Low dietary intake is the principal cause of nutritional deficiencies (Mezey, 1978). Also, decreased intestinal absorption, decreased hepatic storage, metabolic abnormalities, increased nutrient losses, and increased nutrient requirements all contribute to malnutrition. Dietary histories are generally unreliable in alcoholic patients. Nevertheless, a history of grossly substandard diets was reported by 73% of 124 alcoholic patients with cirrhosis and hepatic failure (Patek *et al.*, 1948) and by 64% of 172 alcoholic patients with liver diseases (Leevy *et al.*, 1965). In another study, poor dietary intake, defined as one meal or less per day for 10 days before admission to the hospital, was found in 68% of 56 alcoholic patients with hepatomegaly caused by fatty infiltration of the liver (Mezey and Faillace, 1971).

Table I summarizes five studies of the mean daily caloric intake and the contribution of ethanol and protein to dietary intake in patients with alcoholic hepatitis and cirrhosis. In the first four studies (three in the United States and one in Great Britain), ethanol contributed 47 to 63% of total calories, whereas protein varied between 50 and 64 g/day and contributed 6 to 10% of total calories. In one study, intake of protein and calories by alcoholics without cirrhosis was 13% higher than by those with cirrhosis (Patek *et al.*, 1975). Alcoholics without liver disease had 9% higher intake of calories and 15% higher intake of protein than a group with alcoholic hepatitis (Mendenhall *et al.*, 1984). On the other hand, in a survey of French cirrhotics, ethanol contributed only 22% of calories, and total protein intake was 81 g/day—only slightly lower than that of 89 g/day in a control population (Pequignot and Tuyns, 1980).

In the four studies reporting a relatively low protein intake, intake still exceeded the Recommended Daily Allowance (RDA) for protein. However, it is quite likely that protein requirements increase in alcoholics because of malabsorption, high urinary nitrogen losses, and repair of tissue injury. In patients with decompensated cirrhosis, protein intake of up to 75 g/day was required to maintain nitrogen balance (Gabuzda and Davidson, 1954). In the VA study, an association was found between the intake of nonalcohol calories and protein and the severity of alcoholic hepatitis (Mendenhall *et al.*, 1986).

## III. DIGESTION AND ABSORPTION

Alcoholics with and without liver disease frequently have intestinal malabsorption and pancreatic dysfunction after heavy alcohol ingestion. Substances found to be malabsorbed include D-xylose, amino acids, and vitamins such as thiamine, folic acid, and cobalamin (Mezey, 1975). Mild steatorrhea, a common condition, is caused by decreased pancreatic function and low lipase output rather than by decreased intestinal absorption of fat. An increase in fecal excretion of nitrogen to $>2.75$ g/day was found in 52% of alcoholic patients (Roggin *et al.*, 1969). The abnormalities of intestinal absorption and digestion are readily reversible to normal after institution of abstinence and a normal diet. Both ethanol and dietary deficiencies, such as folic acid deficiency, cause intestinal malabsorption (Halsted *et al.*, 1973). Ethanol also inhibits active transport of low concentrations of thiamine by intestinal loops (Hoyumpa *et al.*, 1975). However, this inhibition can be overcome by administering large concentrations of thiamine, which is then absorbed by passive movement. In advanced cirrhosis, steatorrhea can be more marked and permanent. The principal cause of this steatorrhea is decreased synthesis and excretion of bile acids, which results in a decrease in intestinal bile acids, below the concentration required for the formation of micelles (Badley *et al.*, 1970).

**TABLE I**

**Caloric Intake in Alcoholic Hepatitis and Cirrhosis**

| Numbers of patients | Total | Alcohol | | Nonalcohol | Protein | | |
|---|---|---|---|---|---|---|---|
| | kcal | kcal | % of Intake | kcal | kcal | % of Intake | g/day |
| 195[a] | 3,394 | 1,864 | 55 | 1,530 | 200 | 6.0 | 50 |
| 26[b] | >2,210 | >1,400 | >63 | 810 | 224 | <10.1 | 56 |
| 30[c] | 2,452 | 1,275 | 52 | 1,177 | 234 | 9.5 | 58 |
| 352[d] | 3,409 | 1,595 | 47 | 1,814 | 256 | 7.5 | 64 |
| 184[e] | 3,436 | 770 | 22 | 2,666 | 324 | 9.4 | 81 |

[a]Data from Patek *et al.*, 1975.

[b]All patients reported ingesting >200 g of ethanol/day. Alcohol calories were calculated using a minimum alcohol intake of 200 g/day. (Data from Pichumoni *et al.*, 1980.)

[c]Liver biopsies of all patients revealed fatty liver in 11, cirrhosis in 12, and alcoholic hepatitis in 11. (Data from Mills *et al.*, 1983.)

[d]All patients had alcoholic hepatitis of varying severity. Data were calculated for the entire patient population. (Data from Mendenhall *et al.*, 1984.)

[e]Data from Pequignot and Tuyns, 1980.

## IV. METABOLIC ABNORMALITIES IN LIVER DISEASE

Abnormalities in protein, carbohydrate, lipid, vitamin, and mineral metabolism occur in liver disease. These abnormalities often have significant effects on the nutritional status of patients and on their ability to recover from liver injury.

The basal metabolic rate is normal in compensated, stable cirrhosis. However, the metabolism of dietary constituents is abnormal, and catabolism develops rapidly after an overnight fast. In cirrhotic subjects who fasted overnight, the percentage of energy derived from carbohydrate fell while the percentage derived from fat rose. Similar values are obtained only after 36 to 72 hours of fasting in normal subjects. The percentage of energy derived from protein did not change in the fasted cirrhotic subjects, but it remained remarkably high in view of the marked depletion of muscle mass in many of these patients (Owen *et al.*, 1983).

Inadequate glycogen stores, which result in a low level of readily available glucose, appear to be responsible for these abnormalities in protein and carbohydrate metabolism. Thus, the cirrhotic patient's energy needs appear to be met by increased gluconeogenesis, lipolysis, and fatty acid oxidation. The high demand for protein for gluconeogenesis and repair of liver injury results in enhanced release of amino acids from muscle, which contributes to the muscle wasting commonly observed in patients with cirrhosis.

Preferential catabolism of many amino acids occurs in the liver, whereas branched-chain amino acids are preferentially removed by extrahepatic tissues. In chronic liver disease, the plasma concentrations of amino acids normally removed by the liver tend to rise, while levels of those principally taken up by extrahepatic tissues tend to fall. Therefore, the most common plasma amino acid pattern observed in chronic liver disease consists of increases in aromatic amino acids—tyrosine, phenylalanine, glutamic acid, methionine, and sometimes cystine—and decreases in branched chain amino acids—valine, leucine, and isoleucine (Zinneman *et al.*, 1969; Rosen *et al.*, 1977).

Pyridoxal-5′-phosphate (PLP), the biologically active form of pyridoxine, is a coenzyme in numerous steps of amino acid metabolism. Decreasing levels of plasma PLP were common in alcoholic patients with (Labadarios *et al.*, 1977) and without (Lumeng and Li, 1974) liver dysfunction. The decreases in PLP did not result from decreased production but from accelerated degradation of this vitamin. Acetaldehyde displaced PLP from its binding protein, thereby making PLP susceptible to hydrolysis by membrane-bound alkaline phosphatase (Lumeng and Li, 1974). Accelerated degradation of PLP also occurred in nonalcoholic cirrhotic patients (Labadarios *et al.*, 1977). The mechanism for increased degradation of PLP in liver disease is unknown.

Chronic PLP deficiency changes intermediate metabolism of amino acids and may be a factor in the pathogenesis of alcoholic liver disease. After administration of pyridoxine-deficient diets, rats developed mild fatty liver (French and Castagna, 1967), and monkeys developed cirrhosis (Wizgird *et al.*, 1965). These potentially important observations need further study. No association between chronic pyridoxine deficiency and liver dysfunction has been demonstrated in humans.

## V. INFLUENCE OF LIPOTROPE-DEFICIENT DIETS

Early studies of nutrition and alcoholic liver disease focused on the potential role of dietary deficiencies of lipotropes, which mobilize fat from the liver. Fatty infiltration of the liver and cirrhosis developed in rats fed diets deficient in the lipotropes choline and methionine (Best *et al.*, 1949). However, primates and humans were less susceptible to lipotrope deficiency than rats (Sidranski and Farber, 1960). Species differences in susceptibility to choline deficiency may be explained by differences in choline degradation by the enzyme choline oxidase, which has high activity in rats but very low activity in humans (Sidranski and Farber, 1960). Alcohol administration appeared to increase requirements for choline in the rat (Klatskin *et al.*, 1954). In the first primate model of alcohol-induced liver disease, cirrhosis developed in one-third of baboons fed alcohol and a diet with a choline content of 100 mg/1,000 kcal (Lieber *et al.*, 1975). In two subsequent studies in macaque monkeys fed the same diet, but with a higher choline content of 400 mg/1,000 kcal, chronic alcohol ingestion resulted only in fatty liver without fibrosis or cirrhosis (Rogers *et al.*, 1981; Mezey *et al.*, 1983). In a more recent study of chronic alcoholism in five baboons, a dietary choline content of 500 mg/1,000 kcal did not prevent perivenular fibrosis in two and cirrhosis in one of the experimental animals (Lieber *et al.*, 1985). Species differences in susceptibility to hepatic injury from alcohol, to choline deficiency, and to the combination of the two probably underlie the differences in results of studies of rats, macaque monkeys, and baboons.

## VI. LIVER DISEASE IN MALNOURISHED POPULATIONS

Fatty infiltration of the liver and fibrosis occur in children with kwashiorkor (Cook and Hutt, 1967), and cirrhosis is common in some malnourished populations in underdeveloped countries (Borhanmanesh *et al.*, 1971; Gillman and Gilbert, 1974). However, these observations do not necessarily implicate malnutrition as a cause of liver disease. A toxin or virus could be the actual cause, and malnutrition may be important only in aggravating the disease. Indeed, following World War II, undernourished civilians did not have evidence of hepatocellular damage (Sherlock and Walshe, 1948), whereas heavy drinkers in France developed cirrhosis despite an average daily protein intake of 80 g or more (Pequignot and Tuyns, 1980).

## VII. HISTOPATHOLOGY RESEMBLING ALCOHOLIC LIVER DISEASE IN OTHER DISEASES

The whole spectrum of histopathology characteristic of alcoholic liver disease—fatty liver, pericentral fibrosis, hepatitis, and cirrhosis—has been found after jejunoileal bypass for morbid obesity (Galambos, 1976) and in diabetes mellitus (Itoh *et al.*, 1982).

### A. Morbidly Obese and Jejunoileal Bypass Patients

Even before surgery, patients with morbid obesity often have fatty infiltration of the liver and sometimes mild pericentral and pericellular fibrosis (Galambos, 1976; Marubbio *et al.*, 1976). In the first year following jejunoileal bypass, fatty infiltration increased and fibrosis worsened in 50% of patients (Galambos, 1976). In other studies, cirrhosis developed in 3.4% of 88 patients (Marubbio *et al.*, 1976) and in 9.0% of 45 patients (Campbell *et al.*, 1977) one or two years following surgery. Most of these patients reported no history of significant alcohol consumption, suggesting other factors as the cause of cirrhosis.

Protein malnutrition and production of a hepatotoxic substance by bacteria residing in the bypassed intestinal loop have been suggested as possible causes of the hepatic lesions complicating jejunoileal bypass for morbid obesity.

Changes in plasma amino acids during the rapid weight-loss phase after surgery were similar to those in protein-calorie malnutrition. These amino acid abnormalities disappeared as the patients' weight stabilized. Oral amino acid supplements did not prevent postoperative liver abnormalities (Lockwood *et al.*, 1977). However, intravenous infusion of amino acids reversed severe fatty infiltration and liver dysfunction in a few patients (Heimburger *et al.*, 1975).

In support of the hypotheses that liver abnormalities result from production of a hepatotoxic substance in the bypassed intestinal loop are experiments demonstrating that jejunoileal bypass in dogs resulted in liver dysfunction and death, whereas resection of a similar length of intestine to that of the bypassed intestine did not (Bondar and Pisesky, 1967).

Furthermore, antibiotics prevented fatty infiltration and death after intestinal bypass in dogs (Hollenbeck *et al.*, 1975). Among possible hepatotoxic substances studied have been two produced by intestinal bacteria—lithocholic acid, produced from chenodeoxycholic acid (Sherr *et al.*, 1977), and ethanol, produced from carbohydrate (Mezey *et al.*, 1975). Neither was found to be significantly elevated in the serum of patients after jejunoileal bypass. However, possible elevations in portal vein levels of ethanol and lithocholic acid need to be considered in the pathogenesis of the liver disease.

### B. Diabetes Mellitus Patients

Diabetes mellitus is associated with an increased prevalence of hepatic dysfunction and cirrhosis (Falchuk *et al.*, 1980; Bloodworth, 1961), but the pathogenesis of liver disease in diabetes mellitus is unknown. Hyperglycemia caused by prolonged infusion of hypertonic glucose results in fatty liver in experimental animals (Chang and Silvis, 1974) and in humans (Sheldon *et al.*, 1978). Insulin deficiency is associated with many metabolic abnormalities, including decreased mitochondrial function (Harano *et al.*, 1972) and decreased protein synthesis (Moxley *et al.*, 1974), which may adversely affect the liver (Reaven *et al.*, 1973).

## VIII. EFFECT OF NUTRITIONAL THERAPY ON THE MORBIDITY AND MORTALITY OF ALCOHOLIC LIVER DISEASE

The high prevalence of malnutrition in alcoholic liver disease has led to studies of the effect of nutritional therapy. Early studies indicated that patients with decompensated cirrhosis often improved after receiving a regular or high-protein-supplemented diet—even when alcohol was included (Summerskill *et al.*, 1957; Erenoglu *et al.*, 1964). By contrast, a low-protein diet that included alcohol caused no change or deterioration in clinical state (Erenoglu *et al.*, 1964). Moreover, abstinence from alcohol did not improve clinical status if dietary protein remained low (Phillips *et al.*, 1952).

In a more recent study, parenteral amino acid supplementation for a month in patients with severe alcoholic hepatitis resulted in greater clinical and laboratory improvement and fewer deaths than in a control group (Nasrallah and Galambos, 1980). In this study, patients on a high-calorie, high-protein diet received 70–85 g of amino acids/day intravenously. Serum bilirubin and albumin concentrations improved in patients receiving the amino acid supplements. Four of the 18 control patients died, while all of the 17 patients receiving amino acid supplements survived. In another study, parenteral amino acid supplementation resulted in more rapid clinical improvement in patients with biopsy-proven alcoholic hepatitis (Diehl *et al.*, 1985). However, this early advantage was not sustained at the end of one month. Hepatocellular necrosis and inflammation in initial and final liver biopsies correlated inversely with nitrogen balance at admission. Amino acid therapy resulted in greater improvement in nitrogen balance and greater resolution of fat infiltration but did not otherwise affect hepatic histology.

Oral and enteral administration of formulas providing 40–140 g protein/day improved nutritional status and serum albumin levels in patients with cirrhosis (Smith *et al.*, 1982). Oral administration of up to 80 g/day of branched-chain amino acids improved nitrogen balance without causing encephalopathy in patients with chronic cirrhosis (Horst *et al.*, 1984). Only one of 17 patients receiving branched-chain amino acids developed encephalopathy. By contrast, ingestion of comparable amounts of dietary protein resulted in encephalopathy in 35% of control patients. In another study, enteral administration of branched-chain amino acids to patients with cirrhosis improved their nutritional status, plasma albumin concentrations, and prothrombin time (Bory *et al.*, 1982). In yet another study, however, supplementation with 60 g of enteral or parenteral amino acids—including 20 g of branched-chain amino acids—or with 65 g of conventional protein did not affect clinical or laboratory parameters or mortality in patients with alcoholic hepatitis (Calvey *et al.*, 1985).

## IX. LIVER REGENERATION

There is little information on the relative effects of alcohol, nutrition, or their combination on hepatic regeneration in alcohol-induced hepatic injury. It is well documented that a diet with adequate protein and vitamins such as folic acid, cobalamin, and pyridoxine is required for hepatic regeneration (Leevy, 1967; Stirling *et al.*, 1975). Acute and chronic ethanol administration depressed mitotic activity, [$^3$H]thymidine incorporation into DNA, and protein synthesis in the regenerating rat liver after partial hepatectomy (Frank *et al.*, 1979; Wands *et al.*, 1979). However, despite the inhibition of DNA synthesis by ethanol, total hepatic DNA and liver weight after resection did not differ between ethanol-treated and control animals (Frank *et al.*, 1979; Orrego *et al.*, 1981). In one experiment, parenteral infusion of branched-chain amino acids accelerated incorporation of [$^3$H]thymidine into DNA after partial hepatectomy in the rat, whereas infusion of a standard amino acid solution or dextrose did not (Rigotti *et al.*, 1986). In a study of patients with alcoholic hepatitis and negligible *in vitro* hepatic DNA synthesis, an adequate diet—with supplemental vitamins to correct deficiencies—restored *in vitro* hepatic DNA synthesis in one-fifth of patients (Leevy, 1967).

## X. SUMMARY

The principal factor in the development of alcoholic liver disease is heavy alcohol ingestion. Nutritional deficiencies common in alcoholics may also be important in the pathogenesis of liver disease. An association exists between a low intake of nonalcohol calories and protein and the severity of alcoholic hepatitis. A few studies indicate that providing adequate amounts of protein, either orally or through parenteral amino acid supplements, improves clinical status and possibly lowers mortality in patients with severe alcoholic liver disease.

Future research should be directed toward:

1. determining the interrelationships between specific nutritional deficiencies and alcohol intake in the pathogenesis of liver disease,
2. improving understanding of the mechanisms of hepatic injury and fibrogenesis,
3. studying the regulation of alcohol-metabolizing enzymes to determine potential relationships or markers important to the development of liver disease,
4. developing better markers of hepatic fibrogenesis so that differences in nutritional status and alcohol intake can be more easily correlated with the progression of liver disease, thus avoiding the need for multiple liver biopsies, and
5. establishing additional cooperative clinical trials to determine the effect of nutritional supplement therapy on morbidity and mortality in alcoholic liver disease.

## ACKNOWLEDGMENTS

This work was supported in part by the Alcoholic Beverage Medical Research Foundation, Baltimore, Maryland.

## REFERENCES

Badley, B. W. D., Murphy, G. M., Bouchier, I. A. D., and Sherlock, S. (1970). Diminished micellar phase lipid in patients with chronic nonalcoholic liver disease and steatorrhea. *Gastroenterology* **58**, 781–789.

Best, C. H., Hartroft, W. S., Lucas, C. C., and Ridout, J. H. (1949). Liver damage produced by feeding alcohol or sugar and its prevention by choline. *Brit. Med. J.* **2**, 1001–1006.

Bloodworth, J. M. B., Jr. (1961). Diabetes mellitus and cirrhosis of the liver. *Arch. Intern. Med.* **108**, 695–701.

Bondar, G. F., and Pisesky, W. (1967). Complications of small intestinal short circuiting for obesity. *Arch. Surg.* **94**, 707–716.

Borhanmanesh, F., Ghavami, A., Dutz, W., and Bagheri, S. (1971). Cirrhosis of the liver in Iran: A prospective study of 66 cases. *J. Chronic Dis.* **23**, 891–905.

Bory, F., Kravetz, D., Bruguera, M., Farriol, M., Schwartz, S., and Rodes, J. (1982). Estudio controllado sobre el efecto nutricional de una nueva dieta enteral en la cirrosis hepatica. *Gastroenterologia y Hepatologia* **5**, 371–377.

Calvey, H., Davis, M., and Williams, R. (1985). Controlled trial of nutritional supplementation, with and without branched-chain amino acid enrichment, in treatment of acute alcoholic hepatitis. *J. Hepatol.* **1**, 141–151.

Campbell, J. M., Hunt, T. K., Karam, J. H., and Forsham, P. H. (1977). Jejunoileal bypass as a treatment of morbid obesity. *Arch. Intern. Med.* **137**, 606–610.

Chang, S., and Silvis, S. E. (1974). Fatty liver produced by hyperalimentation of rats. *Amer. J. Gastroenterol.* **62**, 410–418.

Cook, G. C., and Hutt, M. S. R. (1967). The liver after Kwashiorkor. *Brit. Med. J.* **3**, 454–457.

Diehl, A. M., Boitnott, J. K., Herlong, H. F., Potter, J. J., Van Duyn, M. A., Chandler, E., and Mezey, E. (1985). Effect of parenteral amino acid supplementation on alcoholic hepatitis. *Hepatology* **5**, 57–63.

Erenoglu, E., Edreira, J. G., and Patek, A. J., Jr. (1964). Observations on patients with Laennec's cirrhosis receiving alcohol while on controlled diets. *Ann. Intern. Med.* **60**, 814–823.

Falchuk, K. R., Fiske, S. C., Haggitt, R. C., Federman, M., and Trey, C. (1980). Pericentral fibrosis and intracellular hyaline in diabetes mellitus. *Gastroenterology* **78**, 535–541.

Frank, W. O., Rayyes, A. N., Washington, A., and Holt, P. R. (1979). Effect of acute ethanol administration upon hepatic regeneration. *J. Lab. Clin. Med.* **93**, 402–413.

French, S. W., and Castagna, J. (1967). Some effects of chronic ethanol feeding on vitamin $B_6$ deficiency in the rat. *Lab. Invest.* **16**, 526–531.

Gabuzda, G. J., Jr., and Davidson, C. S. (1954). Protein metabolism in patients with cirrhosis of the liver. *Ann. NY Acad. Sci.* **57**, 776–785.

Galambos, J. T. (1976). Jejunoileal bypass and nutritional liver injury. *Arch. Pathol. Lab. Med.* **100**, 229–231.

Gillman, J., and Gilbert, C. (1974). Aspects of nutritional liver disease—Human and experimental. *Ann. NY Acad. Sci.* **57**, 737–749.

Halsted, C. H., Robles, E. A., and Mezey, E. (1973). Intestinal absorption in folate deficient alcoholics. *Gastroenterology* **64**, 526–532.

Harano, Y., DePalma, R. G., Lavine, L., and Miller, M. (1972). Fatty acid oxidation, oxidative phosphorylation and ultrastructure of mitochondria in the diabetic rat liver. Hepatic factors in diabetic ketosis. *Diabetes* **31**, 257–270.

Heimburger, S. L., Steiger, E., Lo Gerfo, A., Biehl, A. G., and Williams, M. J. (1975). Reversal of severe fatty hepatic infiltration after intestinal bypass for morbid obesity by calorie-free amino acid infusion. *Amer. J. Surg.* **129**, 229–235.

Hollenbeck, J. I., O'Leary, J. P., Maher, J. W., and Woodward, E. R. (1975). An etiologic basis for fatty liver after jejunoileal bypass. *J. Surg. Res.* **18**, 83–89.

Horst, D., Grace, N. D., Conn, H. O., Schiff, E., Schenker, S., Viteri, A., Law, D., and Allerbury, C. E. (1984). Comparison of dietary protein with an oral, branched-chain enriched amino acid supplement in chronic portal-systemic encephalopathy: A randomized controlled trial. *Hepatology* **4**, 279–287.

Hoyumpa, A. M., Jr., Breen, K. J., Schenker, S., and Wilson, F. A. (1975). Thiamine transport across the rat intestine. Effect of ethanol. *J. Lab. Clin. Med.* **86**, 803–816.
Itoh, S., Matsuo, S., Ichinoe, A., Yamaba, Y., and Miyazawa, M. (1982). Nonalcoholic steatohepatitis and cirrhosis with Mallory's hyaline. With ultrastructural study in one case. *Dig. Dis. Sci.* **27**, 341–346.
Klatskin, G., Krehl, W. A., and Conn, H. O. (1954). The effect of alcohol on the choline requirement. I. Changes in the rat's liver following prolonged ingestion of alcohol. *J. Exp. Med.* **100**, 604–614.
Labadarios, D., Rossouw, J. E., McConnell, J. B., Davis, M., and Williams, R. (1977). Vitamin $B_6$ deficiency in chronic liver disease—Evidence for increased degradation of pyridoxal 5′-phosphate. *Gut* **18**, 23–27.
Leevy, C. M. (1967). Observations on hepatic regeneration in man. *Adv. Intern. Med.* **13**, 97–126.
Leevy, C. M., Baker, H., ten-Howe, W., Frank, O., and Cherrick, G. R. (1965). B-complex vitamins in liver disease of the alcoholic. *Amer. J. Clin. Nutr.* **16**, 339–346.
Lelbach, W. K. (1972). Dose-effect relationship in alcohol-induced liver damage. *Ger. Med. Monthly* **2**, 116–118.
Lieber, C. S., DeCarli, L. M., and Rubin, E. (1975). Sequential production of fatty liver, hepatitis, and cirrhosis in subhuman primates fed ethanol with adequate diets. *Proc. Nat. Acad. Sci. USA* **72**, 437–441.
Lieber, C. S., Leo, M. A., Mak, K. M., DeCarli, L. M., and Sato, S. (1985). Choline fails to prevent liver fibrosis in ethanol-fed baboons but causes toxicity. *Hepatology* **5**, 561–572.
Lockwood, D. H., Amatruda, J. M., Moxley, R. T., Pozefsky, T., and Boitnott, J. K. (1977). Effect of oral amino acid supplementation on liver disease after jejunoileal bypass for morbid obesity. *Amer. J. Clin. Nutr.* **30**, 58–63.
Lumeng, L., and Li, T. K. (1974). Vitamin $B_6$ metabolism in chronic alcohol abuse. Pyridoxal phosphate levels in plasma and the effects of acetaldehyde on pyridoxal phosphate synthesis and degradation in human erythrocytes. *J. Clin. Invest.* **53**, 693–704.
Marubbio, A. T., Jr., Buchwald, H., Schwartz, M. Z., and Varco, R. (1976). Hepatic lesions of central pericellular fibrosis in morbid obesity, and after jejunoileal bypass. *Amer. J. Clin. Pathol.* **66**, 684–691.
Mendenhall, C. L., Anderson, S., Weesner, R. E., Goldberg, S. J., and Crolic, K. A. (1984). Protein-calorie malnutrition associated with alcoholic hepatitis. Veterans Administration Cooperative Study. *Amer. J. Med.* **76**, 211–222.
Mendenhall, C. L., Tosch, T., Weesner, R. E., Garcia-Pont, P., Goldberg, S. J., Kiernan, T., Seef, L. B., Sorrell, M., Tamburro, C., Zetterman, R., Chedid, A., Chen, T., and Rubin, L. (1986). VA Cooperative Study on alcoholic hepatitis. II. Prognostic significance of protein-calorie malnutrition. *Amer. J. Clin. Nutr.* **43**, 213–218.
Mezey, E. (1975). Intestinal function in chronic alcoholism. *Ann. NY Acad. Sci.* **252**, 215–227.
Mezey, E. (1978). Liver disease and nutrition. *Gastroenterology* **74**, 770–783.
Mezey, E. (1982). Alcoholic liver disease. *Prog. Liver Dis.* **7**, 555–572.
Mezey, E., and Faillace, L. A. (1971). Metabolic impairment and recovery time in acute ethanol intoxication. *J. Nerv. Ment. Dis.* **153**, 445–452.
Mezey, E., Imbembo, A. L., Potter, J. J., Rent, K. C., Lombardo, R., and Holt, P. R. (1975). Endogenous ethanol production and hepatic disease following jejunoileal bypass for morbid obesity. *Amer. J. Clin. Nutr.* **28**, 1277–1283.
Mezey, E., Potter, J. J., French, S. W., Tamura, T., and Halsted, C. H. (1983). Effect of chronic ethanol feeding on hepatic collagen in the monkey. *Hepatology* **3**, 41–44.
Mills, P. R., Shenkin, A., Anthony, R. S., Mclelland, A. S., Main, A. N. H., MacSween, R. N. M., and Russell, R. I. (1983). Assessment of nutritional status and *in vivo* immune responses in alcoholic liver disease. *Amer. J. Clin. Nutr.* **38**, 849–859.

Moxley, R. J., III, Pozefsky, T., and Lockwood, D. H. (1974). Protein nutrition and liver disease after jejunoileal bypass for morbid obesity. *N. Engl. J. Med.* **290**, 921–926.

Nasrallah, S. M., and Galambos, J. T. (1980). Amino acid therapy of alcoholic hepatitis. *Lancet* **2**, 1276–1277.

Orrego, H., Crossley, I. R., Saldivia, V., Medline, A., Varghese, G., and Israel, Y. (1981). Long-term ethanol administration and short- and long-term liver regeneration after partial hepatectomy. *J. Lab. Clin. Med.* **97**, 221–230.

Owen, O. E., Trapp, V. E., Reichard, G. A., Jr., Monzzoli, M. A., Moctezuma, J., Paul, P., Skutches, C. L., and Boden, G. (1983). Nature and quantity of fuels consumed in patients with alcoholic cirrhosis. *J. Clin. Invest.* **72**, 1821–1832.

Patek, A. J., Jr., Post, J., Ratnoff, O. D., Mankin, H., and Hillman, R. W. (1948). Dietary treatment of cirrhosis of the liver. *JAMA-J. Am. Med. Assn.* **138**, 543–549.

Patek, A. J., Jr., Toth, I. G., Saunders, M. G., Castro, G. A. M., and Engel, J. J. (1975). Alcohol and dietary factors in cirrhosis. An epidemiological study of 304 alcoholic patients. *Arch. Intern. Med.* **135**, 1053–1057.

Pequignot, G., and Tuyns, A. J. (1980). Compared toxicity of ethanol on various organs. *In* "Alcohol and the Gastrointestinal Tract" (C. Stock and H. Sarles, eds.), pp. 17–32. INSERM, Paris.

Phillips, G. B., Gabuzda, G. J., Jr., and Davidson, C. S. (1952). Comparative effects of a purified and an adequate diet on the course of fatty cirrhosis in the alcoholic. *J. Clin. Invest.* **31**, 351–356.

Pichumoni, C. S., Sonnenshein, M., Candido, F. M., Panchacharam, P., and Cooperman, J. M. (1980). Nutrition in the pathogenesis of alcoholic pancreatitis. *Amer. J. Clin. Nutr.* **33**, 631–636.

Reaven, E. P., Peterson, D. T., and Reaven, G. M. (1973). The effect of experimental diabetes mellitus and insulin replacement on hepatic ultrastructure and protein synthesis. *J. Clin. Invest.* **52**, 248–262.

Rigotti, P., Peters, J. C., Tranberg, K. G., and Fischer, J. E. (1986). Effects of amino acid infusions in liver regeneration after partial hepatectomy in the rat. *JPEN* **10**, 17–20.

Rogers, A. E., Fox, J. G., and Murphy, J. C. (1981). Ethanol and diet interactions in male rhesus monkeys. *Drug Nutr. Interact.* **1**, 3–14.

Roggin, G. M., Iber, F. L., Kater, R. M. H., and Tobon, F. (1969). Malabsorption in the chronic alcoholic. *Johns Hopkins Med. J.* **125**, 321–330.

Rosen, H. M., Yoshimura, M., Hodgman, J. M., and Fischer, J. E. (1977). Plasma amino acid patterns in hepatic encephalopathy of differing etiology. *Gastroenterology* **72**, 483–487.

Sheldon, G. F., Peterson, S. R., and Sanders, R. (1978). Hepatic dysfunction during hyperalimentation. *Arch. Surg.* **113**, 504–508.

Sherlock, S., and Walshe, V. (1948). Effect of undernutrition in man on hepatic structure and function. *Nature* **161**, 604.

Sherr, H. P., Nair, P. P., White, J. J., Banwell, J. G., and Lockwood, D. H. (1977). Bile acid metabolism and hepatic disease following small bowel bypass for obesity. *Amer. J. Clin. Nutr.* **27**, 1369–1379.

Sidranski, H., and Farber, E. (1960). Liver choline oxidase activity in man and in several species of animals. *Arch. Biochem. Biophys.* **87**, 129–133.

Smith, J., Horowitz, J., Henderson, J. M., and Heymsfield, S. (1982). Enteral hyperalimentation in undernourished patients with cirrhosis and ascites. *Amer. J. Clin. Nutr.* **35**, 56–72.

Stirling, G. A., Bourne, L. D., and Marsh, T. (1975). Effect of protein deprivation and a reduced diet on the regenerating rat liver. *Brit. J. Exp. Pathol.* **56**, 502–509.

Summerskill, W. H. J., Wolfe, S. J., and Davidson, C. S. (1957). Response to alcohol in chronic alcoholics with liver disease. Clinical, pathologic, and metabolic changes. *Lancet* **1**, 335–340.

Wands, J. R., Carter, E. A., Bucher, N. L. R., and Isselbacher, K. J. (1979). Inhibition of hepatic regeneration in rats by acute and chronic ethanol intoxication. *Gastroenterology* **77**, 528–531.

Wizgird, J. P., Greenberg, L. D., and Moon, H. D. (1965). Hepatic lesions in pyridoxine-deficient monkeys. *Arch. Pathol.* **79**, 317–323.

Zinneman, H. H., Seal, U. S., and Doe, P. P. (1969). Plasma and urinary amino acids in Laennec's cirrhosis. *Amer. J. Dig. Dis.* **14**, 118–126.

# 14

# Vitamin A and Alcoholic Liver Disease

Charles S. Lieber
Maria Anna Leo

*Section of Liver Disease and Nutrition*
*Alcohol Research and Treatment Center*
*Bronx Veterans Administration Medical Center*
*Bronx, New York*
*Mount Sinai School of Medicine (CUNY)*
*New York, New York*

# I. INTRODUCTION

Several reviews have described the role of vitamin A in cell differentiation and proliferation as well as in vision (Sporn *et al.*, 1984; Goodman, 1984). The present discussion will focus primarily on the interactions among vitamin A deficiency or excess and hepatic structure and function. The most common cause of vitamin A deficiency in Western countries is liver disease, either obstructive or, more commonly, alcoholic. On the other hand, alterations in liver structure and function are common, but not fully appreciated, undesirable side effects of vitamin A therapy.

# II. PHYSIOLOGY AND REQUIREMENTS OF VITAMIN A

## A. Absorption, Transport and Metabolism of Vitamin A

The major sources of vitamin A are dietary carotenes (such as beta-carotene) and retinyl esters. Beta-carotene is converted to retinol primarily in the intestinal mucosa by cleavage at the central double bond, yielding two molecules of retinaldehyde. The aldehyde is then reduced to retinol (Fig. 1).

Dietary retinyl esters are hydrolyzed in the intestinal lumen to retinol, which is absorbed into mucosal cells. Retinol in the mucosal cell is re-esterified with long-chain fatty acids. Retinyl esters and associated chylomicrons are then transported to the general circulation via the lymph

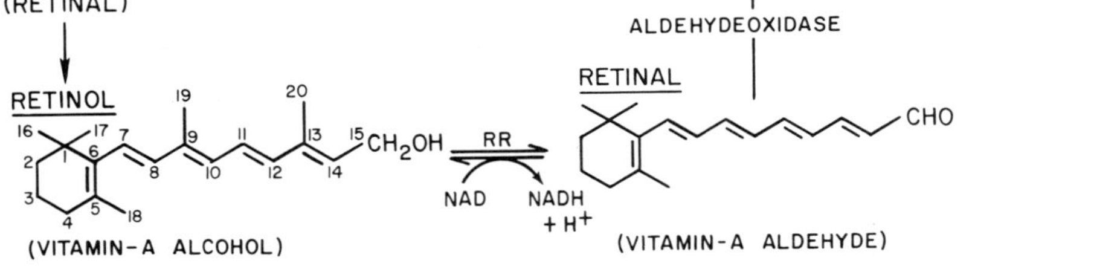


**Fig. 1.** Chemical formulas are shown for retinol, retinal, retinoic acid, and beta-carotene. (From Lieber and Leo, 1985. Reprinted with permission.)

system. The chylomicron remnants formed in the vascular compartment contain essentially all the retinyl esters from the original chylomicrons. The liver removes most of these esters from circulation. Hepatic retinyl esters are stored in parenchymal cells and in nonparenchymal fat-storing cells. Vitamin A is mobilized from these liver storage sites as the free alcohol retinol and is bound to retinol-binding protein (RBP), its plasma transport protein. Retinol exerts all known functions of vitamin A, except the key function of retinal in the visual cycle of the eye.

Retinal is derived intracellularly from retinol or directly from beta-carotene that has escaped intestinal cleavage (Napoli, 1986). In the liver, the classic pathway for conversion of retinol to retinal involves cytosolic retinol dehydrogenase (CRD), an enzyme dependent on nicotinamide-adenine dinucleotide ($NAD^+$). This enzyme is believed to be similar, if not identical, to the liver alcohol dehydrogenase (Figs. 1, 2). The observation that a strain of deermice lacks CRD (Leo and Lieber, 1984) prompted a search for an alternate metabolic pathway for the oxidation of retinol to retinal. Rat liver microsomes converted retinol to polar metabolites in a cytochrome *P*-450-dependent oxidase system, but this microsomal retinol oxidase did not produce retinal (Leo and Lieber, 1985). Recent evidence favors the existence of a microsomal retinol dehydrogenase (MRD) that converts retinol to retinal using $NAD^+$ as a cofactor (Fig. 2). MRD is

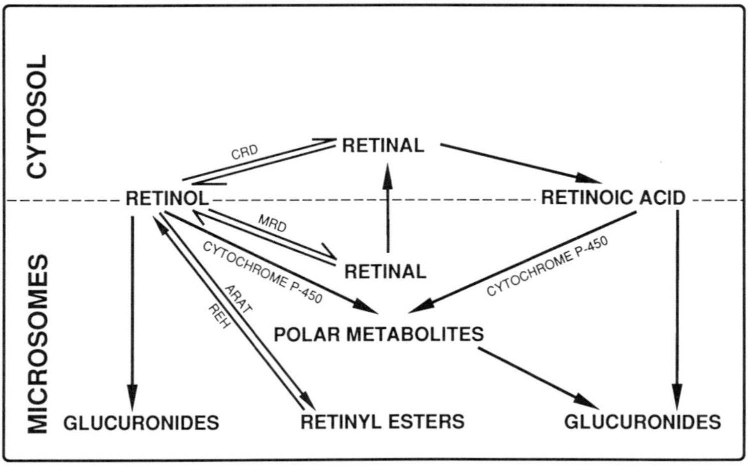


**Fig. 2.** Schematic representation shows the role of cytosolic and microsomal systems in hepatic metabolism of retinol and retinoic acid, where CRD is cytosolic retinol dehydrogenase, MRD is microsomal retinol dehydrogenase, ARAT is acyl-CoA or retinol acyltransferase, and REH is retinyl esters hydrolase. (From Leo *et al.*, 1987a. Reprinted with permission.)

distinct from the microsomal cytochrome *P*-450 system as well as from $NAD^+$-dependent CRD (Leo *et al.*, 1987a). Retinal is further metabolized to retinoic acid by $NAD^+$-dependent cytosolic retinal dehydrogenase, a cytosolic enzyme found in various tissues (Lakshmanan *et al.*, 1964; Moffa *et al.*, 1970; Kishore *et al.*, 1971; Kishore and Boutwell, 1980; Connor and Smit, 1987). Retinoic acid exerts all known functions of vitamin A, except those of retinal in the eye and retinol in the gonads.

## B. Vitamin A Storage and Requirements

The liver has a remarkable capacity to store varying amounts of vitamin A. However, plasma vitamin A levels remain constant over a wide range of dietary intakes and liver stores. Plasma RBP concentrations are low in liver disease and high in chronic renal disease.

Human vitamin A requirements remain uncertain. Few studies have directly assessed human needs, and the enormous capacity of the liver to store vitamin A has hampered efforts to determine precise human requirements. The Sheffield study, in part, forms the basis for currently recommended daily dietary allowances. In this study, human volunteers who were maintained on vitamin A-deficient diets for up to four years developed defective dark adaptation. A daily intake of 390 μg of retinol corrected this defect but was insufficient to restore serum vitamin A to predepletion levels. In two subjects, a daily intake of 750 μg of retinol maintained dark adaptation and serum vitamin A levels (Srikantia, 1976).

The present Recommended Dietary Allowance (RDA) (Recommended Dietary Allowances, 1980) is 1,000 μg for adult males and 800 μg for females. Olson (1987) has recommended lower amounts—700 μg for men and 600 μg for women. In Western countries, the average diet usually contains twice that amount, but in areas where poverty and malnutrition are prevalent, vitamin A deficiency remains a problem, particularly in preschool children.

Although the role of vitamin A in many physiological functions is poorly understood, its role in vision is well established. The most important clinical effects of vitamin A deficiency, grouped under the term "xerophthalmia," are found in the eyes. Clinical symptoms progress from night blindness, to conjunctival xerosis, Bitot's spot, corneal xerosis, and, finally, corneal ulceration or keratomalacia. These latter changes can lead to irreversible damage and blindness. Recent estimates suggest an enormous worldwide problem. Approximately 500,000 new cases of xerophthalmia with active corneal involvement occur annually in southeast Asia, and about half lead to blindness (Sommer, 1982).

In Western countries, dietary vitamin A deficiency does not appear to be a serious public health problem. However, postmortem studies have found low liver reserves of vitamin A in a significant number of people

(Underwood *et al.*, 1970; Raica *et al.*, 1972). These values do not necessarily reflect borderline intake. They could result from metabolic abnormalities, possibly secondary to a high prevalence of alcohol and drug abuse in the populations examined (Underwood *et al.*, 1970; Raica *et al.*, 1972).

## III. EFFECTS OF CHRONIC ETHANOL CONSUMPTION ON HEPATIC VITAMIN A LEVELS

Previous studies of hepatic vitamin A levels in various disease states used only autopsy material and did not include biopsy or alcohol consumption data for the subjects studied (Wolff, 1932; Russell *et al.*, 1978). Low circulating levels of vitamin A were found in patients with alcoholic cirrhosis (Smith *et al.*, 1975; McClain *et al.*, 1979; Russell *et al.*, 1978; Mobarhan *et al.*, 1981), but hepatic vitamin A concentrations were not assessed.

Therefore, we studied both hepatic and serum vitamin A levels in patients at various stages of alcoholic liver disease, in nonalcoholic patients with chronic persistent hepatitis, and in normal subjects (Leo and Lieber, 1982) (Table I; Fig. 3). Patients at all stages of alcoholic liver disease had very low hepatic vitamin A levels. In patients with alcoholic fatty liver, hepatic vitamin A concentrations were about 20% of control values and significantly lower than in patients with chronic persistent hepatitis, even though liver function tests and morphology showed similar degrees of liver damage. Liver vitamin A levels were less than 10% of control values

**TABLE I**

**Serum Vitamin A and Retinol-Binding Protein (RBP) Values in Alcoholic and Nonalcoholic Subjects**[a]

| Group | Vitamin A µg/100 ml | RBP µg/ml |
|---|---|---|
| Normal livers ($n = 6$) | 46.4 ± 7.9 | 50.2 ± 3.2 |
| Chronic persistent hepatitis ($n = 7$) | 43.2 ± 2.2 | 47.0 ± 5.5 |
| Alcoholic fatty liver ($n = 10$) | 48.4 ± 7.3 | 57.8 ± 8.6 |
| Alcoholic hepatitis ($n = 11$) | 35.8 ± 5.0[b] | 41.0 ± 6.0 |
| Alcoholic cirrhosis ($n = 6$) | 20.0 ± 3.0[b] | 23.0 ± 4.0[b] |
| Normal values[c] ($n = 109$) | 50.1 ± 0.5 | 46.2 ± 1.0 |

[a]Data are expressed as means ± SEM. To convert vitamin A values to µ*M*, multiply by 0.03491. (From Leo and Lieber, 1982. Reprinted with permission.)

[b]$p < 0.001$ compared with normal values.

[c]See Smith and Goodman, 1971.

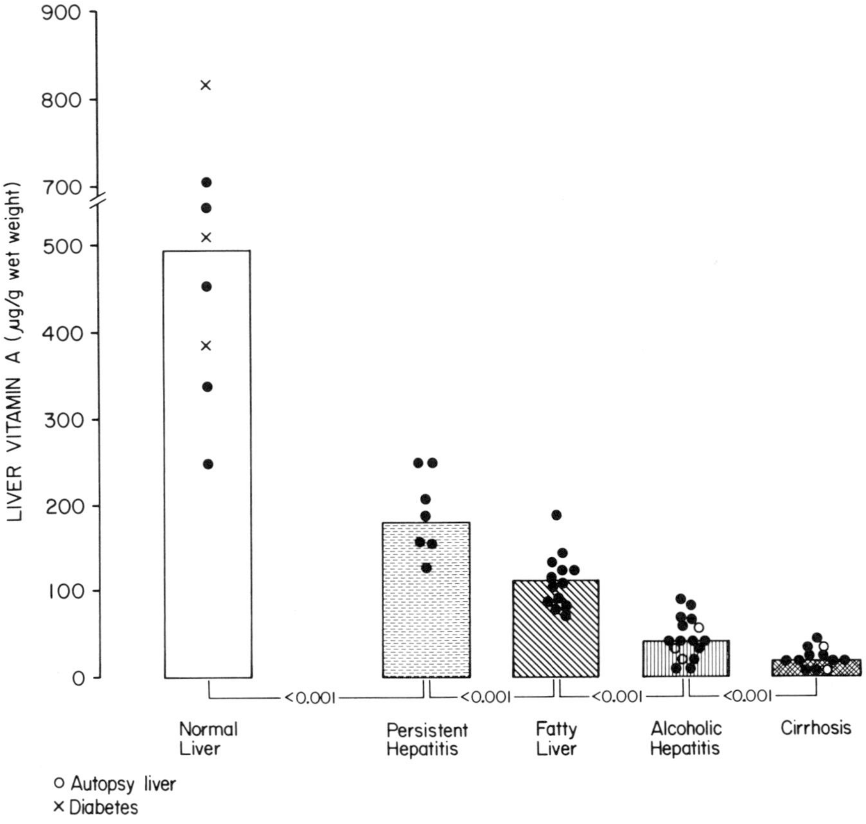


**Fig. 3.** Hepatic vitamin A levels were measured in patients with normal livers, chronic persistent hepatitis, and various stages of alcoholic injury. (From Leo and Lieber, 1983a. Reprinted with permission.)

in patients with alcoholic hepatitis. Even lower hepatic vitamin A levels were observed in patients with cirrhosis (Fig. 3). Thus, alcoholic liver disease is associated with severely decreased hepatic vitamin A levels—even when liver injury is moderate (fatty liver) and blood levels of vitamin A remain normal (Table I). RBP, previously considered a more sensitive index of vitamin A deficiency than dark adaptation (Vahlquist *et al.*, 1978), was also normal in patients with alcoholic fatty liver.

The mechanisms of hepatic vitamin A depletion in alcoholic liver disease are unclear. Malnutrition could contribute to hepatic vitamin A depletion. However, patients with alcoholic fatty liver had low hepatic vitamin A levels but were well nourished and had normal circulating levels of vitamin A and RBP (Table I), and albumin.

To evaluate the effects of alcohol consumption on vitamin A and RBP status, baboons and rats were fed ethanol with diets containing varying amounts of vitamin A (Sato and Lieber, 1981). Pair-fed baboons received a nutritionally adequate liquid diet containing 50% of total energy as ethanol or isocaloric carbohydrate. Fatty liver developed after four months of ethanol feeding, and hepatic vitamin A levels fell 59%. After 24 to 84 months, hepatic vitamin A levels fell 95%, together with development of fibrosis or cirrhosis.

Similarly, rats fed ethanol as 36% of total calories showed a 42% decrease in hepatic vitamin A levels after three weeks and continuing decreases after nine weeks, with no significant change in serum vitamin A and RBP levels. After a fivefold increase in dietary vitamin A, hepatic vitamin A levels still decreased in ethanol-fed rats. With virtual elimination of dietary vitamin A, hepatic vitamin A stores were depleted 2.5 times faster in ethanol-fed rats than in controls.

Although one earlier study found no effect of chronic ethanol consumption on hepatic vitamin A (Suschetet, 1975), others noted decreases in hepatic vitamin A after prolonged ethanol intake (Baumann *et al.*, 1942; Blomstrand *et al.*, 1977). These studies involved rats fed ethanol in drinking water and did not include nutritionally paired controls. However, our study was performed under nutritionally controlled conditions and showed that chronic ethanol consumption lowered hepatic vitamin A (Sato and Lieber, 1981). Hepatic vitamin A depletion became evident at the fatty liver stage and thus did not appear to result from severe hepatic damage. Moreover, plasma vitamin A levels did not change as hepatic vitamin A decreased. Consequently, plasma vitamin A may not be a good marker for hepatic vitamin A storage in alcoholic patients.

The explanation for our finding that hepatic vitamin A stores were significantly lower in ethanol-fed animals than in controls is unclear. Malabsorption of vitamin A appears unlikely because striking differences in hepatic vitamin A levels between ethanol-fed rats and controls were found even when vitamin A was virtually eliminated from the diet (Sato and Lieber, 1981). Two other mechanisms can be considered: increased mobilization of vitamin A from the liver and increased catabolism of vitamin A in the liver or other organs. Experimental evidence favors both.

## IV. EFFECT OF ETHANOL ON HEPATIC VITAMIN A MOBILIZATION

The hypothesis that ethanol causes vitamin A to be mobilized from the liver is supported by the finding that vitamin A levels in the kidney and testis rose two- to threefold in the face of hepatic vitamin A depletion in rats fed ethanol as 36% of total calories for nine weeks (Sato and Lieber, 1981). Similarly, in rats fed ethanol as 36% of total calories for one month, vitamin A levels in the esophageal mucosa increased fivefold, compared to animals pair-fed an isocaloric control diet with the same amount of vitamin A (Fig. 4) (Leo *et al.*, 1986a). Retinoid levels also increased significantly in the lungs and trachea, but not in the eyes. By contrast, another group reported that ethanol-feeding with zinc supplementation of ethanol-fed rats prevented an increase in esophageal retinoids (Mobarhan *et al.*, 1986). However, we found an increase in esophageal retinoids with ethanol feeding even in the presence of zinc supplementation (Leo *et al.*, 1986a). This discrepancy might relate to lower bioavailability of the vitamin A in diets used in the other study (Leo *et al.*, 1987b).

In another investigation, an acute, nonlethal dose of ethanol significantly lowered hepatic vitamin A in rats while increasing serum retinyl esters in the lipoprotein fraction (Sato and Lieber, 1982a). The acute ethanol-induced increase in serum vitamin A was in keeping with earlier observations in animals (Clausen *et al.*, 1942; Crowley and Allen, 1953; Lee and Lucia, 1965; Miller *et al.*, 1969) and humans (Pett, 1940; Clausen *et al.*,

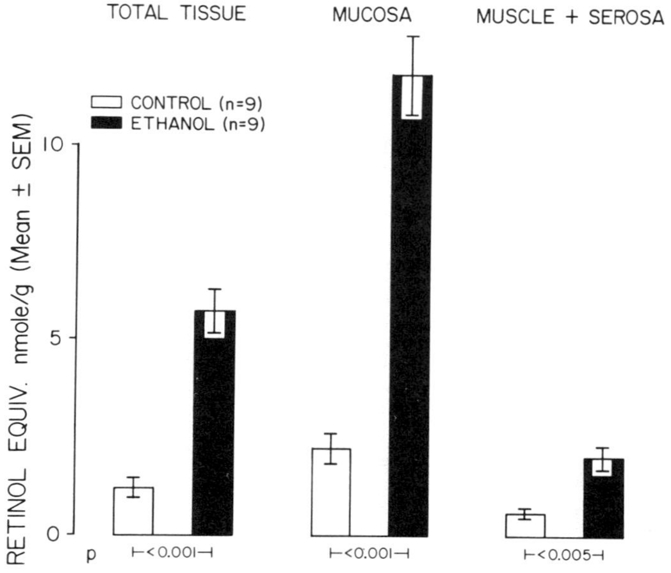


**Fig. 4.** The effect of ethanol feeding on total retinoids in the esophagus was studied in rats fed diets containing 6,000 IU vitamin A plus 7.5 mg zinc/L. Chronic ethanol feeding resulted in increased retinoid concentration in the mucosa as well as in the remainder of the esophagus. (From Leo *et al.*, 1986a. Reprinted with permission.)

1941). Moreover, the concentration of $^{14}$C-labeled vitamin A rose in extrahepatic organs as it fell in the liver (Fig. 5). These results suggest that acute ethanol adminstration shifts vitamin A, via lipoprotein-bound retinyl esters, from the liver to other organs. Prolonged intake of alcohol could conceivably produce the same results. Thus, acute ethanol-induced mobilization of vitamin A from the liver could contribute to significant depletion of hepatic vitamin A stores.

## V. EFFECT OF ETHANOL AND OTHER DRUGS ON HEPATIC VITAMIN A METABOLISM

Traditionally, the main role of the liver in vitamin A metabolism has been perceived to be one of storage. Current studies, however, suggest a more extensive role for the liver in the metabolism of vitamin A.

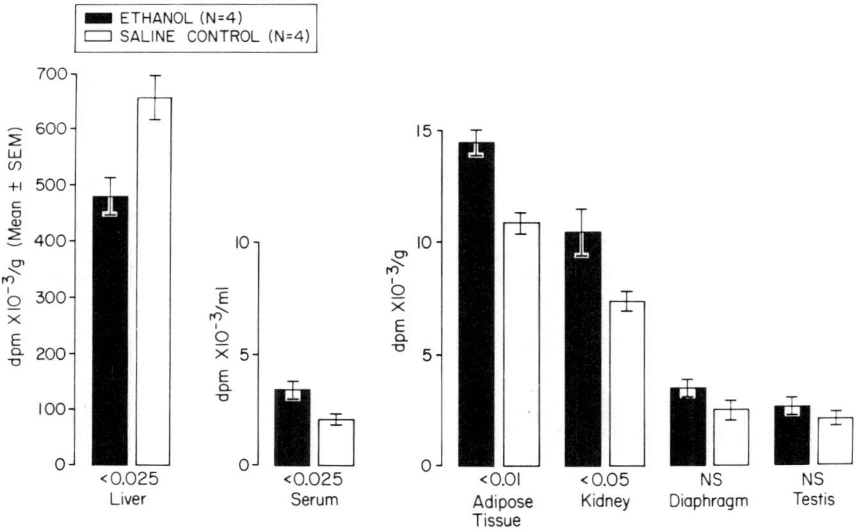


**Fig. 5.** The effect of acute ethanol administration on the distribution of [$^{14}$C]vitamin A in tissues is shown. Rats were given [$^{14}$C]retinol (2 $\mu$Ci, 36 $\mu$g/100 g body weight intravenously) seven days before the experiment to allow for equilibration between injected and endogenous vitamin A. Rats were then fasted 15–18 hours and given saline or 6 g/kg body weight oral ethanol 24 hours before they were killed. [$^{14}$C]vitamin A was assayed in tissue extract. The specific activity of [$^{14}$C]vitamin A (in disintegrations/min/mcg retinol) in serum was 6,995 $\pm$ 599 in the alcohol-treated rats and 6,872 $\pm$ 398 in the saline controls; corresponding liver vitamin A values were 7,454 $\pm$ 939 and 6,949 $\pm$ 328. (From Sato and Lieber, 1982a. Reprinted with permission.)

As previously noted, liver retinol is metabolized to polar metabolites in a cytochrome *P*-450-dependent system or, through the CRD enzyme, to retinal and eventually to retinoic acid (Fig. 2). Retinol or retinoic acid may also be converted to glucuronides. Biliary excretion of glucuronides of retinol and retinoic acid has been demonstrated (Lippel and Olson, 1968; Zile *et al.*, 1980; Swanson *et al.*, 1981). Retinoic acid can also be metabolized through a microsomal cytochrome *P*-450-dependent enzyme system (Roberts *et al.*, 1979; Roberts *et al.*, 1980). Because chronic ethanol consumption can induce a variety of hepatic microsomal cytochrome *P*-450-mediated enzyme activities (Misra *et al.*, 1971; Joly *et al.*, 1973), this may be a mechanism for retinoid depletion in the liver.

## A. Effect of Ethanol on Retinoic Acid Metabolism

Rat liver microsomal activity was compared in animals pair-fed diets containing either ethanol or isocaloric carbohydrate. In normal microsomes, all-*trans*-[11,12-$^{3}$H]retinoic acid was metabolized to polar metabolites in the presence of NADPH, the reduced form of nicotinamide-adenine dinucleotide phosphate (Sato and Lieber, 1982b). One metabolite was coeluted with 4-hydroxy-retinoic acid by reverse-phase high-pressure liquid chromatography (HPLC). This reaction required oxygen and was inhibited by carbon monoxide as well as by aminopyrine, aniline, and ethanol, suggesting the involvement of cytochrome *P*-450. Isolated rat hepatocytes also metabolized all-*trans*-[$^{3}$H]retinoic acid to polar compounds, with elution patterns on HPLC similar to those in the microsomal preparations. After four to six weeks of ethanol feeding, microsomal *P*-450 content and retinoic acid metabolism increased (Sato and Lieber, 1982b). Massive dietary vitamin A supplementation produced a similar outcome (Leo *et al.*, 1984a).

On sodium dodecyl sulfate gel electrophoresis of vitamin A-''induced'' microsomes, one band of increased electrophoretic mobility was identical to that of cytochrome *P*-450f (Ryan *et al.*, 1984). In a system reconstituted with NADPH-cytochrome *P*-450 reductase, NADPH, and phospholipid, purified cytochrome *P*-450f promoted conversion of retinoic acid to its polar metabolites, including 4-hydroxy-retinoic acid. *P*-450f had lower drug metabolizing activity than other forms of cytochrome *P*-450, but it sustained greater metabolism of retinoic acid. Because cytochrome *P*-450-dependent metabolism of retinoic acid in microsomes was postulated as the initial step in the pathway by which retinoic acid is eliminated from the body (Roberts and Frolik, 1979), induction of this metabolism by chronic ethanol consumption may increase catabolism of retinoic acid in the liver, thus reducing hepatic vitamin A stores. However, retinoic acid degradation via this pathway is relatively small.

## B. Effect of Ethanol and Drugs on Retinol Metabolism

We have recently discovered a cytochrome *P*-450-dependent microsomal system that actively converts retinol to its polar metabolites in the presence of NADPH (Leo and Lieber, 1985). This system, reconstituted with purified cytochrome *P*-450, was found to be inducible by ethanol as well as by drugs such as phenobarbital. Microsomes of ethanol- or phenobarbital-treated animals produced strikingly increased amounts of polar metabolites from retinol (Fig. 6). This enhanced catabolism may explain the striking depletion of hepatic vitamin A found in the presence

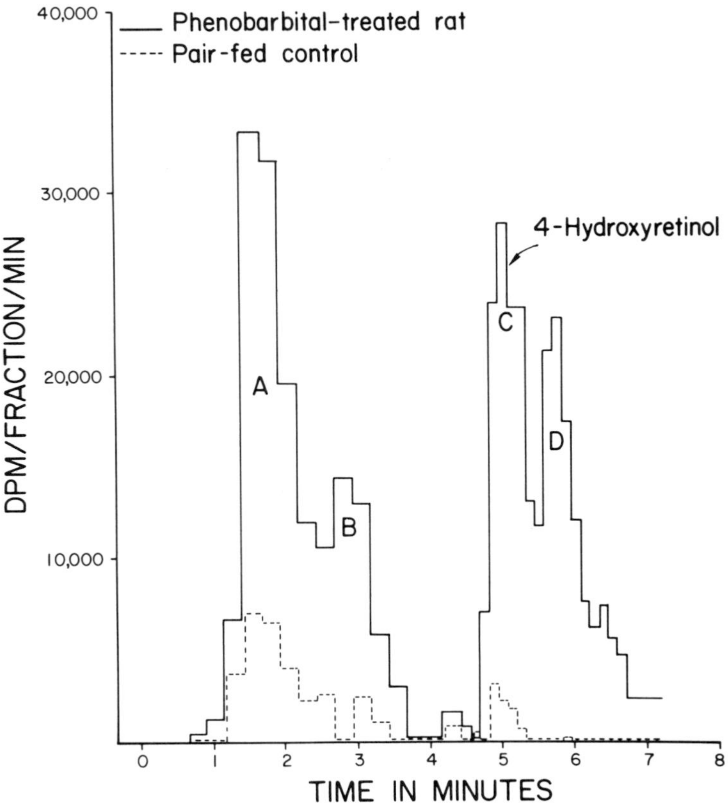


**Fig. 6.** High-pressure liquid chromatography profile shows metabolites produced by microsomes of phenobarbital-treated rats and pair-fed controls after incubation with all-*trans*-[$^{3}H$]retinol. This representative tracing shows that microsomes of animals fed phenobarbital produced more 4-hydroxyretinol and other polar metabolites than controls. (From Leo and Lieber, 1985. Reprinted with permission.)

of ethanol or drugs like phenobarbital. It may also explain why the combination of ethanol and such drugs potentiates this depletion (Fig. 7) (Leo *et al.*, 1987c). Because alcohol and drug abuse often occur together, this potentiation may occur in a much larger population segment than previously recognized.

Clinical results also suggest an association between drug use and hepatic vitamin A depletion. Hepatic vitamin A levels were only 10% of normal values in 11 patients with moderate drug-induced liver changes (Leo *et al.*, 1984b). Hepatic vitamin A levels also fell in experimental animals after administration of carcinogens such as dibenzanthracene (Baumann *et al.*, 1942) and 2-aminoanthraquinone (Reddy and Weisburger, 1980), polychlorinated biphenyls (PCBs) (Innami *et al.*, 1976), and other xenobiotic agents (Kato *et al.*, 1978). Current widespread use of alcohol and/or drugs suggests that hepatic vitamin A depletion may not be uncommon and that concern about its adverse effects on the liver may be warranted. These data also raise the issue of whether the RDA for vitamin A should be raised for psychiatric, epileptic or other patients who require chronic drug treatment.

Another recently described microsomal system is $NAD^+$-dependent and converts retinol to retinal through the action of microsomal retinol dehydrogenase (MRD) in liver microsomes of rats and of a strain of deermice lacking the CRD enzyme (Fig. 2) (Leo *et al.*, 1987a). Unlike CRD, the MRD enzyme is not inhibited by ethanol or 4-methylpyrazole, is insensitive to carbon monoxide, and is not dependent on oxygen. These features

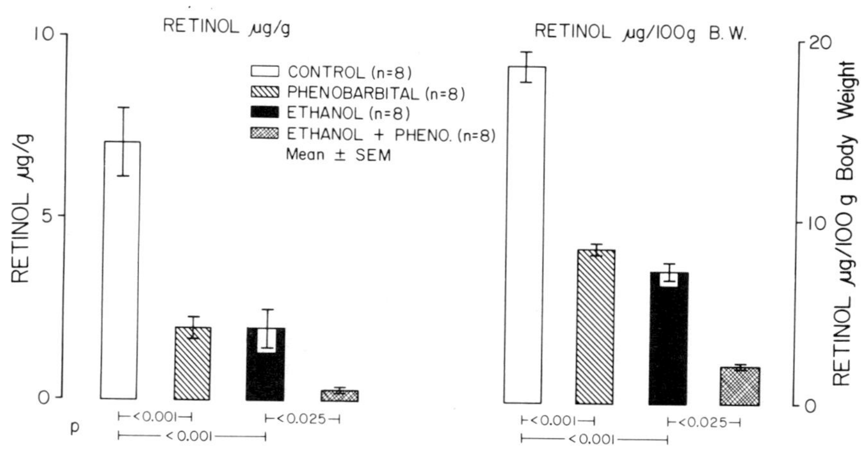


**Fig. 7.** Both phenobarbital and ethanol strikingly depleted hepatic retinol levels. When the two drugs were combined, hepatic retinol levels decreased to 5% of control values. (From Leo *et al.*, 1987c. Reprinted with permission.)

distinguish this $NAD^+$-dependent system from those involving microsomal cytochrome *P*-450 and NADPH-dependent retinol oxidase. Increased MRD activity accompanies chronic ethanol consumption, which, in view of the enzyme's insensitivity to inhibition by ethanol, may contribute to hepatic retinol depletion.

## VI. HEPATIC ABNORMALITIES ASSOCIATED WITH LOW VITAMIN A LEVELS

### A. Multivesicular Lysosomes

Hepatic vitamin A levels were measured in 41 patients with various stages of liver disease and compared to their liver morphology as assessed by light and electron microscopy (Leo *et al.*, 1983). In 25 subjects, multivesicular lysosomes (Fig. 8) were associated with low hepatic vitamin A levels. These organelles, seen primarily in the hepatocytes, were limited by a single membrane with a homogeneous, electron-dense crescent and contained many lipid-like particles of different sizes, some of them reminiscent of lipoprotein particles.

To determine the respective roles of vitamin A and toxins like ethanol in producing this morphological change, we fed rats vitamin A-replete and vitamin A-deficient diets with and without ethanol (Leo *et al.*, 1983). Animals fed vitamin-A deficient diets with or without ethanol developed multivesicular lysosomes (Fig. 9), whereas animals fed vitamin A-replete diets did not. Lesions found in the vitamin A-deficient rats were identical to those in patients with liver disease—they contained round lipid-like particles (Fig. 9B), the smallest of which resembled, in size and shape, the particles found in the secretory vesicles of the Golgi (Fig. 9A). Electron micrographs of very low-density lipoproteins (VLDL) in the plasma of these animals (Fig. 9C) provide indirect support for the lipoprotein nature of these particles. The lysosomal nature of the lesions was substantiated by a clear-cut acid phosphatase reaction. These structures also had a single membrane with a crescent (Figs. 8–9), previously described as characteristic of lysosomes (Tanikawa, 1971).

Although the mechanism by which multivesicular lysosomes develop is unknown, the many lipid-like particles in these organelles suggest a possible abnormality in lipoprotein metabolism (Leo *et al.*, 1983). It is also noteworthy that vitamin A is required for glycosylation of some hepatic export proteins (Wolf *et al.*, 1979). Further studies are needed to clarify the relationships among hepatic vitamin A depletion, the appearance of multivesicular lysosomes, and lipoprotein secretion.

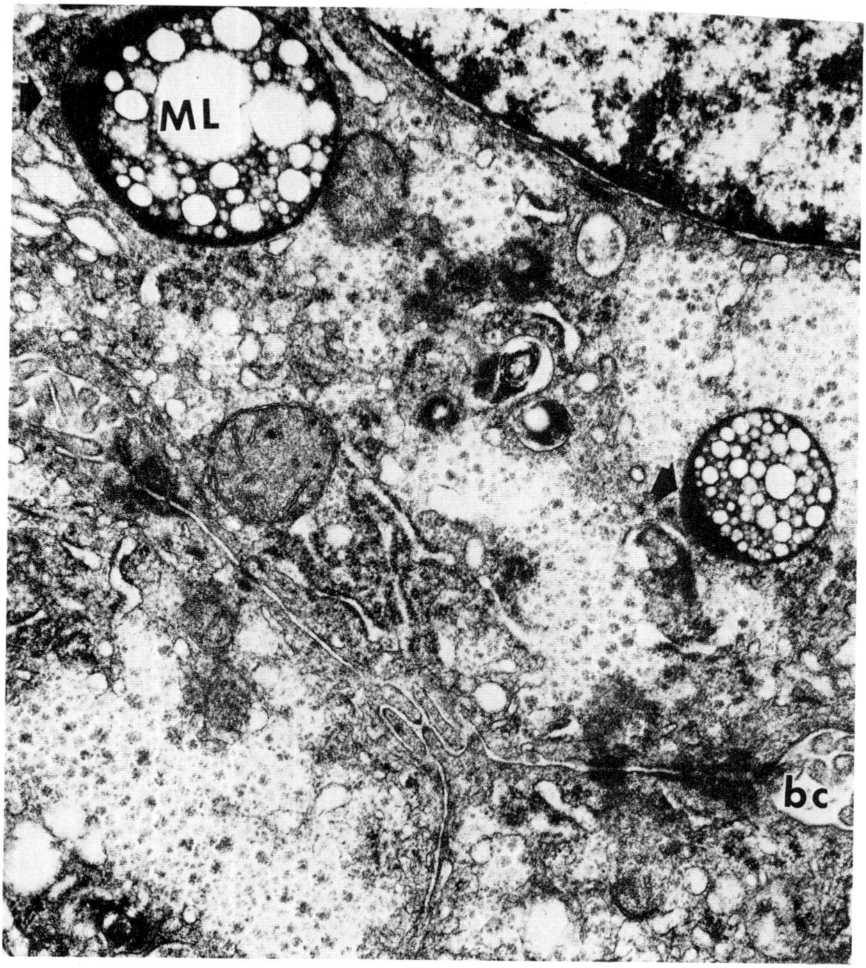


**Fig. 8.** Human hepatocyte (×21,600), showing two multivesicular lysosomes (ML), with a characteristic crescent (arrow) and bile canaliculus (bc). (From Leo *et al.*, 1983. Reprinted with permission.)

## B. Mallory Bodies

Others have postulated that Mallory bodies, a hyaline amorphous, acidophilic material found in hepatocytes in cirrhosis, are caused by low hepatic vitamin A levels (Denk *et al.*, 1979a; Denk *et al.*, 1979b; French, 1981). Mallory bodies were sometimes associated with very low levels of hepatic vitamin A (Leo and Lieber, 1982), but no significant differences in hepatic vitamin A levels were found in patients with and without

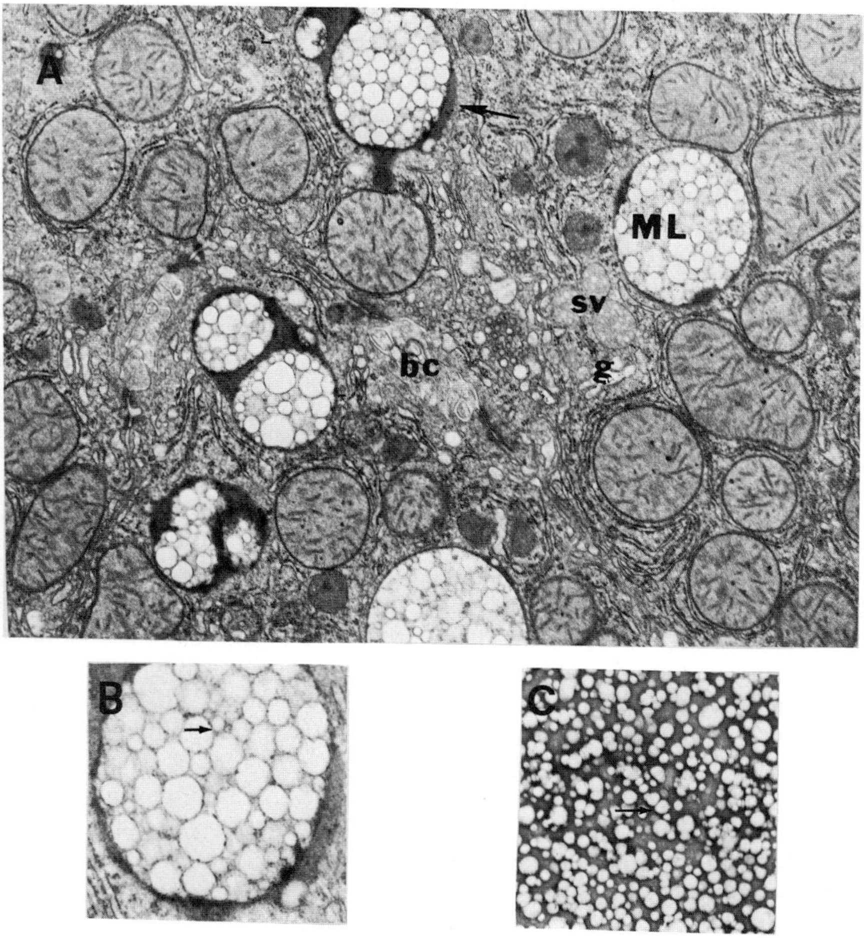


**Fig. 9A.** Periportal area of low vitamin-A control rat (×16,400) shows bile canaliculus (bc) surrounded by several multivesicular lysosomes (ML). Part of the limiting membrane shows a homogeneous, electron-dense crescent (arrow). Secretory vesicles (Sv) and Golgi complex (g) are also shown. **9B.** Inset of Fig. 9A shows a higher magnification (×26,000) of ML with lipoprotein-like particles. **9C.** Negative staining of plasma VLDL fraction (×26,000) in low-vitamin A control rat shows a correspondence in size between the lipoprotein-like particles present in the secretory vesicles (sv) of the Golgi complex (g), the small particles present in ML (arrow), and the negatively stained VLDL particles in the plasma (arrow). (From Leo *et al.*, 1983. Reprinted with permission.)

Mallory bodies. Although our studies have failed to correlate vitamin A levels with Mallory bodies, it remains possible that low vitamin A levels may potentiate the development of Mallory bodies in the presence of ethanol.

### C. Other Hepatic Abnormalities

Vitamin A deficiency may also have other, as yet uncharted, adverse effects on the liver. Alcohol-induced depletion of hepatic vitamin A has been associated with a striking disappearance of vitamin A from plasma membranes (Kim *et al.*, 1988) and a decrease in fluidity (Yamada *et al.*, 1985; Kim *et al.*, 1988), but the mechanisms remain unclear.

## VII. HEPATOTOXICITY OF VITAMIN A AND ITS EFFECT ON FIBROGENESIS

The relationship between vitamin A and fibrogenesis is complex. Although the data support a role for excessive vitamin A in the promotion of fibrogenesis, vitamin A has the opposite effect in certain isolated fibroblasts (Oikarinen *et al.*, 1985) and in carbon tetrachloride-induced hepatic fibrosis (Senoo and Wake, 1985). In view of the low hepatic vitamin A levels in patients with liver disease (Leo and Lieber, 1982) and of the symptoms of vitamin A deficiency reported in alcoholics (Vahlquist *et al.*, 1978), the therapeutic use of vitamin A must be considered. When vitamin A deficiency is corroborated by low serum vitamin A levels, such treatment might particularly be indicated (Russell *et al.*, 1978; Mobarhan *et al.*, 1981). However, liver depletion may even occur in the presence of normal serum levels (Leo and Lieber, 1982). Whether vitamin A should be administered to such patients and, if so, how much is still an open question.

Therapeutic doses of vitamin A have been prescribed to treat alcoholic patients with hypogonadism (McClain *et al.*, 1979) and abnormal dark adaptation (McClain *et al.*, 1979; Russell *et al.*, 1978). The doses of vitamin A, ranging from 10,000 IU/day for up to five months to 50,000 IU/day for one week, were considered safe because no adverse effects at these doses have been reported in normal individuals. However, larger doses than those commonly used to treat severe clinical conditions like xerophthalmia (Sommer *et al.*, 1980) may be hepatotoxic (Russell *et al.*, 1974; Farrell *et al.*, 1977; Herbert, 1982). Studies in experimental animals suggest that vitamin A hepatotoxicity may be potentiated by continual exposure to ethanol (Leo *et al.*, 1982; Leo and Lieber, 1983b).

## A. Animal Studies of Hepatotoxicity

In one study (Leo *et al.*, 1982), rats were fed diets containing normal and five-times-normal amounts of vitamin A with and without ethanol. The normal vitamin A/ethanol diet produced proliferation of smooth endoplasmic reticulum and moderate mitochondrial lesions. The high vitamin A/control diet produced endoplasmic reticulum proliferation, slightly enlarged mitochondria, and moderate decreases in cytochrome oxidase activity and cytochrome $aa_3$ content. The high vitamin A/ethanol diet produced much more severe lesions with giant mitochondria containing paracrystalline inclusions (Fig. 10). There was also depressed oxygen consumption in state-3 respiration with five different substrates,

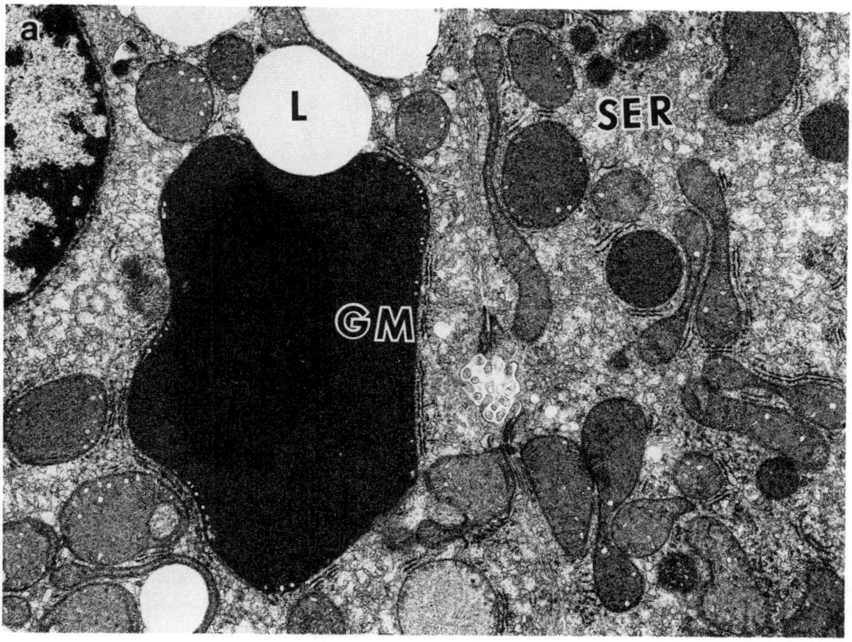


**Fig. 10.** Electron micrographs show pericentral hepatocytes (×11,700) of rats fed high vitamin A diet with or without ethanol. **10A.** In ethanol-fed rat, giant mitochondrion (GM) approaching the size of a nucleus contains an unusually dense matrix with a large fusiform crystalline inclusion. This and adjacent mitochondria display severe disorganization of the cristae. Lipid droplet (L) and proliferated smooth endoplasmic reticulum (SER) are also shown. **10B.** In control rat, mitochondria (M) show slight swelling and clear matrix. Proliferated smooth endoplasmic reticulum (SER) is also shown. (From Leo *et al.*, 1982. Reprinted with permission.)

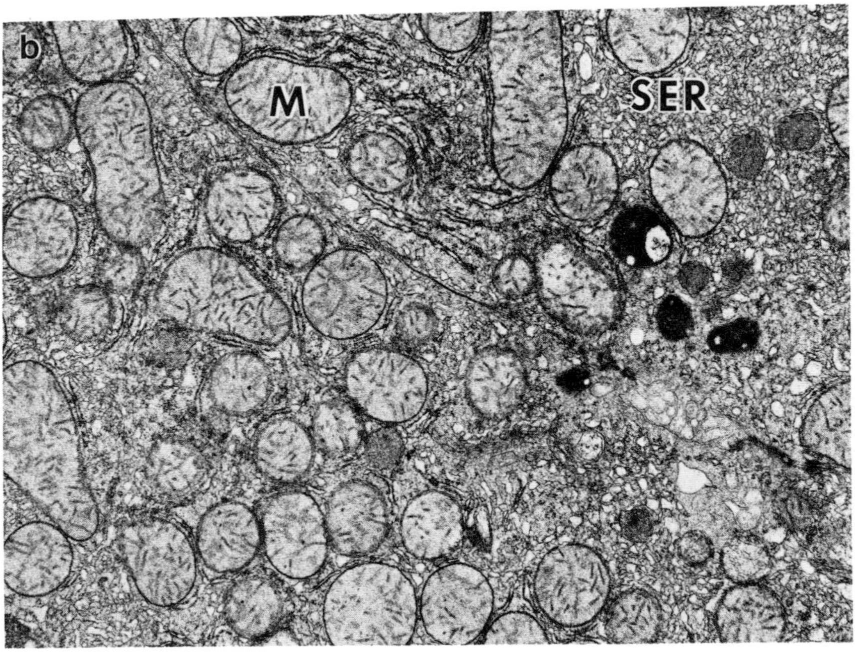


Fig. 10B

including palmitate and palmitoyl coenzyme A (CoA). Depressed fatty acid oxidation may have contributed to lipid accumulation. Mitochondrial toxicity was also reflected in low levels of various cytochromes and in reduced activity of enzymes including glutamate dehydrogenase (GDH). However, serum GDH activity increased (Fig. 11). Plasma vitamin A levels were unaffected in all groups, while liver vitamin A levels rose with the high vitamin A/control diet and fell with each ethanol diet in relation to its pair. As a net result, hepatic vitamin A levels in the high vitamin A/ethanol group were similar to those in the normal vitamin A/control group (Table II). These data suggest that ethanol's potentiation of vitamin A toxicity is mediated by production of a toxic metabolite.

In another study (Leo and Lieber, 1983b), the high vitamin A diet was continued, with and without ethanol, for up to nine months. At that point, necrosis, inflammation, and fibrosis—lesions that ethanol alone does not produce in the rat model—appeared. The anticipated increase in the number of lipocytes or fat storing cells in the high vitamin A/control group correlated significantly with liver vitamin A accumulation (Fig. 12). However, in the high vitamin A/ethanol group, hepatic vitamin A levels and fat-storing cells were decreased compared to controls (Table III)

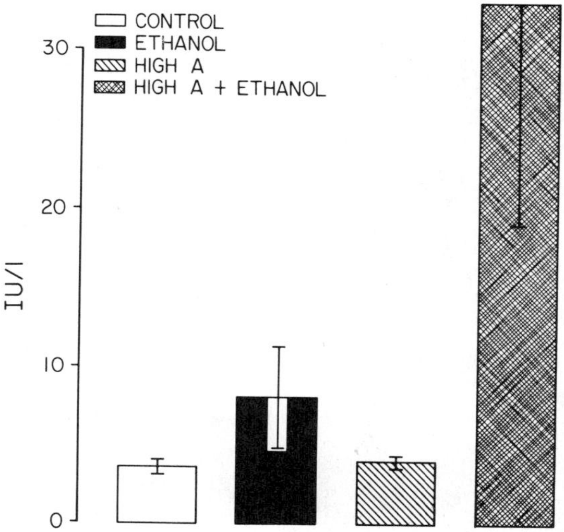


**Fig. 11.** Serum GDH activity was measured in rats fed normal and high vitamin A diets, with and without ethanol, for two months. The most significant increase in serum GDH activity was observed in rats consuming the high vitamin A/ethanol diet. (Data from Leo and Lieber, 1983b.)

**TABLE II**

**Serum and Liver Vitamin A in Rats Fed a Normal or High Vitamin A Diet with or without Ethanol**[a]

| | Serum vitamin A | Liver vitamin A | |
|---|---|---|---|
| Groups | μg/100 ml | μg/g | μg/100 g body weight |
| Normal vitamin A | | | |
| Ethanol-fed rats ($n$ = 5) | 42.5 ± 2.8 | 120 ± 11[b] | 421 ± 43[b] |
| Pair-fed rats ($n$ = 5) | 42.3 ± 2.8 | 303 ± 29[c] | 799 ± 43 |
| | NS | $p < 0.01$ | $p < 0.01$ |
| High vitamin A | | | |
| Ethanol-fed rats ($n$ = 12) | 39.8 ± 1.8 | 235 ± 16 | 907 ± 63 |
| Pair-fed rats ($n$ = 12) | 40.7 ± 2.4 | 636 ± 40 | 1,809 ± 107 |
| | NS | $p < 0.001$ | $p < 0.001$ |

[a]Rats were fed diets with normal or high vitamin A content with or without ethanol for 8 weeks. Values are given as mean ± SEM. (From Leo *et al.*, 1982. Reprinted with permission.)

[b]$p < 0.001$.

[c]$p < 0.05$ when compared to rats fed diets high in vitamin A with ethanol.

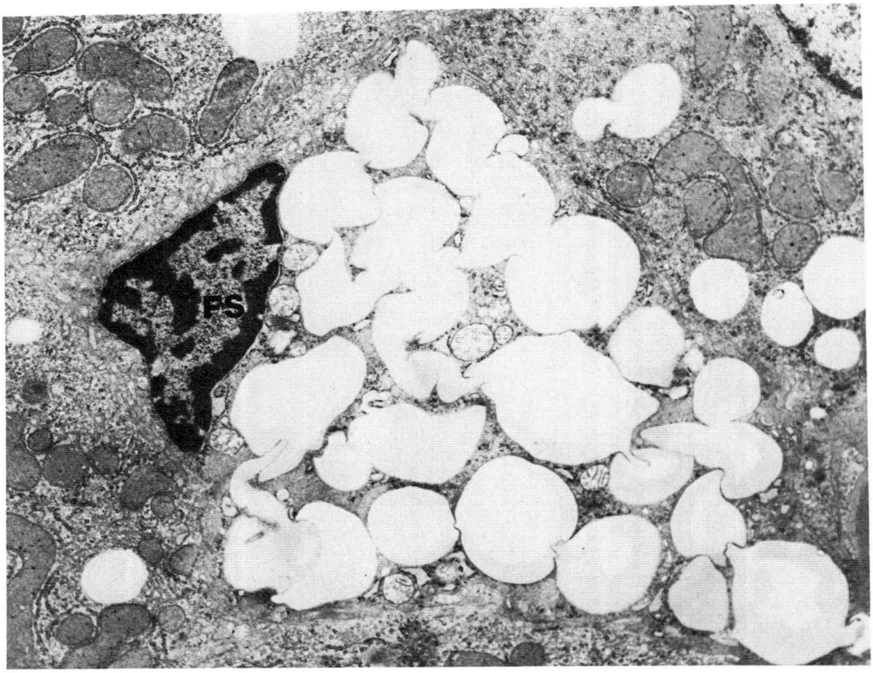


**Fig. 12.** Liver of rat fed high vitamin A/ethanol diet for 9 months shows large fat-storing cell (FS) with numerous lipid droplets (×7,000). (From Leo and Lieber, 1983b. Reprinted with permission.)

together with the appearance of numerous transitional cells (Fig. 13), primarily in the perisinusoidal spaces, and myofibroblasts, primarily in the perivenular areas in association with abundant collagen fibers. Similar increases in myofibroblasts (Lieber *et al.*, 1981; Nakano and Lieber, 1982) and transitional cells (Mak *et al.*, 1984) occurred in baboons after chronic alcohol feeding. The striking hepatic inflammation and necrosis in rats fed the high vitamin A/ethanol diet were accompanied by a rise in serum glutamic-oxaloacetic transaminase (SGOT) and GDH and by a decrease in serum vitamin A and RBP. Thus, this rat study revealed that a level of vitamin A supplementation that does not ordinarily produce significant liver alterations may result in hepatic inflammation, necrosis, and fibrosis in the presence of ethanol—even though the rat is normally refractory to ethanol-induced fibrosis.

We do not know why enhanced liver toxicity occurs when vitamin A supplementation is accompanied by ethanol ingestion. The two rat studies (Leo *et al.*, 1982; Leo and Lieber, 1983b) show that fibrosis does not develop in the presence of vitamin A supplementation alone or ethanol ingestion

TABLE III

**Effect of Vitamin A with or without Ethanol on Hepatic Fat-Storing Cells in Rats[a]**

| Groups | Hepatocytes | Fat-storing cells | |
|---|---|---|---|
| | Per 10,000 $(\mu m)^2$ | Per 10,000 $(\mu m)^2$ | Per 1,000 hepatocytes |
| 2-Month treatment | | | |
| Ethanol-fed rats ($n$ = 7) | 9.8 ± 0.7[b] | 0.7 ± 0.09 | 70 ± 8[d] |
| Pair-fed controls ($n$ = 7) | 11.5 ± 0.6 | 1.4 ± 0.01[c] | 120 ± 10[e] |
| | NS | $p < 0.001$ | $p < 0.005$ |
| 9-Month treatment | | | |
| Ethanol-fed rats ($n$ = 9) | 7.5 ± 0.2 | 0.9 ± 0.04 | 130 ± 4 |
| Pair-fed controls ($n$ = 9) | 10.2 ± 0.1 | 1.4 ± 0.20 | 180 ± 1 |
| | $p < 0.005$ | $p < 0.001$ | $p < 0.005$ |

[a]Long-term vitamin A administration increased the number of fat-storing cells, but ethanol prevented this effect. (From Leo and Lieber, 1983b. Reprinted with permission.)

[b]$p < 0.025$ when compared to the corresponding group treated for 9 months.

[c]$p < 0.02$ when compared to the corresponding group treated for 9 months.

[d]$p < 0.01$ when compared to the corresponding group treated for 9 months.

[e]$p < 0.001$ when compared to the corresponding group treated for 9 months.

alone. Others have postulated that vitamin A-induced toxicity may result from an intrahepatic overflow of the RBP-associated form of vitamin A to its esterified form (Mallia *et al.*, 1975; Smith and Goodman, 1976). Retinol cannot be the sole source of this toxicity because hepatic vitamin A levels in ethanol-fed rats, which showed the most prominent signs of toxicity, were lower than in controls. Because retinol can be further metabolized by liver microsomes, and because ethanol ingestion increases the activity of these microsomal systems (Sato and Lieber, 1982b; Leo *et al.*, 1984a; Leo *et al.*, 1985; Leo *et al.*, 1987a), increased production of certain metabolites may enhance vitamin A toxicity. Thus far, however, no experimental evidence supports this hypothesis.

## B. Clinical Evidence of Hepatotoxicity

Vitamin A hepatotoxicity is well documented clinically (Farrell *et al.*, 1977; Herbert, 1982; Russell *et al.*, 1974). The most common clinical manifestation of liver toxicity is hepatomegaly (Josephs, 1944; Muenter *et al.*, 1971; Stimson, 1961). Cirrhosis (Jacques *et al.*, 1979) and portal hypertension with ascites (Russell *et al.*, 1974) have also been reported. Portal hypertension with ascites has also been observed in the absence of cirrhosis and

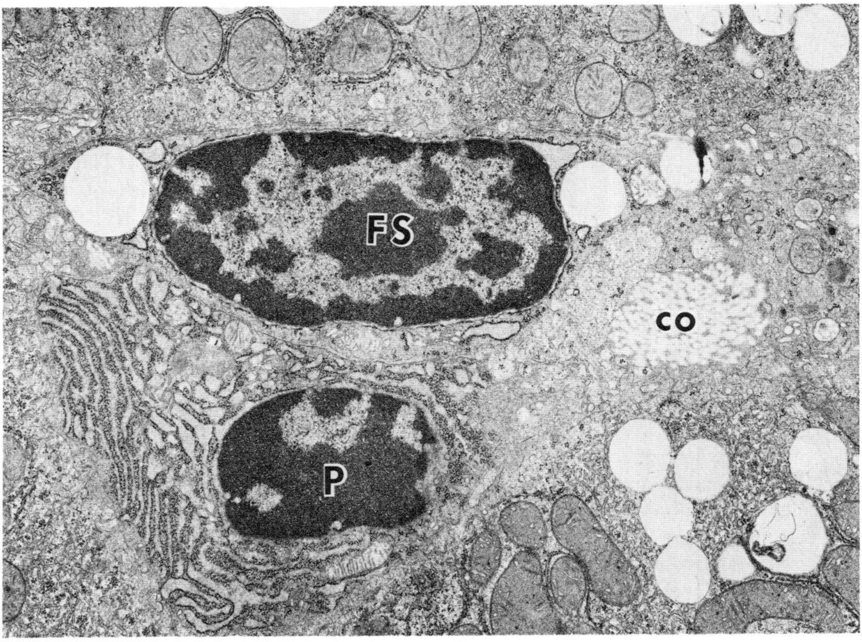


**Fig. 13.** Liver of rat fed high vitamin A/ethanol diet for 9 months shows a fat-storing cell (FS) with dilated, rough endoplasmic reticulum (×8,750). A few fat droplets and adjacent abundant collagen bundles (Co) are present. Plasma cells (P) are also shown. (From Leo and Lieber, 1983b. Reprinted with permission.)

has been attributed to obstruction of sinusoids and terminal venules, to obliteration of the space of Disse by collagen, and to large increases in the number and size of fat-storing cells of Ito (Hruban *et al.*, 1974; Russell *et al.*, 1974). In some of these studies, particularly those related to food faddism, vitamin A intake greatly exceeded normal therapeutic doses.

Because vitamin A supplementation, when combined with ethanol or drug abuse, potentiates vitamin A toxicity in rats, extrapolation of rat data to humans suggests that signs of toxicity may appear in individuals who combine normally safe amounts of vitamin A with alcohol or drugs. In addition, over-the-counter availability of capsules containing 25,000 IU of vitamin A may encourage a relatively high vitamin A intake. Excessive supplementation may also be influenced by lay media reports of vitamin A therapy used for dermatological conditions (Elias and Williams, 1981) or for cancer therapy and prevention (Anonymous, 1980).

Traditionally, vitamin A toxicity has been reported following doses of about 100,000 IU/day for periods ranging from weeks to months (Jeghers and Marraro, 1958; Korner and Vollm, 1975). However, severe toxicity with a plasma vitamin A level 10 times higher than normal was reported in a 16-year-old who ingested 50,000 IU/day for more than two years (Farris and Erdman, 1982). Liver damage from massive vitamin A deposition has also been reported in association with a subnormal serum vitamin A level (Weber *et al.*, 1982). In this instance, the low serum level may have been caused by protein deficiency or liver damage (Leo and Lieber, 1988).

## VIII. VITAMIN A AND CANCER

A major physiologic role of vitamin A is control of cell differentiation. Because loss of this control is a basic feature of cancer, there is ample reason to suspect that vitamin A intake and cancer incidence are related.

A general description of the role of vitamin A and ethanol in carcinogenesis is beyond the scope of this discussion; the role of ethanol in promoting carcinogenesis is discussed in detail elsewhere (Lieber *et al.*, 1986). This discussion centers on possible mechanisms by which ethanol may favor hepatic carcinogenesis in vitamin A-linked disorders.

Membrane lesions and other changes give clues to possible mechanisms that predispose cells to became cancerous. Vitamin A depletion is associated with striking increases in the sialic acid, galactose and mannose content of membranes (Kim *et al.*, 1988). An increase in sialic acid content has frequently been observed in malignant cell surfaces (Van Beek *et al.*, 1973; Litin and Girimes, 1983). Vitamin A deficiency *per se* has produced precancerous metaplasia in epithelial linings (Mak *et al.*, 1984; Mak *et al.*, 1987). Moreover, squamous metaplasia of the trachea caused by vitamin A deficiency was strikingly potentiated in the rat by concomitant ethanol ingestion, which resulted in lysosomal and ciliary abnormalities in the tracheal ciliated cells (Mak *et al.*, 1984).

Ethanol may also act as a cocarcinogen via its effects on enzyme systems that activate and detoxify carcinogens. Ethanol is a potent inducer of the cytochrome *P*-450-dependent microsomal system. Although this enzyme system functions primarily to detoxify xenobiotics, it is also involved in converting many structurally diverse chemicals to electrophilic mutagens and carcinogens (Miller and Miller, 1977).

The effect of ethanol on activation of microsomal cytochrome *P*-450-dependent procarcinogens was examined using microsomes from various tissues: the liver, the principal site of xenobiotic metabolism; the lungs and intestines, major portals of entry for tobacco smoke and dietary carcinogens; and the esophagus, a site at which ethanol consumption poses a major cancer risk (Garro *et al.*, 1981). These studies used isolated microsomal preparations from tissues of pair-fed or acute ethanol-exposed rats, hamsters, or mice. Preparations were analyzed for their ability to activate procarcinogens to mutagens detectable in the Ames *Salmonella* mutagenesis assay (Ames *et al.*, 1975) or to produce defined products.

We found that ethanol is unique in its ability to increase hepatic dimethylnitrosamine (DMN) demethylase activity, which was detectable at DMN concentrations of 0.3–100 m*M*. By contrast, other microsomal enzyme inducers, such as phenobarbital, 3-methylcholanthrene, and PCBs, increased the activity of DMN demethylase isozymes at relatively high DMN concentrations of >40m*M* and repressed the activity of low $K_m$ DMN demethylases (Venkatesan *et al.*, 1968; Czygan *et al.*, 1973; Guttenplan and Garro, 1976).

Some of these effects may result from the induction by ethanol of a unique species of cytochrome *P*-450 (Ohnishi and Lieber, 1977; Koop *et al.*, 1982; Lasker *et al.*, 1987), which differentially affects activation of various carcinogens. For example, a selective affinity for DMN has been demonstrated for ethanol-induced cytochrome *P*-450 (Yang *et al.*, 1985). This DMN activation by liver microsomes was competitively inhibited by retinol (Fig. 14), presumably because of a partially shared microsomal metabolic system (Leo *et al.*, 1986b). Because both DMN and retinol can be metabolized by a microsomal *P*-450 system, retinol may exert a beneficial effect by directly interfering with microsomal activation of chemical

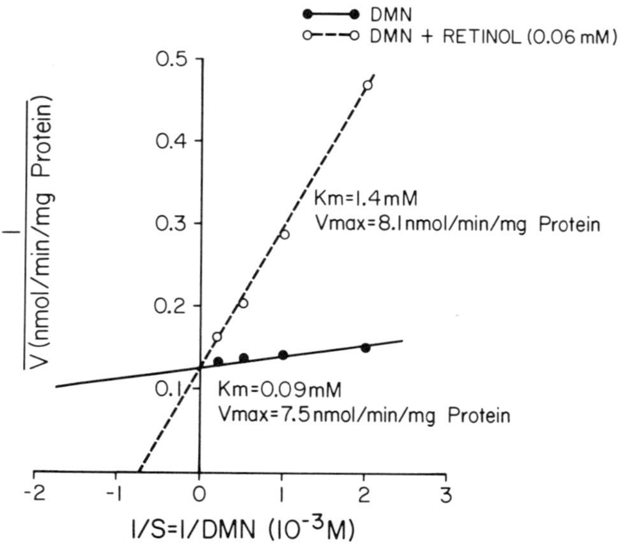


**Fig. 14.** Liver microsomes of rats fed ethanol were incubated with various concentrations of DMN, with or without retinol. Retinol was shown to be a competitive inhibitor of hepatic microsomal dimethylnitrosamine (DMN) demethylation. (From Leo *et al.*, 1986b. Reprinted with permission.)

carcinogens. Low hepatic Vitamin A stores might diminish this inhibition and thus indirectly favor chemical carcinogenesis.

Vitamin A may protect against cancer in other ways. Because carcinogenesis involves immunologic factors (Lieber *et al.*, 1986), the decline in immune response secondary to vitamin A deficiency (Smith *et al.*, 1987) may have far-reaching consequences in the pathogenesis of both cancer and infectious diseases. The possible anticarcinogenic role of carotene, independent of its role as a vitamin A precursor, is presently under study (Hennekens, 1986).

## IX. THERAPEUTIC IMPLICATIONS

The amount of vitamin A needed to correct or prevent hypovitaminosis A lesions without producing toxicity must be determined. Careful monitoring of patients is mandatory but difficult because early signs of toxicity cannot readily be measured. Data presented here clearly indicate that serum vitamin A measurements are unreliable indicators of hepatic vitamin A stores or toxicity in patients with liver disease. Increases in serum GDH and SGOT may reflect hepatotoxicity, but these measurements may be of limited use in alcoholics because they do not differentiate between the enzyme changes caused by vitamin A toxicity and those caused by the direct hepatotoxic effects of alcohol. Liver biopsies may be similarly unrevealing because they cannot show whether hepatic vitamin A levels have decreased as a result of ethanol consumption or increased as a result of vitamin A therapy. In the absence of early clinical indicators of vitamin A toxicity, great caution is required when selecting doses to be used in treating the vitamin A abnormalities associated with alcoholism. In the alcoholic, the beneficial range of vitamin A supplementation may fall within a narrow therapeutic window.

In contrast with retinol, carotenoids—even when chronically ingested in large amounts—have not been known to produce toxic manifestations (Heywood *et al.*, 1985; Olson, 1987). Moreover, blood carotenoid levels have been found to be sensitive to beta-carotene intake, whereas blood retinol levels are not affected over a wide range of intake (Urbach *et al.*, 1952; Willett *et al.*, 1983). Whether carotene may serve as an effective but less toxic substitute for retinol is under investigation.

## X. SUMMARY

In Western countries, vitamin A deficiency is most commonly associated with liver disease. In addition to its occurrence in alcoholic hepatitis or cirrhosis, vitamin A depletion occurs at early stages of liver injury, such as the fatty liver of alcoholism. Experimental administration of either alcohol or other drugs results in hepatic vitamin A depletion, in part because of mobilization of vitamin A to peripheral tissues and also because of enhanced microsomal degradation via induction of newly described pathways of vitamin A metabolism. These include retinol oxidation by a cytochrome *P*-450-dependent system and retinol dehydrogenation by an enzyme distinct from CRD.

Vitamin A depletion can be readily overlooked because, at its early stages, serum vitamin A may still be normal. Patients with severe hepatic vitamin A depletion display a hepatic lesion characterized by the appearance of giant lysosomes filled with lipoprotein-like particles. The causal relationship between these lesions and vitamin A depletion was established in animals fed diets low in vitamin A. Ethanol feeding also resulted in vitamin A depletion in plasma membranes, which was associated with decreased microviscosity. An increasing body of experimental and epidemiological evidence links cancer and hypovitaminosis A, particularly when the latter occurs in alcoholism. In addition to mucosal alterations, mechanisms include relative lack of protection by retinoids against chemical carcinogenesis. Correction of vitamin A deficiency may need to be contemplated not only for the traditional indications of night blindness and sexual dysfunction but also for treatment of patients with alcoholic liver injury and for prevention of carcinogenesis.

However, retinoid treatment must take into account that large amounts of vitamin A can be hepatotoxic. Experimental administration of ethanol enhances the hepatotoxicity of vitamin A. When associated with alcohol consumption, amounts of vitamin A equivalent to those commonly used in therapeutic supplements were found in rats to result in mitochondrial dysfunction with decreased respiration, leakage of GDH and other mitochondrial enzymes into the bloodstream, and striking ultrastructural lesions. Eventually, hepatocellular necrosis developed, with inflammation and an increase in the number of cells transitional between Ito cells and fibroblasts, both of which appeared to contribute to the associated fibrosis. These lesions represent the experimental counterpart of fibrosis and cirrhosis clinically associated with long-term vitamin A excess.

Both alcohol and drug abuse promote vitamin A depletion, and vitamin A administration is indicated to prevent liver lesions and possibly carcinogenesis. Treatment, however, must stay within a narrow therapeutic window when associated with alcohol or drug abuse. Thus, both hepatic vitamin A depletion and excess are associated with significant liver injury in the alcoholic.

## ACKNOWLEDGMENTS

Original studies were supported by DHHS grants AA 03508 and DK 32810 and the Veterans Adminstration.

## REFERENCES

Ames, B. N., McCann, J., and Yamasaki, E. (1975). Methods for detecting carcinogens and mutagens with the *Salmonella*/mammalian-microsome mutagenicity test. *Mutat. Res.* **31**, 347–364.

Baumann, C. A., Foster, E. G., and Moore, P. R. (1942). The effect of dibenzanthracene, of alcohol, and other agents on vitamin A in the rat. *J. Biol. Chem.* **142**, 597–608.

Blomstrand, R., Lof, A., and Osling, H. (1977). Studies on the metabolic effects of long-term administration of ethanol and 4-methylpyrazole in the rat. *Nutr. Metab.* **21**, 149–151.

Clausen, S. W., Breese, B. B., Baum, W. S., McCoord, A. B., and Rydeen, J. O. (1941). Effect of alcohol on vitamin A content of blood in human subjects. *Science* **93**, 21–22.

Clausen, S. W., Baum, W. S., McCoord, A. B., Rydeen, J. O., and Breese, B. B. (1942). The mobilization by alcohols of vitamin A from its stores in the tissues. *J. Nutr.* **24**, 1–14.

Connor, M. J., and Smit, M. H. (1987). Terminal-group oxidation of retinol by mouse epidermis. *Biochem. J.* **244**, 489–493.

Crowley, J. W., and Allen, N. N. (1953). The effect of ethyl alcohol on the plasma vitamin A levels of calves and goats. *J. Dairy Sci.* **36**, 156–160.

Czygan, P., Greim, H., Garro, A. J., Hutterer, F., Schaffner, H., Popper, O., Rosenthal, O., and Cooper, D. Y. (1973). Microsomal metabolism of dimethylnitrosamine and the cytochrome *P*-450 dependence of its activation to a mutagen. *Cancer Res.* **33**, 2983–2986.

Denk, H., Franke, W. W., Eckerstorfer, R., Schmid, E., and Kerjaschki, D. (1979a). Formation and involution of Mallory bodies ("alcoholic hyalin") in murine and human liver revealed by immunofluorescence microscopy with antibodies to prekeratin. *Proc. Nat. Acad. Sci. USA* **76**, 4112–4116.

Denk, H., Franke, W. W., Kerjaschki, D., and Eckerstorfer, R. (1979b). Mallory bodies in experimental animals and man. *Int. Rev. Exp. Pathol.* **20**, 77–121.

Anonymous. (1980). Vitamin A, retinol, carotene, and cancer prevention (Editorial). *Brit. Med. J.* **281**, 957–958.

Elias, P. M., and Williams, M. L. (1981). Retinoids, cancer, and the skin. *Arch. Dermatol.* **117**, 160–180.

Farrell, G. C., Bathal, P. S., and Powell, L. W. (1977). Abnormal liver function in chronic hypervitaminosis A. *Dig. Dis. Sci.* **22**, 724–728.

Farris, W., and Erdman, J. (1982). Protracted hypervitaminosis A following long-term low-level intake. *JAMA-J. Am. Med. Assn.* **247**, 1317–1318.

French, S. W. (1981). The Mallory body: Structure, composition, and pathogenesis. *Hepatology* **1**, 76–83.

Garro, A. J., Seitz, H. K., and Lieber, C. S. (1981). Enhancement of dimethylnitrosamine metabolism and activation to a mutagen following chronic ethanol consumption. *Cancer Res.* **41**, 120–124.

Goodman, D. S. (1984). Vitamin A and retinoids in health and disease. *N. Engl. J. Med.* **310**, 1023–1031.

Guttenplan, J. B., and Garro, A.J . (1976). Factors affecting the induction of dimethylnitrosamine by Aroclor 1254. *Cancer Res.* **37**, 329–330.

Hennekens, C. H. (1986). Micronutrients and cancer prevention. *N. Engl. J. Med.* **315**, 1288–1289.

Herbert, V. (1982). Toxicity of 25,000 IU vitamin A supplements in "health" food users. *Amer. J. Clin. Nutr.* **36**, 185–186.

Heywood, R., Palmer, A. K., Gregson, R. L., and Hummler, H. (1985). The toxicity of beta-carotene. *Toxicology* **36**, 91–100.

Hruban, Z., Russell, R. M., Boyer, J. L., Glagov, S., and Bagheri, S. A. (1974). Ultrastructural changes in livers of two patients with hypervitaminosis A. *Amer. J. Pathol.* **76**, 451–468.

Innami, S., Nakamura, A., Miyazaki, M., Nagayama, S., and Nishide, E. (1976). Further studies on the reduction of vitamin A content in the livers of rats given polychlorinated biphenyls. *J. Nutr. Sci. Vitaminol.* **2**, 409–418.

Jacques, E. A., Buschmann, R. J., and Layden, T. J. (1979). The histopathologic progression of vitamin A-induced hepatic injury. *Gastroenterology* **76**, 599–602.

Jeghers, H., and Marraro, H. (1958). Hypervitaminosis A: Its broadening spectrum. *Amer. J. Clin. Nutr.* **6**, 335–339.

Joly, J.-G., Ishii, H., Teschke, R., Hasumura, Y., and Lieber, C. S. (1973). Effect of chronic ethanol feeding on the activities and submicrosomal distribution of reduced nicotinamide adenine dinucleotide phosphate (NADPH)-cytochrome *P*-450 reductase and the demethylases for aminopyrine and ethylmorphine. *Biochem. Pharmacol.* **22**, 1532–1535.

Josephs, H. W. (1944). Hypervitaminosis A and carotenemia. *Amer. J. Dis. Child.* **67**, 33–43.

Kato, N., Kato, M., Kimura, T., and Yoshida, A. (1978). Effect of dietary addition of PCB, DDT or DHT and dietary protein on vitamin A and cholesterol metabolism. *Nutr. Rep. Int.* **18**, 437–445.

Kim, C., Leo, M. A., Lowe, N., and Lieber, C. S. (1988). Effects of vitamin A and ethanol on liver plasma membrane fluidity. *Hepatology* **8**, 735–741.

Kishore, G. S., and Boutwell, R. K. (1980). Enzymatic oxidation and reduction of retinal by mouse epidermis. *Biochem. Biophys. Res. Commun.* **94**, 1381–1386.

Kishore, G. S., Perumal, A. S., and Cama, H. R. (1971). The effect of thyroid activity on the enzymes of vitamin A metabolism and on the stability of lysosomes. *Int. J. Vit. Nutr. Res.* **41**, 171–179.

Koop, D. R., Morgan, E. T., Tarr, G. E., and Coon, M. J. (1982). Purification and characterization of a unique isozyme of cytochrome *P*-450 from liver microsomes of ethanol-treated rabbits. *J. Biol. Chem.* **257**, 8472–8480.

Korner, W. F., and Vollm, J. (1975). New aspects of the tolerance of retinol in humans. *Int. J. Vit. Nutr. Res.* **45**, 363–372.

Lakshmanan, M. R., Vaidyanathan, C. S., and Cama, H. R. (1964). Oxidation of vitamin $A_1$ aldehyde and vitamin $A_2$ aldehyde to the corresponding acids by aldehyde oxidase from different species. *Biochem. J.* **90**, 569–573.

Lasker, J. M., Raucy, J., Kubota, S., Bloswick, B. P., Black, M., and Lieber, C. S. (1987). Purification and characterization of human liver cytochrome *P*-450-ALC. *Biochem. Biophys. Res. Commun.* **148**, 232–238.

Lee, M., and Lucia, S. P. (1965). Effect of ethanol on the mobilization of vitamin A in the dog and in the rat. *J. Stud. Alcohol* **26**, 1–9.

Leo, M. A., and Lieber, C. S. (1982). Hepatic vitamin A depletion in alcoholic liver injury in man. *N. Engl. J. Med.* **307**, 597–601.

Leo, M. A., and Lieber, C. S. (1983a). Interaction of ethanol with vitamin A. *Alcoholism: Clin. Exp. Res.* **7**, 15–21.

Leo, M. A., and Lieber, C. S. (1983b). Hepatic fibrosis after long term administration of ethanol and moderate vitamin A supplementation in the rat. *Hepatology* **2**, 1–11.

Leo, M. A., and Lieber, C. S. (1984). Interaction of ethanol with vitamin A. *Alcoholism: Clin. Exp. Res.* **7**, 15–21.

Leo, M. A., and Lieber, C. S. (1985). New pathway for retinol metabolism in liver microsomes. *J. Biol. Chem.* **260**, 5228–5231.

Leo, M. A., and Lieber, C. S. (1988). Hypervitaminosis: A liver lover's lament. *Hepatology* **8**, 412–417.

Leo, M. A., Arai, M., Sato, M., and Lieber, C. S. (1982). Hepatotoxicity of vitamin A and ethanol in the rat. *Gastroenterology* **82**, 194–205.

Leo, M. A., Sato, M., and Lieber, C. S. (1983). Effect of hepatic vitamin A depletion on the liver in humans and rats. *Gastroenterology* **84**, 562–572.

Leo, M. A., Iida, S., and Lieber, C. S. (1984a). Retinoic acid metabolism by a system reconstituted with cytochrome *P*-450. *Arch. Biochem. Biophys.* **234**, 305–312.

Leo, M. A., Lowe, N., and Lieber, C. S. (1984b). Decreased hepatic vitamin A after drug administration in men and in rats. *Amer. J. Clin. Nutr.* **40**, 1131–1136.

Leo, M. A., Mak, K. M., Savolainen, E. R., and Lieber, C. S. (1985). Isolation and culture of myofibroblasts from rat liver. *Proc. Soc. Exp. Biol. Med.* **180**, 382–391.

Leo, M. A., Kim, C., and Lieber, C. S. (1986a). Increased vitamin A in esophagus and other extrahepatic tissues after chronic ethanol consumption in the rat. *Alcoholism: Clin. Exp. Res.* **10**, 487–492.

Leo, M. A., Lowe, N., and Lieber, C. S. (1986b). Interaction of drugs and retinol. *Biochem. Pharmacol.* **35**, 3949–3953.

Leo, M. A., Kim, C., and Lieber, C. S. (1987a). $NAD^+$-dependent retinol dehydrogenase in liver microsomes. *Arch. Biochem. Biophys.* **259**, 241–249.

Leo, M. A., Kim, C., and Lieber, C. S. (1987b). Alcohol, vitamin A and zinc. *Nutr. Rev.* **45**, 253–254.

Leo, M. A., Lowe, N., and Lieber, C. S. (1987c). Potentiation of ethanol-induced hepatic vitamin A depletion by phenobarbital and butylated hydroxytoluene. *J. Nutr.* **117**, 70–76.

Lieber, C. S., and Leo, M. A. (1985). Role of vitamin A deficiency and excess in liver disease. *In* "Metabolism and Nutrition in Liver Disease, Falk Symposium 41" (E. Holm and H. Kasper, eds.), pp. 157–179. MTP Press Ltd., Lancaster, England.

Lieber, C. S., Nakano, M., and Worner, T. M. (1981). Ultrastructure of the initial stages of hepatic perivenular fibrosis after alcohol. *Trans. Assn. Amer. Phys.* **94**, 292–330.

Lieber, C. S., Garro, A., Leo, M. A., Mak, K. M., and Worner, T. (1986). Alcohol and cancer. *Hepatology* **6**, 1005–1009.

Lippel, K., and Olson, J. A. (1968). Biosynthesis of beta-glucuronides of retinol and retinoic acid *in vivo* and *in vitro*. *J. Lipid Res.* **9**, 168–175.

Litin, B. S., and Girimes, W. J. (1983). Heterogeneity of sialoglycoproteins purified from normal and malignant cells. *Cancer Res.* **43**, 2131–2139.

Mak, K. M., Leo, M. A., and Lieber, C. S. (1984). Alcoholic liver injury in baboons: transformation of lipocytes to transitional cells. *Gastroenterology* **87**, 188–200.

Mak, K. M., Leo, M. A., and Lieber, C. S. (1987). Potentiation by ethanol consumption of tracheal squamous metaplasia caused by vitamin A deficiency in rats. *J. Nat. Cancer Inst.* **93**, 362–370.

Mallia, A. K., Smith, J. E., and Goodman, D. W. S. (1975). Metabolism of retinol binding protein and vitamin A during hypervitaminosis A in the rat. *J. Lipid Res.* **16**, 180–188.

McClain, C. J., Van Thiel, D. H., Parker, S., Badzin, L. K., and Gilbert, H. (1979). Alteration in zinc, vitamin A and retinol-binding protein in chronic alcoholics: A possible mechanism for night blindness and hypogonadism. *Alcoholism: Clin. Exp. Res.* **3**, 135–140.

Miller, J. A., and Miller, E. C. (1977). Ultimate chemical carcinogens as reactive mutagenic electrophiles. *In* "Origin of Human Cancer" (H. H. Hiatt, J. D. Watson, and J. A. Winston, eds.), pp. 605–628. Cold Spring Harbor Laboratory, New York.

Miller, R. W., Hemken, R. W., Waldo, D. R., and Moore, L. A. (1969). Effect of ethyl alcohol on the vitamin A status of Holstein heifers. *J. Dairy Sci.* **52**, 1998–2000.

Misra, P. S., Lefevre, A., Ishii, H., Rubin, E., and Lieber, C. S. (1971). Increase of ethanol, meprobamate, and phenobarbital metabolism after chronic ethanol administration in man and in rats. *Amer. J. Med.* **51**, 346–351.

Mobarhan, S., Russell, R. M., Underwood, B. A., Wallingford, J., Mathieson, R. D., and Al-Midani, H. (1981). Evaluation of the relative dose response test for vitamin A in cirrhotics. *Amer. J. Clin. Nutr.* **34**, 2264–2270.

Mobarhan, S., Lagden, T. J., Friedman, H. Kunigk, A., and Donahue, P. I. (1986). Depletion of liver and esophageal epithelium vitamin A after chronic moderate ethanol consumption in rats: Inverse relation to zinc nutriture. *Hepatology* **6**, 615–621.

Moffa, D. J., Lotspeich, F. J., and Krause, R. F. (1970). Preparation of properties of retinal-oxidizing enzyme from rat intestinal mucosa. *J. Biol. Chem.* **245**, 439–447.

Muenter, M. D., Perry, H. O., and Ludwig, J. (1971). Chronic vitamin A intoxication in adults: Hepatic, neurologic and dermatologic complications. *Amer. J. Med.* **50**, 129–136.

Nakano, M., and Lieber, C. S. (1982). Ultrastructure of initial stages of perivenular fibrosis in alcohol-fed baboons. *Amer. J. Pathol.* **106**, 145–155.

Napoli, J. L. (1986). Retinol metabolism in LLC-$PK_1$ cells. *J. Biol. Chem.* **261**, 13592–13597.

Ohnishi, K, and Lieber, C. S. (1977). Reconstitution of the microsomal ethanol-oxidizing system: Qualitative and quantitative changes of cytochrome *P*-450 after chronic alcohol consumption. *J. Biol. Chem.* **252**, 7124–7131.

Oikarinen, H., Oikarinen, A. I., Tan, E. M. L., Abergel, R. P., Meeker, C. A., Chu, M.-L., Prockop, D. J., and Uitto, J. (1985). Modulation of procollagen gene expression by retinoids. *J. Clin. Invest.* **75**, 1545–1553.

Olson, J. A. (1987). Recommended dietary intakes (RDI) of vitamin A in humans. *Amer. J. Clin. Nutr.* **45**, 704–716.

Pett, L. B. (1940). Mobilization of vitamin A by alcohol. *Science* **92**, 63.

Raica, N., Jr., Scott, J., and Lowry, L. (1972). Vitamin A concentration in human tissues collected from five areas in the United States. *Amer. J. Clin. Nutr.* **25**, 291–296.

"Recommended Dietary Allowances" (1980). 9th edition. Food and Nutrition Board, National Academy of Sciences, National Research Council, Washington, D.C.

Reddy, T. V., and Weisburger, E. K. (1980). Hepatic vitamin A status of rats during feeding of hepatocarcinogen 2-aminoanthraquinone. *Cancer Lett.* **10**, 39–44.

Roberts, A. B., and Frolik, C. A. (1979). Recent advances in the *in vivo* and *in vitro* metabolism of retinoic acid. *Fed. Proc.* **38**, 2524–2527.

Roberts, A. B., Nichols, M. D., Newton, D. L., and Sporn, M. B. (1979). *In vitro* metabolism of retinoic acid in hamster intestine and liver. *J. Biol. Chem.* **254**, 6296–6303.

Roberts, A. B., Lamb, L. C., and Sporn, M. B. (1980). Metabolism of all-*trans*-retinoic acid in hamster liver microsomes: Oxidation of 4-hydroxy- to 4-keto-retinoic acid. *Arch. Biochem. Biophys.* **199**, 374–383.

Russell, R. M., Boyer, J. L., Bagheri, S. A., and Hruban, Z. (1974). Hepatic injury from chronic hypervitaminosis A resulting in portal hypertension and ascites. *N. Engl. J. Med.* **291**, 435–440.

Russell, R. M., Morrison, S. A., Smith, F. R., Oaks, E. V., and Carney, E. A. (1978). Vitamin-A reversal of abnormal dark adaptation in cirrhosis. Study of effects on the plasma retinol transport system. *Ann. Intern. Med.* **88**, 622–626.

Ryan, D. E., Iida, S., Wood, A. W., Thomas, P. E., Lieber, C. S., and Levin, W. (1984). Characterization of three highly purified cytochromes *P*-450 from hepatic microsomes of adult male rats. *J. Biol. Chem.* **259**, 1239–1250.

Sato, M., and Lieber, C. S. (1981). Hepatic vitamin A depletion after chronic ethanol consumption in baboons and rats. *J. Nutr.* **111**, 2015–2023.

Sato, M., and Lieber, C. S. (1982a). Changes in vitamin A status after acute ethanol administration in the rat. *J. Nutr.* **112**, 1188–1196.

Sato, M., and Lieber, C. S. (1982b). Increased metabolism of retinoic acid after chronic ethanol consumption in rat liver microsomes. *Arch. Biochem. Biophys.* **213**, 557–564.

Senoo, H., and Wake, K. (1985). Suppression of experimental hepatic fibrosis by administration of vitamin A. *Lab. Invest.* **52**, 182–194.

Smith, F. R., and Goodman, D. S. (1971). The effects of diseases of the liver, thyroid, and kidneys on the transport of vitamin A in human plasma. *J. Clin. Invest.* **50**, 2426–2436.

Smith, F. R., and Goodman, D. W. S. (1976). Vitamin A transport in human vitamin A toxicity. *N. Engl. J. Med.* **294**, 805–808.

Smith, J. C., Brown, E. D., White, S. C., and Finkelson, J. D. (1975). Plasma vitamin A and zinc concentration in patients with alcoholic cirrhosis. *Lancet* **1**, 1251–1252.

Smith, S. A., Levy, N. S., and Hayes, C. E. (1987). Impaired immunity in vitamin A-deficient mice. *J. Nutr.* **117**, 857–865.

Sommer, A. (1982). "Nutritional Blindness: Xerophthalmia and Keratomalacia." University

Press Oxford, New York.

Sommer, A., Tarwotjo, I., Djunadedi, M. E., and Glover, J. (1980). Oral versus intramuscular vitamin A in the treatment of xerophthalmia. *Lancet* **1**, 557–559.

Sporn, M. B., Roberts, A. B., and Goodman, D. S. (eds.) (1984). "The Retinoids." Academic Press, New York.

Srikantia, S. G. (1976). Human vitamin A deficiency. *World Rev. Nutr. Diet.* **20**, 184–230.

Stimson, W. H. (1961). Vitamin A intoxication in adults. Report of a case with a summary of the literature. *N. Engl. J. Med.* **265**, 369–373.

Suschetet, M. (1975). Incidence d'une ingestion prolongee d'acide tannique, de metabisulfite de potassium et d'ethanol administres isolement ou en association, sur la tenuer du foie en vitamine A chez le rat. *J. Int. Vit. Nutr.* **45**, 129–137.

Swanson, B. N., Frolik, C. A., Zahrevitz, D. W., Roller, P. P., and Sporn, M. B. (1981). Dose-dependent kinetics of all-*trans*-retinoic acid in rats. Plasma levels and excretion into bile, urine, and faeces. *Biochem. Pharmacol.* **30**, 107–113.

Tanikawa, K. (1971). Liver diseases. "Ultrastructural Aspects of the Liver and its Disorders," 2nd edition, pp. 283–284. Igaku-shoin Ltd., New York.

Underwood, B. A., Siegel, H., Weisell, R. C., and Dolinksi, M. (1970). Liver stores of vitamin A in a normal population dying suddenly or rapidly from unnatural causes in New York City. *Amer. J. Clin. Nutr.* **23**, 1037–1042.

Urbach, C., Hickman, K., and Harris, P. L. (1952). Effect of individual vitamins A, C, E, and carotene administered at high levels on their concentration in the blood. *Exp. Med. Surg.* **10**, 7–20.

Vahlquist, A., Sjolund, K., Norden, A., Pererson, P. A., Stigmar, G., and Johansson, B. (1978). Plasma vitamin A transport and visual dark adaptation in diseases of the intestine and liver. *Scand. J. Clin. Lab. Invest.* **38**, 301–308.

Van Beek, W. P., Smets, L. A., and Emmelot, P. (1973). Increased sialic acid density in surface glycoprotein of transformed and malignant cells—a general phenomenon? *Cancer Res.* **33**, 2913–2922.

Venkatesan, N., Arcos, J. C., and Argus, M. F. (1968). Differential effect of polycyclic hydrocarbons on the demethylation of the carcinogen dimethylnitrosamine by rat tissues. *Life Sci.* **7**, 1111–1119.

Weber, F. L., Mitchell, G. E., Jr., Powell, D. E., Reiser, B. J., and Banwell, J. G. (1982). Reversible hepatotoxicity associated with hepatic vitamin A accumulation in a protein-deficient patient. *Gastroenterology* **82**, 118–123.

Willett, W. C., Stampfer, M. J., Underwood, B. A., Taylor, J. O., and Hennekens, C. H. (1983). Vitamin A, E, and carotene: Effects of supplementation on their plasma levels. *Amer. J. Clin. Nutr.* **38**, 559–566.

Wolf, G., Kiorpes, T. C., Masushige, S., Schreiber, J. B., Smith, M. J., and Anderson, R. S. (1979). Recent evidence for the participation of vitamin A in glycoprotein synthesis. *Fed. Proc.* **38**, 2540–2543.

Wolff, K. L. (1932). On the quantity of vitamin A present in the human liver. *Lancet* **223**, 617–620.

Yamada, S., Mak, K. M., and Lieber, C. S. (1985). Chronic ethanol consumption alters rat liver plasma membranes and potentiates release of alkaline phosphatase. *Gastroenterology* **88**, 1799–1806.

Yang, C. S., Tu, Y. Y., Koop, D. R., and Coon, J. J. (1985). Metabolism of nitrosamines by purified rabbit liver cytochrome *P*-450 isozymes. *Cancer Res.* **45**, 1140–1145.

Zile, M. H., Schnoes, H. K., and DeLuca, H. F. (1980). Characterization of retinyl beta-glucuronide as a minor metabolite of retinoic acid in bile. *Proc. Nat. Acad. Sci. USA* **77**, 3230–3233.

# 15

# Alcoholism and Folate Homeostasis

Charles H. Halsted

*Division of Clinical Nutrition*
*Department of Internal Medicine*
*University of California, Davis*
*School of Medicine*
*Davis, California*



## I. INTRODUCTION: NUTRITIONAL REQUIREMENTS AND BIOCHEMICAL ROLES OF FOLATES

Folates are a family of water-soluble compounds found in green vegetables and bound to animal protein. Folates are mainly required for nucleic acid synthesis and cell regeneration.

Present in the diet as reduced, methylated, and formylated pteroylpolyglutamates ($PteGlu_n$), folates undergo hydrolysis in the upper intestine and, after intestinal transport, reach the liver in the form of pteroylmonoglutamates (PteGlu). Within hepatocytes, folates are reconverted to the $PteGlu_n$ form, in which they are stored and function in various carbon-transfer reactions. Folates undergo enterohepatic cycling and circulate systemically as reduced and methylated pteroylmonoglutamate ($CH_3H_4PteGlu$). The principal route of elimination is via the kidney, where $CH_3H_4PteGlu$ is filtered at the glomerulus and reabsorbed across the tubular membrane. A smaller, indeterminate amount of folate escapes the enterohepatic circulation and is excreted in the feces.

The daily requirement of folate has recently been reevaluated and, based on knowledge of efficiency of absorption, tissue requirements, storage, and elimination, is estimated at 3 $\mu$g/kg body weight (Herbert, 1987).

Important biochemical functions of folates include methionine synthesis from homocysteine in a transmethylation reaction, which requires vitamin $B_{12}$, and thymidine synthesis, which is essential for DNA and cellular regeneration. The metabolic interaction of folate with vitamin $B_{12}$ and the requirement for folate in DNA synthesis explain the common clinical manifestation of vitamin $B_{12}$ and folate deficiency in inducing megaloblastic anemia and macrocytosis of the intestinal epithelium.

## II. INCIDENCE OF FOLATE DEFICIENCY IN ALCOHOLISM

Folate deficiency is described clinically in patients consuming inadequate diets (e.g., unattended chronically ill), in patients with intestinal malabsorption (e.g., celiac or tropical sprue), in patients with increased requirements (e.g., pregnancy), in patients treated with drugs that affect folate absorption (e.g., sulfasalazine) and in chronic alcoholism.

In the United States, chronic alcoholism is probably the leading cause of folate deficiency (Halsted, 1980). Surveys indicate that folate deficiency is more common in derelict than employed alcoholics, and more prevalent in alcoholics with than without liver disease (Halsted and Tamura, 1978). According to these data, low levels of serum folate may be found in as many as 80% of recently drinking alcoholics (Herbert *et al.*, 1963), whereas low red-cell folate levels and clinical expression of megaloblastic anemia occur in about 40% of derelict alcoholics (Hines and Cowan, 1974). Less is known about the incidence of folate deficiency in otherwise well-nourished and well-to-do alcoholics.

## III. CLINICAL SIGNIFICANCE OF FOLATE DEFICIENCY IN ALCOHOLISM

### A. Anemia

Anemia, or low circulating hemoglobin levels, is common in alcoholic patients and is attributed to combined deficiencies of iron, pyridoxine, and folate. In a prospective series of 65 consecutive alcoholic patients, 75% were anemic; in these, bone marrow examinations revealed the megaloblastosis of folate deficiency in 40% and ring sideroblasts of pyridoxine deficiency in 30% (Eichner and Hillman, 1971). In the remaining patients, anemia was ascribed to overt or occult gastrointestinal blood loss, hemolysis caused by hypersplenism, or other causes. Although sideroblastosis is usually associated with folate deficiency, folate and pyridoxine metabolism are not directly linked.

The relationship of folate deficiency to megaloblastosis of the bone marrow in alcoholism was established about 30 years ago in two classical studies. In the earlier study by Jandl and Lear (1956), megaloblastic anemia in chronic alcoholic patients was described as morphologically identical to that of pernicious anemia, but the patients had normal or increased serum vitamin $B_{12}$ levels and the anemia was responsive to oral folic acid therapy. In a subsequent study of three cirrhotic alcoholics, megaloblastic anemia responded to low doses of 75 $\mu$g/day of oral or parenteral folic acid with reticulocytosis and reversion of bone marrow red cells to normal morphology (Sullivan and Herbert, 1964). The coadministration of 150–200 g ethanol/day prevented or reversed the responsiveness of the bone marrow to oral and parenteral folic acid, thus establishing for the first time an inhibitory effect of ethanol on the tissue availability of folate.

### B. Intestinal Mucosa

Like the bone marrow, the intestinal mucosal epithelium is a tissue with rapid cellular turnover—its regeneration occurs in 4 to 6 days. Diseases such as tropical sprue are associated with nuclear enlargement of intestinal mucosal crypt cells that respond somewhat to folic acid therapy (Swanson and Thomassen, 1965). Two separate observers reported on individual alcoholic patients with severe megaloblastic anemia, including enlarged crypt cell nuclei and epithelial cells; both patients responded to folic acid therapy (Bianchi *et al.*, 1970; Hermos *et al.*, 1972). Similar changes, produced experimentally in rats fed folate-deficient diets, were associated with decreased tissue folate levels (Klipstein *et al.*, 1973). The functional significance of these changes is uncertain.

However, induction of folate deficiency by poor diet together with ethanol administration was associated with abnormal absorption of water, electrolytes, glucose, and folic acid in two patient volunteers (Halsted *et al.*, 1973). In other human volunteers, ingestion of low-folate diets with ethanol lowered intestinal fluid absorption (Mekhjian and May, 1977). In rats fed folate-deficient diets, jejunal fluid transport reverted from absorption to a net secretory state (Goetsch and Klipstein, 1977). These data suggest that intestinal transport of fluid, and perhaps absorption of some water-soluble nutrients, may be influenced by the tissue folate level and its effect on cell turnover. The broader, untested hypothesis is that folate deficiency may contribute significantly to the diarrhea, malabsorption, and malnutrition prevalent among chronic alcoholics.

## C. Hepatic Injury and Regeneration

Measurements in liver biopsies show that hepatic folate stores decrease in patients with alcoholic cirrhosis (Baker *et al.*, 1964). Because folates play a central role in DNA and methionine metabolism, low hepatic folate levels could affect cell regeneration and pathways of tissue repair that depend on an adequate tissue supply of methionine. Hepatic DNA synthesis, measured by [$^3$H]thymidine uptake *in vitro*, correlated with poor prognosis in alcoholic hepatitis and increased with folic acid therapy (Leevy, 1966).

Several lines of evidence point to the methionine/glutathione pathway as essential in protecting against free-radical-mediated hepatic injury. Acute and/or chronic ethanol exposure in experimental animals and alcoholic patients is followed by hepatic lipid peroxidation, assessed by diene conjugate production, together with decreased hepatic glutathione (GSH) (Shaw *et al.*, 1981; Shaw *et al.*, 1983). The lipid peroxidizing effect of acute ethanol was attenuated by concurrent administration of methionine in experimental rats (Shaw *et al.*, 1981). The suppressive effect of alcohol on rat hepatic GSH levels was confirmed by two other groups, who differ as to whether the alcohol affects only hepatic GSH synthesis from methionine (Lauterburg *et al.*, 1984) or whether it promotes both hepatic GSH synthesis and cellular GSH efflux (Fernandez-Checa *et al.*, 1987). Because folate is required for endogenous methionine synthesis via the methyltransferase reaction, the supply of hepatic folate in the chronically malnourished alcoholic could conceivably limit the level of methionine essential for GSH synthesis, thus promoting ethanol-induced lipid peroxidative injury. This hypothesis awaits testing.

## IV. PATHOGENESIS OF FOLATE DEFICIENCY IN ALCOHOLISM

### A. Acute Effects of Alcoholism

A hypothesis for the pathogenesis of folate deficiency in alcoholism must account for several diverse observations. Ethanol administration to folate-deficient patients (Sullivan and Herbert, 1964) or to volunteers consuming a folate-deficient diet (Eichner and Hillman, 1971) is rapidly followed by tissue folate deficiency with megaloblastosis of the bone marrow. Furthermore, acute administration of ethanol to normal subjects or to chronic alcoholic patients is followed within hours by a fall in the serum folate level (Eichner and Hillman, 1971; Eichner and Hillman, 1973). These data imply an acute inhibitory effect of ethanol on folate metabolism and/or tissue availability. Recent *in vitro* studies suggest that superoxide ion, generated by the metabolism of ethanol and acetaldehyde, cleaves and inactivates the $CH_3H_4$PteGlu molecule (Shaw *et al.*, 1987). If confirmed *in vivo,* this observation might explain the acute suppressive effect of ethanol ingestion on the serum folate level.

### B. Chronic Alcoholism and Folate Deficiency

A variety of mechanisms account for depletion of folate stores during chronic exposure to ethanol. These include inadequate diet, intestinal malabsorption, decreased storage in the liver, and increased urinary excretion. Each possibility appears to occur in chronic alcoholism.

#### 1. *Dietary Inadequacy*

Based on self-experimentation and reasonable estimates of hepatic folate stores, Herbert (1962) showed that tissue folate deficiency—megaloblastic anemia—could be induced by a folate-free diet in 150 days, with a calculated minimal daily requirement of 50 $\mu$g. In detailed studies of chronic alcoholic patients, megaloblastosis of the bone marrow was induced by a folate-free diet with daily ethanol in 24 to 52 days (Eichner and Hillman, 1971). In the same patients restudied without ethanol, dietary induction of folate deficiency required 35 to 70 days (Eichner *et al.*, 1971). Another study of a cirrhotic patient confirmed that megaloblastosis could be induced by diet without ethanol in about 70 days (Halsted *et al.*, 1973). These studies indicate that chronic alcoholic patients are at greater risk for folate deficiency from dietary inadequacy, presumably because their hepatic folate stores are much lower than normal (Herbert, 1971). Indeed, low hepatic levels of folate have been correlated with the severity of alcoholic liver injury (Baker, 1964). Surveys that relied on retrospective diet histories found a rough correlation between poor diet and folate deficiency in chronic alcoholics (Eichner and Hillman, 1971; Halsted and Tamura, 1978).

### 2. *Intestinal Malabsorption*

Intestinal absorption of dietary folates requires hydrolysis of $PteGlu_n$ to PteGlu, followed by binding and transport of PteGlu to and across epithelial cell membranes. Recent *in vitro* models indicate that binding and transport of PteGlu are the rate-limiting steps in the process of folate absorption (Reisenauer and Halsted, 1987). Data from clinical studies and animal models show that chronic ethanol exposure inhibits intestinal uptake of PteGlu, but little information is available on the effect of acute or chronic ethanol on the intestinal hydrolysis of $PteGlu_n$.

In a study of folate absorption in binge drinkers, triple-lumen perfusion of physiologic amounts of tritium-labeled PteGlu ([$^3$H]PteGlu) was used to measure the jejunal mucosal uptake of the vitamin (Halsted *et al.*, 1971). Low uptake was reported in eight poorly nourished derelict patients, whereas normal uptake occurred in three well-nourished alcoholics. After two weeks of abstinence and adequate hospital diet, [$^3$H]PteGlu uptake increased to normal in the eight malnourished patients and was subsequently unaffected by in-hospital ethanol ingestion for 2 weeks.

A subsequent study evaluated the effects of drinking and malnutrition on folate absorption (Halsted, 1973). Three alcoholic patients underwent jejunal perfusion of [$^3$H]PteGlu before and after induction of folate deficiency by inadequate diet. In two patients who consumed $>250$ g ethanol/day in conjunction with the folate-deficient diet, induction of megaloblastic anemia was associated with significantly lower intestinal uptake of [$^3$H]PteGlu, glucose, and fluid; this was rapidly corrected by treatment with oral folic acid (Fig. 1). Intestinal uptake of fluid, [$^3$H]PteGlu, and glucose were unchanged after dietary induction of folate deficiency without added ethanol in a third patient. Failure to induce malabsorption by folate-deficient diet alone is consistent with Herbert's self-experimentation (1962). A fourth patient had a normal perfusion test after consuming 300 g ethanol/day with a folate-replete normal hospital diet for 3 weeks.

These clinical studies suggested a synergistic effect of folate deficiency and ethanol exposure on small intestinal mucosal function. Of interest, the morphology of the small intestinal mucosa remained normal in spite

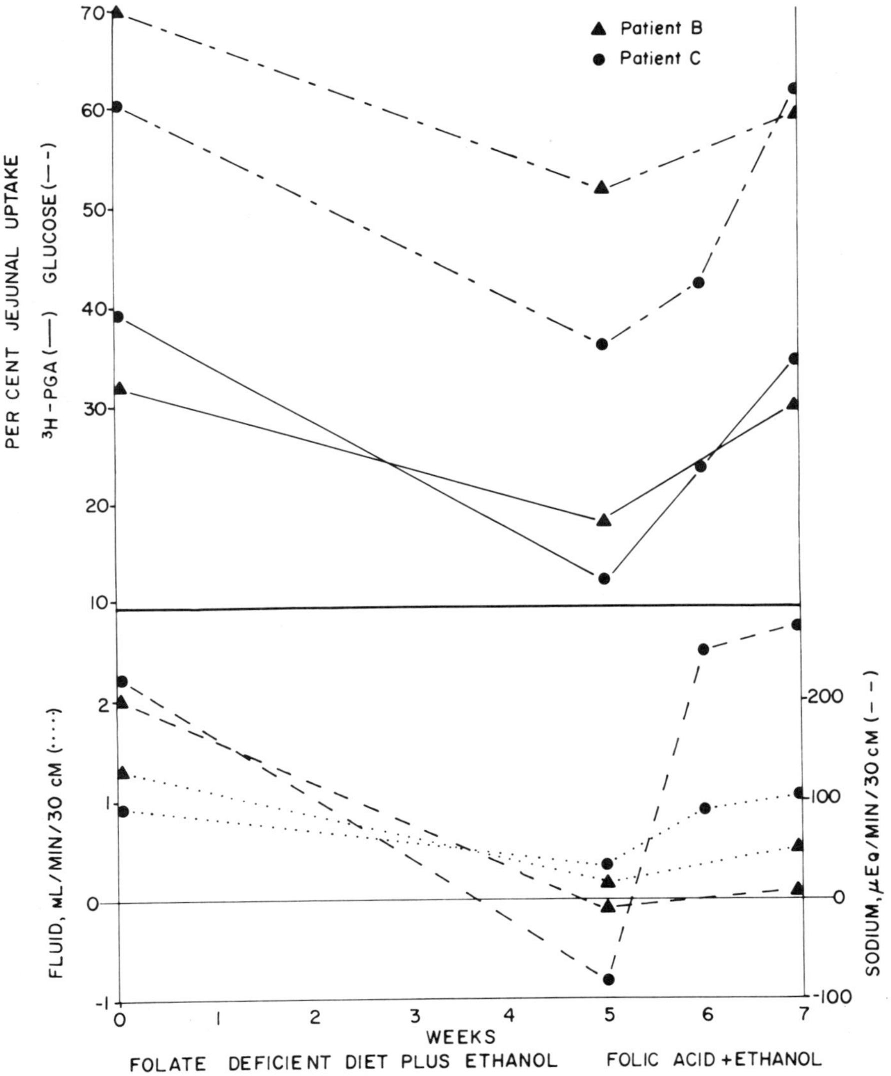


**Fig. 1.** Jejunal uptakes of glucose, [$^3$H]folic acid, fluid, and sodium were measured in two chronic alcoholic patients to determine the effect of prolonged feeding of a folate-deficient diet with 200 g ethanol/day. Dietary folate deficiency was induced after 5 weeks and was proven by development of megaloblastic bone marrow in each patient. Folic acid therapy corrected the intestinal malabsorption even though alcohol consumption continued. (From Halsted *et al.*, 1973. Reprinted with permission.)

of functional changes induced by folate deficiency and ethanol. Subsequent data in experimental monkeys (described below) suggest that malabsorption of [$^3$H]PteGlu can be induced by longer daily exposure to ethanol, even with adequate dietary folate intake.

### 3. *Hepatobiliary Metabolism*

After intestinal absorption, folate appears in the portal vein as $CH_3H_4$PteGlu and is cleared by hepatic parenchymal cells in a sequence of membrane binding and active transport. Once in the hepatocyte, $CH_3H_4$PteGlu is polyglutamated and then bound to a cytosolic folate-binding protein (Wagner, 1982). Thus, acute or chronic ethanol exposure could affect hepatic folate metabolism at three points: membrane transport, polyglutamation by a specific synthetase, and binding of polyglutamate folate to a cytosolic protein.

*In vitro*, ethanol metabolism stimulates the transport of $CH_3H_4$PteGlu by hepatocytes, which possibly results from an increased cellular NADH/NAD ratio because pyrazole blocks this effect (Horne *et al.*, 1979). Three separate studies with animal models have failed to show an effect of chronic ethanol exposure on hepatic polyglutamation of parenterally administered [$^3$H]PteGlu (Wilkinson and Shane, 1982; Keating *et al.*, 1985; Tamura *et al.*, 1981).

The existence of an enterohepatic folate circulation has been established in humans and rats. Patients who have had cholecystectomy with T-tube drainage excreted a significant fraction of parenterally administered [$^3$H]PteGlu in the bile (Pratt and Cooper, 1971). In the rat, placement of physiologic concentrations of labeled $CH_3H_4$PteGlu in isolated loops of intestine was followed by recovery of about 10% of the label in bile drainage, whereas continuous biliary drainage resulted in a rapid fall in serum folate (Steinberg *et al.*, 1979). Short-term exposure to ethanol may affect enterohepatic folate cycling (Hillman *et al.*, 1977). After parenteral [$^3$H]PteGlu administration, the excretion of label decreased in the bile of rats fed 10% ethanol in drinking water for 3 days, while hepatic incorporation of the label was nearly twice that found in control rats. Using these data, these authors postulated that ethanol-associated low serum folate levels result from diversion of folate from the enterohepatic cycle to the hepatic pool. However, these findings conflict with our studies described below, which showed that the hepatic folate pool decreased in monkeys chronically fed ethanol (Tamura and Halsted, 1983).

### 4. *Urinary Folate Excretion*

Circulating folate as $CH_3H_4$PteGlu undergoes glomerular filtration and partial reabsorption in the distal renal tubule (Williams and Hueng, 1982;

Selhub *et al.*, 1987). Tubular reabsorption requires a folate-binding protein and a transport mechanism across the brush-border membrane (Selhub and Rosenberg, 1978). Clinical studies of patient volunteers suggest that chronic ethanol feeding promotes urinary folate excretion. In one study, 17 days of ethanol administration augmented urinary folate excretion in 4 of 5 chronic alcoholic patients (Russell *et al.*, 1983). Another group showed that acute intoxicating doses of ethanol increased urinary folate concentrations in human volunteers (McMartin *et al.*, 1986). Urinary folate excretion increased during ethanol feeding in rats by a mechanism unrelated to ethanol metabolism (McMartin and Collins, 1983). The mechanism by which ethanol affects renal folate excretion and its significance in terms of folate economy are uncertain.

## V. STUDIES IN ANIMAL MODELS OF FOLATE DEFICIENCY IN ALCOHOLISM

To study the mechanisms of folate deficiency in alcoholism, our laboratory has used two experimental animal species fed controlled diets with and without the substitution of ethanol for carbohydrate.

### A. Ethanol-Fed Monkeys

In the first set of experiments 10 monkeys (*Macaque radiata*, 3–6 kg) were paired by sex and weight and fed the Lieber–DeCarli monkey diet containing 50% of calories as ethanol (average intake 6.2 ± 0.3 g/kg body weight/day) or isocaloric control diets. Each diet contained all essential nutrients, including 50 $\mu$g folic acid/100 kcal. During 4 years of feeding, daily energy intake, weight gain, nitrogen balance, fecal fat excretion, and serum and red-cell folate levels were similar in each group (Romero *et al.*, 1981; Tamura *et al.*, 1983). Minimal histologic changes in the livers of the ethanol-fed animals included mild steatosis and mitochondrial enlargement. In contrast to these findings, decreases in liver folate levels were highly significant and progressive in the ethanol-fed monkeys. Several mechanisms accounted for the development of hepatic folate deficiency in the ethanol-fed animals.

#### 1. *Intestinal Malabsorption*

After two years of feeding ethanol-containing and control diets, folate absorption was measured by comparing isotope recovery in urine and feces after oral administration of [$^3$H]PteGlu (Romero *et al.*, 1981). In the ethanol-fed animals, isotope recovery in urine fell by one-half while fecal isotope recovery increased sixfold (Fig. 2). The net result was significantly lower total retention of the labeled folate. When the studies were repeated after a tissue-saturating dose of parenteral folic acid, similar differences occurred in fecal isotope recovery, and urinary isotope recovery increased somewhat in each group. These data are consistent with the concept that chronic ethanol feeding decreases intestinal uptake of orally administered PteGlu, as shown by greater fecal loss and lower urinary excretion of the radiolabel.

## 2. *Hepatic Folate Metabolism*

After two years of feeding ethanol or control diets, [$^3$H]PteGlu was parenterally injected, and, using open liver biopsies, its hepatic uptake and metabolism were measured (Tamura *et al.*, 1981). Total folate concentrations/g/wet weight of liver tissue, measured by microbiologic assay and tritium recovery, were significantly lower in the ethanol-fed monkeys (Table I). Using chromatographic techniques with appropriate markers, we determined that the labeled folates were similarly distributed in liver tissue in both groups of monkeys. In each group, more than 80% of the labeled dose was converted to polyglutamyl derivatives (Table I), with no significant differences between groups. Using differential microbiologic assays of chromatogram eluates of deconjugated folates, we also determined that

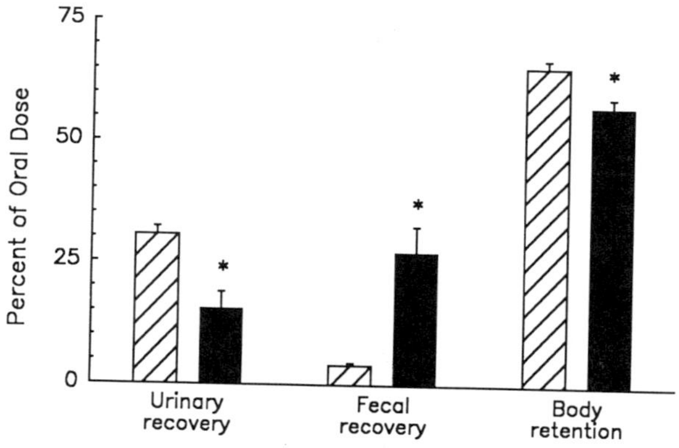


**Fig. 2.** Tritium recovery was measured in 5-day collections of urine and feces after oral administration of 33 mcg [$^3$H]PteGlu/kg body weight in control and ethanol-fed (solid-bar) monkeys. Body retention was calculated as difference between administered dose and the sums of urine and fecal excretions of tritium. Intestinal malabsorption of [$^3$H]PteGlu was shown by decreased urinary recovery and increased fecal recovery of [$^3$H]PteGlu in the ethanol-fed monkeys; the net effect was decreased body retention of the administered dose ($p < 0.05$). (Data from Romero *et al.*, 1981.)

TABLE I

**Hepatic Folate Concentrations and Tissue Uptake of [$^3$H]PteGlu in Monkeys After 2 Years of Control and Ethanol-Containing Diets[a]**

| Group | Folate concentration[b] | [$^3$H]PteGlu uptake[c] | [$^3$H]PteGlu$_n$[d] |
|---|---|---|---|
| Control | 6.0 ± 1.2 | 0.12 ± 0.03 | 0.90 ± 0.04 |
| Ethanol-fed | 4.2 ± 1.0 | 0.08 ± 0.02 | 0.85 ± 0.04 |
| | $p < 0.05$ | $p < 0.05$ | NS |

[a]Data from Tamura *et al.*, 1981.
[b]Data stated as μg/g wet weight.
[c]Data stated as % of parenteral dose/g wet weight.
[d]Data stated as % of total labeled folate.

the pattern of formyl, methyl, and reduced-folate derivatives was similar in each group. These studies showed that chronic ethanol feeding results in hepatic folate depletion, partly as a consequence of decreased hepatic uptake of circulating PteGlu, with no apparent effect on hepatic folate metabolism.

### 3. *Turnover of Folates*

To measure the effect of chronic alcoholism on folate turnover after four years of feeding, each monkey received a parenteral tracer dose of [$^3$H]PteGlu to label the endogenous folate pool (Tamura and Halsted, 1983). The cumulative percentage excretion of tritium in both urine and feces was measured daily for 25 days. The percentage of the dose retained in the body each day was calculated by subtraction of each day's cumulative excretion from the administered dose of the radiolabel. Chromatography of urine on the third day indicated similar labeling of folate metabolites in each group. Results of the turnover study (Fig. 3) are summarized below.

Maximal urinary excretion of tritium occurred in the first three days, and at least twice as much labeled folate was lost in the urine from the ethanol group as from the control group (Fig. 3A). Fecal excretion of the label was about one-tenth that of urinary excretion in each group, but was significantly greater in the ethanol-fed monkeys. Plotting total body elimination as the log value of the percentage of retained dose, two separate phases were obtained (Fig. 3A). The early rapid phase was significantly shorter in the ethanol-fed group, with a half-life of 1.1 ± 0.2 days, than in the control group, with a half-life of 1.8 ± 0.3 days ($p < 0.05$). Similar half-lives were obtained for the slow-elimination phase in each group.

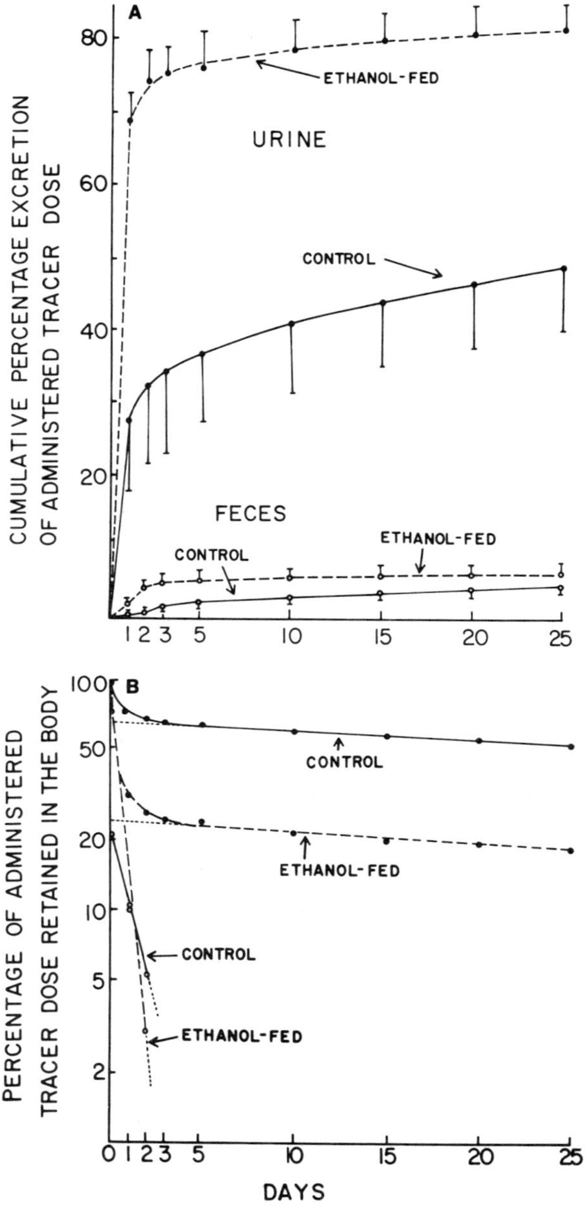
A
80
60
40
20
ETHANOL-FED
URINE
CONTROL
FECES
ETHANOL-FED
CONTROL
CUMULATIVE PERCENTAGE EXCRETION
OF ADMINISTERED TRACER DOSE
1 2 3 5 10 15 20 25
B
100
50
20
10
5
2
CONTROL
ETHANOL-FED
CONTROL
ETHANOL-FED
PERCENTAGE OF ADMINISTERED
TRACER DOSE RETAINED IN THE BODY
0 1 2 3 5 10 15 20 25
DAYS

Table II shows the concentrations of folate and residual tritium recovery in the liver after the monkeys were killed. The livers of the ethanol-fed monkeys showed significantly lower hepatic folate concentration and residual hepatic tritium recovery.

In summary, chronic feeding of ethanol as 50% of calories to monkeys resulted in minimal hepatic pathology but a significant decrease in hepatic folate concentration. Factors contributing to low hepatic folate levels included intestinal malabsorption and decreased hepatic uptake of PteGlu, which were associated with increased urinary and fecal excretion of folate metabolites. Assuming that hepatic uptake and renal excretion of $CH_3H_4$PteGlu and [$^3$H]PteGlu are similar, we can conclude that hepatic folate depletion in chronically ethanol-fed animals causes rapid turnover of circulating exogenous folates without affecting the hepatic metabolism or turnover rate of endogenous storage folate. These phenomena could be ascribed to a common effect of chronic ethanol exposure—inhibition of membrane transport of folate across three different tissues, the intestinal epithelium, the hepatic parenchyma, and the renal tubular epithelium. The observation of decreased hepatic folate levels with increased fecal folate excretion opposes the previous hypothesis that alcoholism increases the hepatic folate pool as it decreases the enterohepatic folate circulation (Hillman *et al.*, 1977). The finding of increased fecal tritium excretion (Fig. 2) could reflect either increased biliary folate excretion and/or intestinal malabsorption of biliary folate.

## B. The Miniature Pig Model

The miniature pig is a suitable model for study of the effects of alcoholism on folate metabolism. Others have shown that this species will drink intoxicating amounts of ethanol daily *ad libitum* (Dexter *et al.*, 1976). In a species-comparison study, we found that the intestine of the pig (unlike that of the rat or monkey) contains the same distribution of $PteGlu_n$ hydrolases as the human intestine (Wang *et al.*, 1985), thereby

---

**Fig. 3A.** Cumulative recoveries of tritium in the urine and feces of control and ethanol-fed monkeys are expressed as a percentage of the administered dose. The percentage excretion of tritium in the urine was significantly greater in ethanol-fed monkeys than in controls at each time point. Significantly greater fecal excretion was also observed during the first 3 days in the ethanol-fed group. **3B.** Tritium elimination during the 25-day experiment is plotted as log values of the percentage of administered dose retained in the body vs. time. Two elimination phases are shown by the straight solid and broken lines. The half-time of elimination in the early phase was significantly shorter in the ethanol-fed group than in controls, whereas the slow-phase half-time of elimination was similar in each group. (From Tamura and Halsted, 1983. Reprinted with permission.)

TABLE II

**Hepatic Folate Concentration and Tritium Recovery 25 days after Parenteral [$^3$H]PteGlu in Monkeys Fed Control and Ethanol-Containing Diets for 4 Years[a]**

| Group | Folate concentration[b] | Whole-liver tritium recovery[c] |
|---|---|---|
| Control | 5.3 ± 0.8 | 18.6 ± 3.0 |
| Ethanol-fed | 2.7 ± 0.6 | 5.1 ± 1.6 |
| | $p < 0.025$ | $p < 0.025$ |

[a]Data from Tamura and Halsted, 1983.
[b]Data stated as μg/g wet weight.
[c]Data stated as % of injected dose.

permitting more detailed study of the effects of chronic ethanol exposure on the processes of hydrolysis, binding, and transport by the intestinal membrane. In previous studies of the properties of the pig intestinal mucosa, we purified and characterized the brush-border hydrolase for $PteGlu_n$ (Chandler *et al.*, 1986) and characterized the binding of [$^3$H]PteGlu by isolated brush-border membrane vesicles (Reisenauer *et al.*, 1986). In ongoing studies in the pig, we are examining the effect of chronic ethanol feeding on the mechanisms of intestinal hydrolysis and absorption of the predominant dietary $PteGlu_n$ and on the mechanism of renal excretion of circulating PteGlu.

Ten pigs with initial weights of 60 to 80 kg were paired by sex and weight to receive diets (Purina Minipig Chow) at 6.4 g/kg body weight, supplemented with ethanol at 4 g/kg body weight or 60% of total calories or a caloric equivalent of sucrose. The chow diet contains all essential vitamins and minerals and provides protein at 1.3 g/kg body weight and folate (assayed with *L. casei*) at 6.0 μg/kg body weight. After the addition of ethanol or sucrose, caloric intake is 50 kcal/kg/day, including 10% of calories as protein, 5% as fat, 25% as complex carbohydrate, and the remainder ethanol or sucrose. Pigs are fed twice daily, and blood ethanol levels range from 70 to 140 mg/dl during the 6 hours after each feeding. Over 8 months, control animals gained 26 ± 9.8 kg, and ethanol-fed animals gained 6.1 ± 3.6 kg ($p < 0.05$ after 3 months). During 10 months of feeding, there were no changes in serum or red-cell folate levels. Significant elevations were found in serum alanine amino transaminase (ALT) and aspartate amino transaminase (AST) in the ethanol-fed animals. Measurements of serum phospholipid fatty acids showed significant decreases in arachidonic acid (20:4 omega 6) and eicosapentaenoic acid (20:5 omega 3) in the ethanol-fed animals ($p < 0.05$; $p < 0.05$), suggesting an ethanol-induced defect in fatty acid desaturation (Phinney *et al.*, 1988). After killing at 8 to 10 months, liver folate levels were similar in both groups. Failure to induce folate deficiency in this model may reflect insufficient duration of ethanol feeding together with an abundant folate level in the diet. Liver histology demonstrated fatty changes in the ethanol-fed pigs.

### 1. *Urinary Folate Excretion*

After 8 months of feeding, each pig was housed in a metabolic cage; urine was collected for 5 days and radioassayed for creatinine and folate. Both groups had similar 24-hour urinary folate excretion and creatinine clearance. These data, which suggest no demonstrable effect of chronic ethanol feeding on folate excretion in the pig, are consistent with the similar slow-elimination phases of folate excretion described in our ethanol- and control-fed monkeys (Fig. 3B).

### 2. *Intestinal Folate Absorption*

Intestinal perfusion was used to study labeled $PteGlu_n$ hydrolysis and PteGlu uptake *in vivo*. Double-lumen tubes were surgically implanted in the proximal jejunum and perfusions performed 10 days later in the fully recovered animals. Uptake of [$^3$H]PteGlu over a range of concentrations in an ethanol-fed animal was one-third to one-half that in a control. Addition of ethanol to the perfusate in concentrations of 0.5 to 2 g/dl had no acute effect on [$^3$H]PteGlu uptake in either animal. After animals were killed, brush-border vesicles were prepared for studies of enzyme activities and of *in vitro* uptake of folic acid. Folate hydrolase, measured with [$^{14}$C]$PteGlu_3$ substrate, was significantly lower in vesicles from ethanol-fed pigs ($p < 0.05$) than in controls. Using a rapid filtration method, the vesicular uptake of [$^3$H]PteGlu was measured over time and at varied concentrations. The affinity for uptake of [$^3$H]PteGlu was increased in ileal vesicles prepared from the ethanol-fed pigs, while uptake by jejunal vesicles was unaffected (Naughton *et al.*, 1988). These *in vitro* studies suggest that chronic ethanol feeding inhibits the synthesis of folate hydrolase in this experimental model. A primary effect of chronic alcohol consumption on fatty acid metabolism may also contribute to altered structure and function of the intestinal brush-border membrane. Further measurements of changes in membrane lipid composition and viscosity will be used to evaluate this hypothesis.

## VI. SUMMARY

Folate deficiency occurs in the majority of binge-drinking derelict alcoholics and is the leading cause of anemia in this population. In addition, folate deficiency affects the morphology and function of the small intestine and may play a role in intestinal malabsorption in chronic alcoholism. As cofactors for amino acid and nucleic acid metabolism, folates may be important in the regulation of ethanol-induced hepatic injury and regeneration. The etiology of folate deficiency in alcoholism is multifactorial, including possible acute effects on degradation of the folate molecule and on chronic dietary inadequacy as well as chronic effects on intestinal absorption, hepatic uptake, biliary excretion, and renal excretion. Data from animal models suggest that the folate deficiency that occurs during chronic ethanol exposure may be mediated by impaired transport of the vitamin across intestinal, hepatic, and renal membranes.

## ACKNOWLEDGMENTS

These studies were supported in part by grants from the National Institutes of Health (DK 35747), the National Institute of Alcohol Abuse and Alcoholism (AA 06938), Bristol-Myers Company, and the Alcoholic Beverage Medical Research Foundation.

## REFERENCES

Baker, H., Frank, O., Ziffer, H., Goldfarb, S., Leevy, C. M., and Sobotka, H. (1964). Effect of hepatic disease on liver beta-complex vitamin titers. *Amer. J. Clin. Nutr.* **14**, 1–6.

Bianchi, A., Chipman, D. W., Dreskia, A., and Rosensweig, N. (1970). Nutritional folic acid deficiency with megaloblastic changes in the small bowel epithelium. *N. Engl. J. Med.* **282**, 859–861.

Chandler, C. J., Wang, T. T. Y., and Halsted, C. H. (1986). Brush border pteroylpolyglutamate hydrolase in pig jejunum. *In* "Chemistry and Biology of Pteridines" (B.A. Cooper and V.M. Whitehead, eds.), pp. 539–542. Walter de Gruyter & Co., New York.

Dexter, J. D., Tumbleson, M. E., Hutcheson, D. P., and Middleton, C. C. (1976). Sinclair (S-1) miniature swine as a model for the study of human alcoholism. *Ann. NY Acad. Sci.* **273**, 188–193.

Eichner, E. R., and Hillman, R. S. (1971). The evolution of anemia in alcoholic patients. *Amer. J. Med.* **50**, 218–232.

Eichner, E. R., and Hillman, R. S. (1973). Effect of alcohol on serum folate level. *J. Clin. Invest.* **52**, 584–591.

Eichner, E. R. Pierce, H. I., and Hillman, R. S. (1971). Folate balance in dietary induced megaloblastic anemia. *N. Engl. J. Med.* **284**, 933–938.

Fernandez-Checa, J. C., Ookhtens, M., and Kaplowitz, N. (1987). Effect of chronic ethanol feeding on rat hepatocytic glutathione. *J. Clin. Invest.* **80**, 57–62.

Goetsch, C. A., and Klipstein, F. A. (1977). Effect of folate deficiency of the intestinal mucosa on jejunal transport in the rat. *J. Lab. Clin. Med.* **89**, 1002–1008.

Halsted, C. H. (1980). Folate deficiency in alcoholism. *Amer. J. Clin. Nutr.* **33**, 2736–2740.

Halsted, C. H., and Tamura, T. (1978). Folate deficiency in liver disease. *In* "Problems in Liver Disease" (C. S. Davidson, ed.), pp. 91–100. Stratton Intercontinental Medical Book Co., New York.

Halsted, C. H., Robles, E. A., and Mezey, E. (1971). Decreased jejunal uptake of labeled folic acid ($^3$H-PGA) in alcoholic patients: Roles of alcohol and malnutrition. *N. Engl. J. Med.* **285**, 701–706.

Halsted, C. H., Robles, E. A., and Mezey, E. (1973). Intestinal malabsorption in folate-deficient alcoholics. *Gastroenterology* **64**, 526–532.

Herbert, V. (1962). Experimental nutritional folate deficiency in man. *Trans. Assoc. Amer. Physicians* **75**, 307–320.

Herbert, V. (1971). Predicting nutrient deficiency by formula. *N. Engl. J. Med.* **284**, 976–977.

Herbert, V. (1987). Recommended dietary intakes (RDI) of folate in humans. *Amer. J. Clin. Nutr.* **45**, 661–670.

Herbert, V., Zalusky, R., and Davidson, C. S. (1963). Correlation of folate deficiency with alcoholism and associated macrocytosis, anemia, and liver disease. *Ann. Intern. Med.* **58**, 977–988.

Hermos, J. A., Adams, W. H., Lin, Y. C., and Tries, J. (1972). Mucosa of the small intestine in folate deficient alcoholics. *Ann. Intern. Med.* **76**, 957–965.

Hillman, R. S., McGuffin, R., and Campbell, C. (1977). Alcohol interference with the folate enterohepatic cycle. *Trans. Assoc. Amer. Physicians* **90**, 145–156.

Hines, J. D., and Cowan, D. H. (1974). Anemia in alcoholism. *In* "Drugs and Hematopoietic Reactions" (N.V. Dimitrov and J.H. Nodine, eds.), pp. 141–153. Grune & Stratton, New York.

Horne, D. W., Briggs, W. T., and Wagner, C. (1979). Studies on the transport mechanism of 5-methyltetrahydrofolic acid in freshly isolated hepatocytes: Effect of ethanol. *Arch. Biochem. Biophys.* **196**, 557–565.

Jandl, J. H., and Lear, A. A. (1956). The metabolism of folic acid in cirrhosis. *Ann. Intern. Med.* **45**, 1027–1044.

Keating, J. N., Weir, D. G., and Scott, J. M. (1985). The effect of ethanol consumption on folate polyglutamate biosynthesis in the rat. *Biochem. Pharmacol.* **34**, 1913–1916.

Klipstein, F. A., Lipton, S. D., and Schenk, E. A. (1973). Folate deficiency of the intestinal mucosa. *Amer. J. Clin. Nutr.* **26**, 728–737.

Lauterburg, B. H., Davies, S., and Mitchell, J. R. (1984). Ethanol suppresses hepatic glutathione synthesis in rats *in vivo*. *J. Pharmacol. Exp. Ther.* **230**, 7–11.

Leevy, C. M. (1966). Abnormalities of hepatic DNA synthesis in man. *Medicine* **45**, 423–433.

McMartin, K. E., and Collins, T. D. (1983). Relationship of alcohol metabolism to folate deficiency produced by ethanol in the rat. *Pharmacol. Biochem. Behav.* **18**, 257–262.

McMartin, K. E., Collins, T. D., Shiao, C. Q., Vidrine, L., and Redefski, H. M. (1986). Study of dose-dependence and urinary folate excretion produced by ethanol in humans and rats. *Alcoholism* **10**, 419–424.

Mekhjian, H., and May, E. S. (1977). Acute and chronic effects of ethanol on fluid transport in the small intestine. *Gastroenterology* **72**, 1280–1226.

Naughton, C. A., Reisenauer, A. M., Chandler, C. J., and Halsted, C. H. (1988). Intestinal absorption of folates in alcoholic pigs [Abstract]. *FASEB J* **2**, A1614.

Phinney, S. D., Johnson, S. B., Holman, R. T., Reisenauer, A. M., and Halsted, C. H. (1988). Reduced arachidonate in serum lipid fractions of alcohol-fed pigs [Abstract]. *Amer. J. Clin. Nutr.* (In press.)

Pratt, R. F., and Cooper, B. A. (1971). Folates in plasma and bile of man after feeding [$^3$H] folic acid and 5-formyltetrahydrofolate (folinic acid). *J. Clin. Invest.* **50**, 455–462.

Reisenauer, A. M., and Halsted, C. H. (1987). Issues and opinions in nutrition: Human folate requirements. *J. Nutr.* **117**, 600–602.

Reisenauer, A. M., Chandler, C. J., and Halsted, C. H. (1986). Folate binding and hydrolysis by pig intestinal brush border membranes. *Amer. J. Physiol.* **251**, G481–G486.

Romero, J. J., Tamura, T., and Halsted, C. H. (1981). Intestinal absorption of [$^3$H]folic acid in the chronic alcoholic monkey. *Gastroenterology* **80**, 99–102.

Russell, R. M., Rosenberg, I. M., Wilson, P. D., Iber, F. L., Oaks, E. V., Giovetti, A. C., Otradovec, C. L., Karwoski, P. A., and Press, A. W. (1983). Increased urinary excretion and prolonged turnover time of folic acid during ethanol ingestion. *Amer. J. Clin. Nutr.* **38**, 64–70.

Selhub, J., and Rosenberg, I. H. (1978). Demonstration of a high affinity folate binding activity associated with the brush border membranes of rat kidney. *Proc. Nat. Acad. Sci. USA* **75**, 3090–3093.

Shaw, S., Jayatilleke, E., Ross, A., Gordon, E. R., and Lieber, C. S. (1981). Ethanol induced lipid peroxidation: Potentiation by long-term alcohol feeding and attenuation by methionine. *J. Lab. Clin. Med.* **98**, 417–424.

Shaw, S., Rubin, K. P., and Lieber, C. S. (1983). Depressed hepatic glutathionine and increased diene conjugates in alcoholic liver disease: Evidence of lipid peroxidation. *Dig. Dis. Sci.* **28**, 585–589.

Shaw, S., Jayatilleke, E., Herbert, V., and Colman, N. (1987). Cleavage of 5-methyltetrahydrofolate during ethanol metabolism: Role of acetaldehyde-xanthine oxidase generated superoxidase [Abstract]. *Clin. Res.* **35**, 644A.

Steinberg, S. E., Campbell, C. L., and Hillman, R. S. (1979). Kinetics of the normal folate enterohepatic cycle. *J. Clin. Invest.* **64**, 83–88.

Sullivan, L. W., and Herbert, V. (1964). Suppression of hematopoiesis by ethanol. *J. Clin. Invest.* **43**, 2048–2062.

Swanson, V. L., and Thomassen, R. W. (1965). Pathology of the jejunal mucosa in tropical sprue. *Amer. J. Pathol.* **46**, 511–551.

Tamura, T., and Halsted, C. H. (1983). Folate turnover in chronically alcoholic monkeys. *J. Lab. Clin. Med.* **101**, 623–628.

Tamura, T., Romero, J. J., Watson, J. E., Gong, E. J., and Halsted, C. H. (1981). Hepatic folate metabolism in the chronic alcoholic monkey. *J. Lab. Clin. Med.* **97**, 654–661.

Wagner, C. (1982). Cellular folate binding proteins; function and significance. *Ann. Rev. Nutr.* **2**, 229–248.

Wang, T. T. Y., Reisenauer, A. M., and Halsted, C. H. (1985). Comparison of folate conjugase activities in human, pig, rat and monkey intestine. *J. Nutr.* **115**, 814–819.

Wilkinson, J., and Shane, B. (1982). Folate metabolism in the ethanol-fed rat. *J. Nutr.* **112**, 604–609.

Williams, W. M., and Hueng, K. C. (1982). Renal tubular transport of folic acid and methotrexate in the monkey. *Amer. J. Physiol.* **242**, F484–F490.

# 16

# Glutathione, Alcohol, and Hepatotoxicity

Neil Kaplowitz, Jose Fernandez-Checa, and Murad Ookhtens

*Department of Medicine*
*University of California, Los Angeles*
*School of Medicine and*
*Liver Research Laboratory*
*Wadsworth Veterans Administration Hospital Center*
*Los Angeles, California*

## I. INTRODUCTION

Glutathione (GSH) is a tripeptide, gamma-glutamyl-cysteinyl-glycine that plays a critical role in detoxification. We will describe its functions and regulation with particular attention to the liver. Because of its importance in cellular defense, we will also discuss the potential role of GSH in the pathophysiology of alcoholic liver disease and the influence of alcohol on the regulation of hepatic GSH.

## II. FUNCTIONS OF GLUTATHIONE (GSH)

Glutathione is a unique, specific substrate for two classes of enzymes that catalyze detoxification: selenium-dependent GSH peroxidase and GSH *S*-transferases (Fig. 1).

### A. GSH Peroxidase

GSH peroxidase catalyzes the reduction of hydrogen peroxide and organic peroxides (Stadtman, 1980) and is found in cytosol and mitochondria. GSH functions primarily as a substrate for GSH peroxidase in the conversion of hydrogen peroxide to water or in the reduction of lipid peroxidases.

### B. GSH *S*-Transferases

GSH *S*-transferases are a family of enzymes that catalyze important detoxification reactions (Kaplowitz, 1980). Substrates for these enzymes are electrophiles that react with the nucleophilic GSH group (Ketterer, 1986). Products of lipid peroxidation can be reduced by GSH (organic peroxides) or conjugated with GSH (hydroxy-alkenals) (Alin *et al.*, 1985). The most significant of the few known physiologic substrates is leukotriene $LTA_4$, which, conjugated with GSH, yields $LTC_4$ (Pace-Asciak *et al.*, 1986).

The *N*-acetyl-*p*-benzoquinoneimine metabolite of acetaminophen and other electrophilic toxins that are substrates for GSH *S*-transferases exhibit a GSH threshold (Kaplowitz *et al.*, 1986). These electrophiles can react with protein or GSH thiols *in vitro*. However, transferases catalyze a preferential reaction with GSH. Thus, an attack on protein thiols is only observed at the GSH threshold, when cytosolic GSH is fully depleted.

### C. GSH Oxidation–Reduction Cycle

The oxidation of GSH by peroxidase yields the oxidized form, GSSG. GSSG is efficiently reduced to GSH by NADPH-dependent GSSG reductase (Babson *et al.*, 1981). The normal GSH/GSSG ratio in hepatocytes

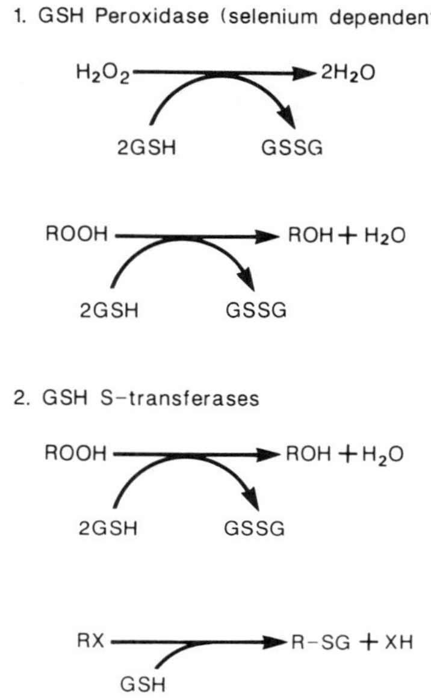


**Fig. 1.** Glutathione (GSH) functions as a specific and unique substrate for detoxifying enzymes. Oxidation of GSH by peroxidase reactions yields its oxidized form, GSSG. The action of GSH and its enzymes on hydrogen peroxide ($H_2O_2$), organic peroxides (ROOH), and electrophiles with a leaving group (RX) is shown.

is 300, but the concentration of GSSG may increase during oxidant stress. Secondary changes in the thiol-disulfide status of proteins may adversely affect cell function (Bellomo and Orrenius, 1985).

## III. REGULATION OF HEPATIC GSH

### A. Cellular and Zonal Compartmentation

Although 90% of GSH is located in cytosol, the 10% in mitochondria is believed to be critical in maintaining cell viability and mitochondrial integrity (Meredith and Reed, 1983). Because mitochondria do not synthesize GSH, mitochondrial GSH is sequestered, via an unknown mechanism, from cytosol. The half-life of GSH is about 36 hours in mitochondria and about 2 hours in cytosol.

Superoxide and hydrogen peroxide are normally formed in mitochondria during aerobic respiration. Because an estimated 5% of oxygen consumption leads to formation of oxyradicals (Jones, 1982), GSH and GSH peroxidase are critical in protecting mitochondria from oxidant stress.

The liver acinus may have a gradient of GSH; its content in periportal cells appears to be as much as twice that in pericentral cells (Smith *et al.*, 1979; Vaananen, 1986). This may result from low levels of precursor amino acids or adenosine triphosphate (ATP) required for GSH synthesis in pericentral cells. A low GSH level in pericentral cells may affect their susceptibility to toxins and may, in part, account for the preferential centrilobular necrosis caused by many toxins.

## B. GSH Synthesis

GSH synthesis from amino acids in cytosol requires the sequential activity of two ATP-dependent enzymes (Kaplowitz *et al.*, 1985). The first step is catalyzed by gamma-glutamyl-cysteine synthetase. A GSH feedback mechanism nonallosterically regulates this enzyme by competitive inhibition of substrate binding (Richman and Meister, 1975). Thus, GSH depletion enhances its synthesis. The second enzyme, glutathione synthetase, adds glycine.

Amino acid availability is crucial for GSH synthesis via this pathway. Glycine and glutamate are abundant, whereas cysteine is limited (Vina *et al.*, 1978). Normal cysteine concentrations in cytosol are in the range of the $K_m$ for gamma-glutamyl-cysteine synthetase (Richman and Meister, 1975). One source of cysteine is carrier-mediated uptake from plasma. Another is trans-sulfuration or conversion of methionine to cysteine in hepatocytes (Beatty and Reed, 1980). Cystine, the disulfide and major circulating form of cysteine, is not taken up by hepatocytes. However, an unusual exchange process has been demonstrated in incubations of isolated hepatocytes (Reed and Orrenius, 1977; Aw *et al.*, 1986b). In these studies, GSH released from hepatocytes underwent thiol-disulfide exchange, and the liberated cysteine was taken up (Table I). The importance of this process *in vivo* remains to be defined.

## C. Degradation of Hepatic GSH

### 1. *Intracellular Loss of GSH*

The only intracellular mechanisms for degradation or loss of GSH are conjugation with electrophiles and oxidation. Conjugation is normally infrequent, and oxidation is efficiently reversed by NADP-dependent GSSG reductase. However, GSSG is exported into bile and further concentrated in proportion to its cellular concentration. Although GSSG losses during export are normally small, oxidant stress can significantly affect GSH turnover.

TABLE I

**Dependence of Cysteine Uptake from Cystine By Isolated Hepatocytes on GSH Reflux[a]**

| | Control[b] | 100 $\mu M$ [$^{35}$S]Cystine Incubation[b] | |
|---|---|---|---|
| Experiment | GSH Released | GSH-Cysteine | Cysteine Uptake |
| A | 3.1 | 2.8 | 3.0 |
| B | 3.8 | 4.3 | 4.2 |

[a]Two different preparations (A and B) of hepatocytes ($10^6$/ml) were incubated in Krebs Henseleit buffer alone or in the presence of 100 $\mu M$ cystine. Cell GSH was about 50 nmol/$10^6$ cells. We found a close parallel between GSH released in 10 minutes in control cells and both the GSH-cysteine mixed disulfide formed and cell uptake of cysteine equivalents in the medium with excess cystine. (Data from Aw *et al.*, 1986a.)

[b]Data are stated as nmol/$10^6$ cells/10 min.

## 2. *GSH Efflux*

Loss or turnover of cellular GSH occurs primarily during export from the hepatocyte. Carrier-mediated transport appears to be the mechanism by which GSH is released into plasma and bile (Kaplowitz *et al.*, 1985). Release into sinusoidal plasma represents the bulk of GSH turnover (Lauterburg *et al.*, 1984a). GSH release into bile was previously underestimated because its degradation by gamma-glutamyltransferase in the biliary tree was not taken into account (Abbott and Meister, 1986; Ballatori *et al.*, 1986). This enzyme acts on luminal GSH in the canalicular membrane and ducts. Its inhibition by retrograde biliary infusion of acivicin indicates that release into bile represents about one-third of total GSH turnover (Abbott and Meister, 1986).

GSH transport kinetics have been studied extensively in perfused liver (Ookhtens *et al.*, 1985), isolated hepatocytes (Aw *et al.*, 1986a), and sinusoidal membranes (Inoue *et al.*, 1984; Aw *et al.*, 1987). Saturable transport has been demonstrated in all systems, but trans-stimulation has only been demonstrated in sinusoidal membrane vesicles (Aw *et al.*, 1987).

Membrane potential seems critical to GSH transport in both isolated hepatocytes and membrane vesicles. Because GSH has a net negative charge, hyperpolarization increases transport and depolarization inhibits transport (unpublished observations). Thus, hormones, stress and other physiological factors that affect membrane potential may also influence GSH transport. Exhaustive exercise (Lew *et al.*, 1985; Pyke *et al.*, 1986) and fasting (Lauterburg and Mitchell, 1981; Lauterburg *et al.*, 1984a) appear to promote the release of hepatic GSH.

Carrier-mediated transport of GSH is affected by saturability, by trans-stimulation, and by two forms of competitive inhibition. In isolated cell models of competitive inhibition, intracellular GSH content did not affect uptake of the inhibitor but did affect its ability to inhibit GSH efflux. In one study, methionine inhibited GSH efflux (Aw *et al.*, 1984; Aw *et al.*, 1986b). This inhibition was overcome by raising intracellular GSH content but not by blocking methionine uptake. The evidence suggests that extracellular methionine allosterically inhibits the GSH carrier, changing the affinity but not the capacity for GSH within the cell. The action of methionine in promoting GSH synthesis and inhibiting GSH efflux may lead to more rapid recovery from hepatic GSH depletion.

In another study, organic anions like bilirubin also inhibited GSH efflux (unpublished observations). However, this inhibition was overcome by raising intracellular GSH or by blocking bilirubin uptake, which occurs in an organic anion transport system independent of GSH. This latter finding suggests that bilirubin inhibits GSH efflux by competing with GSH for a shared transport pathway within the cell.

## D. Interorgan GSH Homeostasis

Almost all plasma GSH is derived from the liver and turns over very rapidly (Griffith and Meister, 1979; Hahn *et al.*, 1978). About two-thirds of GSH is cleared by the kidney, but the intestine, lungs and other organs may also clear GSH (Fig. 2). Clearance occurs primarily through the activity of gamma-glutamyltransferase and peptidases that break down GSH into its component amino acids. Sodium-dependent GSH uptake in a transport system shared with gamma-glutamyl amino acids has been described in the kidney (Lash and Jones, 1984), in the intestine (Lash *et al.*, 1986; Hagen and Jones, 1987), and in alveolar type II cells (Hagen *et al.*, 1986). However, the high millimolar $K_m$ of this system suggests that it is not important—plasma GSH concentrations are 10–20 $\mu M$ and intraluminal GSH in the intestine is usually greatly diluted. Nevertheless, millimolar concentrations of GSH infused into the intestine can be absorbed intact (Hagen and Jones, 1987). This finding suggests exciting possibilities for treating toxic and oxidant injuries in the lung, kidney, and intestine. However, the liver does not clear GSH absorbed into portal blood (Ookhtens *et al.*, 1985).

Although the precise role of the interorgan GSH homeostatic system remains unclear, sinusoidal GSH efflux may have several important functions:

1. The liver has the unique ability to convert methionine to cysteine, which is packaged as GSH for export to other tissues. GSH can then be hydrolyzed by extrahepatic cells that express abundant gamma-glutamyltransferase and dipeptidases. This process may be a mechanism by which cysteine is transferred to other tissues.

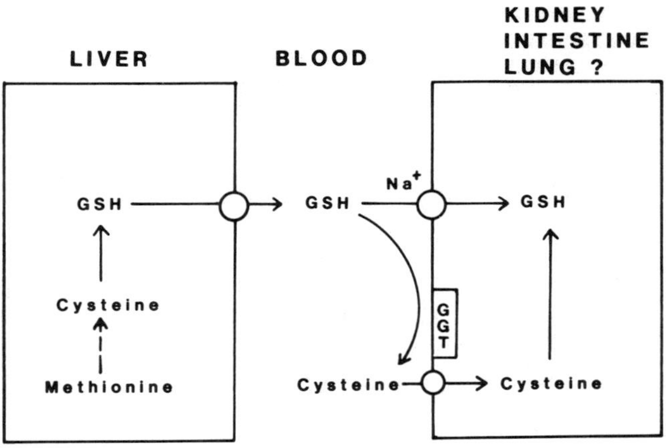


**Fig. 2.** Schematic drawing of interorgan GSH homeostasis depicts the packaging of cysteine derived from methionine in the form of GSH in hepatocytes. Hepatic GSH is transported into plasma and cleared by other organs through hydrolysis or uptake.

2. Intact GSH released from the liver may support detoxification when it is absorbed in other tissues.
3. The release of GSH in the sinusoidal plasma may liberate cysteine from cystine by thiol-disulfide exchange, thus enhancing hepatic cysteine availability.
4. GSH release may also maintain extracellular thiol status.

## IV. IMPORTANCE OF GSH IN ALCOHOLISM

Glutathione is a critical substrate for detoxification reactions, and chronic ethanol exposure may affect its regulation. Disturbances in GSH regulation may be important in the pathophysiology of alcoholic liver disease and in the enhanced susceptibility to hepatotoxins in chronic alcoholics. As the substrate for GSH peroxidases (GP) and GSH *S*-transferases (GST), GSH detoxifies hydrogen peroxide (GP), fatty acid peroxides (GP or GST), hydroxy-alkenals (GST), and *N*-acetyl-*p*-benzoquinoneimine, an electrophilic metabolite of acetaminophen (GST).

### A. Effect of Ethanol on Susceptibility to Hepatotoxins

Ethanol exposure influences hepatotoxicity and other hepatic biotransformation processes. Its effects on hepatotoxicity have been observed in studies of acetaminophen (Moldeus *et al.*, 1980; Sato *et al.*, 1981) and other toxins in rodents and have been suggested by the unusual susceptibility of chronic alcoholic patients to acetaminophen toxicity (Black and Raucy, 1986). Ethanol appears to exert its principal effects on the cytochrome *P*-450 system. Chronic ethanol exposure induces a specific form of *P*-450 in rodents that appears to oxidize ethanol, aniline, and acetaminophen (Koop and Coon, 1986). Conversely, acute ethanol exposure inhibits the *P*-450 system, either by limiting the availability of NADPH or by competitively inhibiting *P*-450.

Acetaminophen is safe in therapeutic doses up to 8 g/day in normal individuals because the cytochrome *P*-450 system converts only a small portion of the drug to an electrophilic metabolite that is preferentially detoxified by GSH. Detoxification of this metabolite depends on an adequate GSH pool and on the capacity for synthesis of GSH. Necrosis occurs when an acute overdose of $>10$ g of acetaminophen depletes the existing pool of GSH, overwhelms the capacity to synthesize GSH, and permits covalent binding of the reactive metabolite to protein thiol groups (Black and Raucy, 1986). Although this metabolite can react with any thiol group, its preferential reaction with GSH can only be explained by the catalytic action of GSH *S*-transferases. The point at which GSH is almost completely depleted is the threshold for toxicity.

Chronic ethanol exposure induces a form of *P*-450 that preferentially activates acetaminophen (Koop and Coon, 1986) and metabolizes a greater fraction of any dose of the drug. Thus, a smaller than normal dose of acetaminophen can deplete GSH in the presence of ethanol. Chronic ethanol exposure may also lower GSH levels, thus potentiating acetaminophen toxicity. Cytosolic GSH levels decreased moderately in well-nourished animals exposed to ethanol (Fernandez-Checa *et al.*, 1987), but greater decreases may occur in poorly nourished or starved animals exposed to ethanol. Thus, a low hepatic GSH level may also be important in determining susceptibility to acetaminophen toxicity.

Many have reported acetaminophen toxicity in alcoholic patients who ingested moderate to large doses of 2.5 to 10 g/day for 1 to 14 days for analgesia (McClain *et al.*, 1980; Leist *et al.*, 1985; Lesser *et al.*, 1986; Seef *et al.*, 1986). It appears that ingestion of up to 2 g/day of acetaminophen in alcoholic patients is safe but that larger doses are risky.

### B. Ethanol and Lipid Peroxidation

One theory of the pathogenesis of alcoholic liver disease implicates lipid peroxidation as a cause of hepatocellular injury after acute and chronic alcohol ingestion. Substantial evidence now suggests that ethanol consumption does increase lipid peroxidation. However, we do not know whether lipid peroxidation is a byproduct of alcohol metabolism or whether it is a cause or a consequence of hepatic injury. Lipid peroxidation may be a symptom of general oxidant stress mediated by oxyradicals. Oxidant stress affects the structure and composition of membranes and the function of membrane proteins. It may also affect gene expression, the extracellular matrix, and critical enzymes. Lipid, protein, carbohydrate, and nucleic acid can all be oxidized, but lipid oxidation is easiest to measure.

In studies with mice and rats, acute (DiLuzio, 1966) and chronic (Shaw *et al.*, 1981) ethanol adminstration induced lipid peroxidation, as demonstrated in assays of malondialdehyde and conjugated dienes (MacDonald, 1973; Shaw *et al.*, 1981; Videla *et al.*, 1981; Stege, 1982); ethane (Muller and Sies, 1982; Muller and Sies, 1983); and chemiluminescence (Boveris *et al.*, 1983; Videla *et al.*, 1983). Findings are similar in baboons (Shaw *et al.*, 1981) and humans (Fink *et al.*, 1985; Shaw *et al.*, 1983; Tanner *et al.*, 1986).

Oxyradical formation, initiated by superoxide formation, is clearly critical in ethanol-induced lipid peroxidation. A number of superoxide sources, some stimulated by the action of ethanol or acetaldehyde, are conceivable (Fig. 3):

1. Chronic ethanol exposure leads to increased microsomal production of superoxide in hepatocytes, which probably results from increased induction of NADPH—*P*-450 reductase (Reitz, 1975; Decker and Cederbaum, 1987).

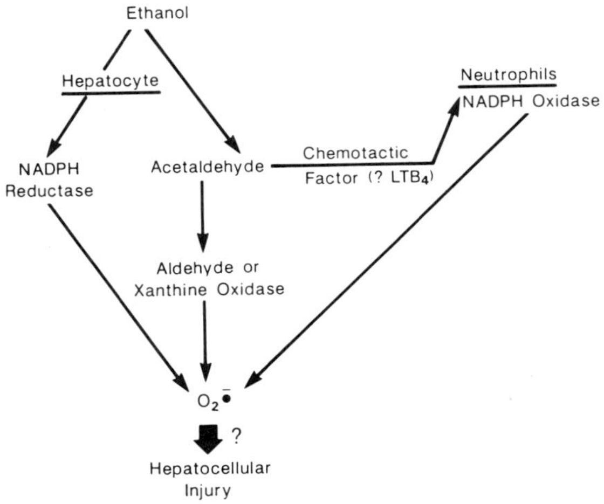


**Fig. 3.** Superoxide from several sources may produce hepatocellular injury after ethanol exposure.

2. Acetaldehyde is a substrate for peroxisomal enzymes like xanthine and aldehyde oxidases (Shaw and Jayatilleke, 1987), which also generate superoxide by oxidizing ethanol.

3. Neutrophilic infiltration is a characteristic of alcoholic hepatitis. Activated neutrophils release superoxide through the activity of their NADPH oxidase.

Superoxide is rapidly converted to hydrogen peroxide by superoxide dismutase, and hydrogen peroxide is reduced to water by GSH peroxidase (Fig. 4). This process may deplete the GSH pool and hinder detoxification, especially in mitochondria. In the presence of $Fe^{2+}$, hydrogen peroxide can be converted to the potent hydroxyl radical, which initiates lipid peroxidation. Higher than normal levels of iron, stored as $Fe^{3+}$ in ferritin, are found in livers exposed to ethanol. Superoxide stimulates the release of $Fe^{2+}$ from ferritin (Shaw and Jayatilleke, 1987). Superoxide may have several critical roles in ethanol-induced peroxidation:

1. It is the initial oxyradical produced in most biological systems and, as such, the obligatory precursor of the more toxic free radicals.

2. It can release $Fe^{2+}$, a catalyst in the formation of hydroxyl radicals.

3. Ethanol metabolism in cultured hepatocytes leads to the release of a superoxide-stimulated chemotactic lipid, possibly $LTB_4$ (Perez *et al.*, 1984; Roll *et al.*, 1986). The acetaldehyde-dependent formation of $LTB_4$ by hepatocytes might also be stimulated by superoxide.

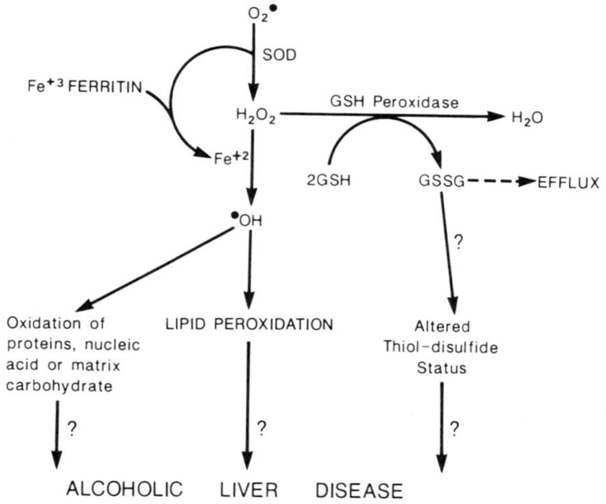


**Fig. 4.** Ethanol-induced superoxide formation may have several possible roles in the pathogenesis of alcoholic liver disease.

## V. EFFECTS OF ALCOHOL ON HEPATIC GSH

### A. Acute Ethanol Exposure

Many studies show that administration of a single large dose—approximately 3 g/kg—of ethanol results in a progressive decline in hepatic GSH over six hours, with significant decreases seen after three hours (MacDonald *et al.*, 1977; Videla *et al.*, 1980; Videla *et al.*, 1981; Lauterburg *et al.*, 1984b; Speisky *et al.*, 1985). There are conflicting explanations for this phenomenon.

Our studies demonstrated that acute ethanol and acetaldehyde administration do not directly affect cytosolic or mitochondrial GSH or GSH or GSSG efflux. This lack of effect in ethanol-fed rats and pair-fed controls was shown in studies of GSH efflux from *in situ* perfused livers and in studies of freshly isolated hepatocytes (Fernandez-Checa *et al.*, 1987) (Table II). We therefore concluded that the *in vivo* effects of ethanol are indirect and possibly nonspecific. Proposed mechanisms for GSH depletion after acute ethanol administration *in vivo* include:

1. Oxidant stress and lipid peroxidation may increase formation and loss of GSSG through active canalicular transport of GSSG into bile, but studies of bile GSSG have not confirmed this theory (Lauterburg *et al.*, 1984b). The oxidant stress may have been insufficient to deplete GSH.

2. Formation of an adduct of acetaldehyde and GSH may lead to loss of GSH (Vina *et al.*, 1980), but this is unconfirmed (Speisky *et al.*, 1985; Fernandez-Checa *et al.*, 1987).

**TABLE II**

**Sinusoidal GSH Efflux from *in situ* Perfused Livers of Ethanol-Fed Rats After Incubation with Ethanol[a]**

| | Hepatic GSH[b] | Sinusoidal GSH efflux[c] | | | |
|---|---|---|---|---|---|
| | | Without ethanol | | 50 m*M* Ethanol | |
| Pair-fed control | 5.96 | 18.7 | 0.18 | 19.6 | 0.19 |
| Ethanol-fed | 3.70 | 25.9 | 0.42 | 25.0 | 0.40 |
| | $p < 0.01$ | $p < 0.01$ | $p < 0.001$ | $p < 0.01$ | $p < 0.001$ |

[a] *In situ* perfused livers of ethanol-fed rats and pair-fed controls were examined after 6 weeks in the presence or absence of 50 m*M* ethanol. (From Fernandez-Checa *et al.*, 1987. Reprinted with permission.)

[b] Data are stated as microm/g.

[c] Data are stated as nmol/min/g (columns 1 and 3) or as fractional efflux per hour (columns 2 and 4).

3. Formation of an adduct between acetaldehyde and cysteine may limit GSH synthesis, but this is unconfirmed (Speisky *et al.*, 1985; Fernandez-Checa *et al.*, 1987).

4. Stress mediated by catecholamines (James *et al.*, 1983) or hormones may deplete hepatic GSH by increasing GSH efflux into plasma. Epinephrine, whose release is stimulated by ethanol, and dibutyryl cAMP deplete hepatic GSH by an unknown mechanism. One hypothesis is that increased sinusoidal efflux of GSH occurs in response to increased membrane potential resulting from hormonal action on hepatocytes.

5. Tracer-kinetic turnover studies have attributed decreased GSH turnover to decreases in GSH synthesis and in plasma GSH (Lauterburg *et al.*, 1984b), but others found no apparent change in turnover after increased sinusoidal release and decreased synthesis (Speisky *et al.*, 1985). Thus, the drop in GSH may be caused by decreased synthesis alone or by decreased synthesis combined with increased release. The decreasing hepatic GSH pool during the turnover studies and other problems in study design complicate interpretation of results.

## B. Chronic Ethanol Exposure

Chronic ethanol exposure affects hepatic GSH by decreasing cytosolic GSH, by increasing sinusoidal GSH efflux, by increasing GSH synthesis and turnover, and by markedly depleting mitochondrial GSH.

Chronic ethanol exposure lowered hepatic GSH before other evidence of liver disease was present in humans (Shaw *et al.*, 1983; Jewell *et al.*, 1986) and in baboons (Shaw *et al.*, 1981). However, studies of hepatic GSH levels in chronic ethanol-fed rats have shown decreases (Fernandez-Checa *et al.*, 1987), no change (Vendemiale *et al.*, 1984; Pierson and Mitchell, 1986), or increases (Hétu *et al.*, 1982; Morton and Mitchell, 1985). The increased hepatic GSH turnover described by Morton and Mitchell (1985) appears to have resulted from increased sinusoidal efflux (Pierson and Mitchell, 1986). Lieber and colleagues have confirmed increased GSH synthesis (Vendemiale *et al.*, 1984), and we have confirmed increased GSH efflux and synthesis (Fernandez-Checa *et al.*, 1987).

As with acute ethanol exposure, early reports of increased biliary GSSG excretion after chronic ethanol exposure (Sies *et al.*, 1979) have not been confirmed (Vendemiale *et al.*, 1984; Morton and Mitchell, 1985). Again, as with acute ethanol exposure, lipid peroxidation may occur, but this oxidant stress alone appears insufficient to deplete GSH through loss of GSSG.

Overall, studies of chronic ethanol exposure suggest a modest depletion of total hepatic GSH, along with increased synthesis to keep up with

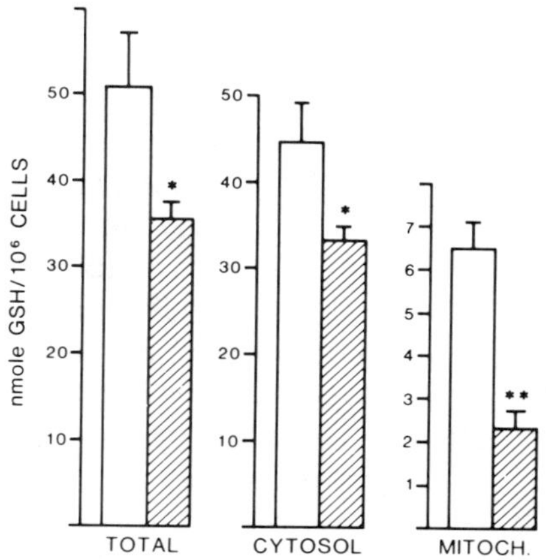


**Fig. 5.** The effects of 6 weeks of chronic ethanol administration on total hepatocellular, cytoplasmic, and mitochondrial GSH were studied in isolated hepatocytes from ethanol-fed rats (cross-hatched bars) and pair-fed controls (Lieber-DeCarli diet). Cells were isolated by collagenase perfusion. Plasma membrane was disrupted by digitonin to separate the soluble (cytosol) and particulate (including mitochondria) fractions. Values are mean ± SD; $p < 0.01$; $p < 0.001$. (From Fernandez-Checa *et al.*, 1987. Reprinted with permission.)

increased efflux. Paradoxically, although net synthesis may increase, this gain may be insufficient to maintain the normal hepatic GSH pool. Thus, GSH levels apparently fall to achieve a balance between GSH synthesis and efflux. Below $V_{max}$ for efflux, cytosolic GSH concentration determines the efflux rate (Kaplowitz *et al.*, 1985). A drop in cytosolic concentration, therefore, leads to a lower efflux rate. We assume that this occurs in hepatocytes from ethanol-fed and control rats. However, the effect of chronic ethanol exposure on the kinetics of GSH efflux is unknown.

Chronic ethanol consumption also produces structural and functional changes in hepatic mitochondria, where about 10% of cell GSH is stored. We have noted a selective 65% decrease in hepatic mitochondrial GSH after 6 to 8 weeks of ethanol feeding in rats (Fernandez-Checa *et al.*, 1987) (Fig. 5). The cause and implications of this decrease in mitochondrial GSH are unclear, but it probably reflects the effects of ethanol on mitochondrial structure and function. It is also tempting to speculate that this decrease may explain the markedly enhanced susceptibility to oxidant stress that occurs in alcoholism. Indeed, increased mitochondrial sensitivity to peroxidation has been demonstrated after only four days' exposure to ethanol (Rouach *et al.*, 1983).

## VI. SUMMARY

Glutathione is a vital peptide, 90% of which is found in cytosol and 10% in mitochondria. It serves as a substrate for detoxification reactions catalyzed by GSH peroxidase and transferases, and it participates in metabolism of sulfur amino acids. Cytosolic GSH turnover occurs primarily by efflux into sinusoidal plasma and bile. This efflux is controlled by a putative membrane carrier because GSH transport is saturable. Competitive inhibition of efflux has been shown in isolated perfused rat liver and in freshly isolated hepatocytes, and trans-stimulation has been shown in membrane vesicles. Various studies have described the key elements of the complex interorgan system for GSH homeostasis.

In our studies of the importance of GSH in alcoholism, hepatocytes from rats fed ethanol for 6 to 8 weeks showed cytosolic GSH levels 24% lower than controls and mitochondrial GSH levels 65% lower than controls. Fractional GSH efflux and synthesis increased after chronic alcohol feeding while cellular GSH concentration fell. Incubation of hepatocytes with ethanol showed no direct, acute effect on hepatic GSH homeostasis.

## ACKNOWLEDGMENTS

The secretarial assistance of Anita Starlight is gratefully appreciated. This work was supported by Veterans Administration medical research funds and NIH grant DK 30312. Dr. Fernandez-Checa is a recipient of a postdoctoral fellowship awards from the American Liver Foundation and Smith-Kline-Beckman.

## REFERENCES

Abbott, W. A., and Meister, A. (1986). Intrahepatic transport and utilization of biliary glutathione and its metabolites. *Proc. Nat. Acad. Sci. USA* **83**, 1246–1250.

Alin, P., Danielson, U. H., and Mannervik, B. (1985). 4-hydroxyalk-2-enals are substrates for glutathione transferase. *FEBS Lett.* **179**, 267–270.

Aw, T. Y., Ookhtens, M., and Kaplowitz, N. (1984). Inhibition of glutathione efflux from isolated rat hepatocytes by methionine. *J. Biol. Chem.* **259**, 9355–9358.

Aw, T. Y., Ookhtens, M., Ren, C., and Kaplowitz, N. (1986a). Kinetics of glutathione efflux from isolated rat hepatocytes. *Amer. J. Physiol.* **250**, G236–G243.

Aw, T. Y., Ookhtens, M., and Kaplowitz, N. (1986b). Mechanism of inhibition of glutathione efflux by methionine from isolated rat hepatocytes. *Amer. J. Physiol.* **251**, G354–G361.

Aw, T. Y., Ookhtens, M., Kuhlenkamp, J. F., and Kaplowitz, N. (1987). Trans-stimulation and driving forces for GSH transport in sinusoidal membrane vesicles from rat liver. *Biochem. Biophys. Res. Commun.* **143**, 377–382.

Babson, J. R., Abell, N. S., and Reed, D. J. (1981). Protective role of the glutathione redox cycle against adriamycin-mediated toxicity in isolated hepatocytes. *Biochem. Pharmacol.* **30**, 2299–2304.

Ballatori, N., Jacob, R., and Boyer, J. L. (1986). Intrabiliary glutathione hydrolysis: a source of glutamate in bile. *J. Biol. Chem.* **261**, 7860–7865.

Beatty, P. W., and Reed, D. J. (1980). Involvement of the cystathionine pathway in the biosynthesis of glutathione by isolated rat hepatocytes. *Arch. Biochem. Biophys.* **204**, 80–87.

Bellomo, G., and Orrenius, S. (1985). Altered thiol and calcium homeostasis in oxidative hepatocellular injury. *Hepatology* **5**, 876–882.

Black, M., and Raucy, J. (1986). Acetaminophen, alcohol, and cytochrome *P*-450. *Ann. Intern. Med.* **104**, 487–492.

Boveris, A., Fraga, C. G., Varsavsky, A. I., and Koch, O. R. (1983). Increased chemiluminescence and superoxide production in the liver of chronically ethanol-treated rats. *Arch. Biochem. Biophys.* **227**, 534–541.

Decker, E., and Cederbaum, A. I. (1987). Hydroxyl radical generation by microsomes after chronic ethanol consumption. *Alcoholism* **11**, 309–314.

DiLuzio, N. R. (1966). A mechanism of the acute ethanol-induced fatty liver and the modification of liver injury by antioxidants. *Lab. Invest.* **15**, 50–64.

Fernandez-Checa, J. C., Ookhtens, M., and Kaplowitz, N. (1987). Effect of chronic ethanol feeding on rat hepatocytic glutathione: Compartmentation, efflux, and response to incubation with ethanol. *J. Clin. Invest.* **80**, 57–62.

Fink, R., Marjot, D. H., Cawood, P., Iversen, S. A., Clemens, M. R., Patsalos, P., Norden, A. G., and Dormandy, T. L. (1985). Increased free-radical activity in alcoholics. *Lancet* **2**, 291–294.

Griffith, O. W., and Meister, A. (1979). Interorgan translocation, turnover and metabolism. *Proc. Nat. Acad. Sci. USA* **76**, 5606–5610.

Hagen, T. M., and Jones, D. P. (1987). Transepithelial transport of glutathione in vascularly perfused small intestine of rat. *Amer. J. Physiol.* **252**, G607–G613.

Hagen, T. M., Brown, L. A., and Jones, D. P. (1986). Protection against paraquat-induced injury by exogenous GSH in pulmonary alveolar type II cells. *Biochem. Pharmacol.* **35**, 4537–4542.

Hahn, R., Wendel, A., and Flohe, L. (1978). The fate of extracellular glutathione in the rat. *Biochim. Biophys. Acta* **539**, 324–337.

Hétu, C., Yelle, L., and Joly, J.-G. (1982). Influence of ethanol on hepatic glutathione content and on the activity of glutathione *S*-transferases and epoxide hydrase in the rat. *Drug Metab. Dispos.* **10**, 246–250.

Inoue, M., Kinne, R., Tran, T., and Arias, I. M. (1984). Glutathione transport across hepatocyte plasma membranes: Analysis using isolated rat-liver sinusoidal vesicles. *Eur. J. Biochem.* **138**, 491–495.

James, R. C., Roberts, S. M., and Harbison, R. D. (1983). The perturbation of hepatic glutathione by gamma$_2$-adrenergic agonists. *Fund. Appl. Toxicol.* **3**, 303–308.

Jewell, S. A., DiMonte, D., Gentile, A., Guglielmi, A., Altomare, E., and Albano, O. (1986). Decreased hepatic glutathione in chronic alcoholic patients. *J. Hepatology* **3**, 1–6.

Jones, D. P. (1982). Intracellular catalase function: Analysis of catalatic activity by-product formation in isolated liver cells. *Arch. Biochem. Biophys.* **214**, 806–814.

Kaplowitz, N. (1980). Physiologic significance of the glutathione *S*-transferases. *Amer. J. Physiol.* **239**, G439–G444.

Kaplowitz, N., Aw, T. Y., and Ookhtens, M. (1985). The regulation of hepatic glutathione. *Ann. Rev. Pharmacol. Toxicol.* **25**, 715–744.

Kaplowitz, N., Aw, T. Y., Simon, F. R., and Stolz, A. (1986). Drug-induced hepatotoxicity. *Ann. Intern. Med.* **104**, 826–839.

Ketterer, B. (1986). Detoxication reactors of glutathione and glutathione transferases. *Xenobiotica* **16**, 957–973.

Koop, D. R., and Coon, M. J. (1986). Ethanol oxidation and toxicity: Role of alcohol *P*-450 oxygenase. *Alcoholism* **10**, 44S–49S.

Lash, L. H., and Jones, D. P. (1984). Renal glutathione transport: Characteristics of the sodium-dependent system in the basal-lateral membrane. *J. Biol. Chem.* **259**, 14508–14514.

Lash, L. H., Hagen, T. M., and Jones, D. P. (1986). Exogenous glutathione protects intestinal epithelial cells from oxidative injury. *Proc. Nat. Acad. Sci. USA* **83**, 4641–4645.

Lauterburg, B. H., and Mitchell, J. R. (1981). Regulation of hepatic glutathione turnover in rats *in vivo* and evidence for kinetic homogeneity of the hepatic glutathione pool. *J. Clin. Invest.* **67**, 1415–1424.

Lauterburg, B. H., Adams, J. D., and Mitchell, J. R. (1984a). Hepatic glutathione homeostasis in the rat: Efflux accounts for glutathione turnover. *Hepatology* **4**, 586–590.

Lauterburg, B. H., Davies, S., and Mitchell, J. R. (1984b). Ethanol suppresses hepatic glutathione synthesis in rats *in vivo*. *J. Pharmacol. Exp. Ther.* **230**, 7–11.

Leist, M. H., Gluskin, L. E., and Payne, J. A. (1985). Enhanced toxicity of acetaminophen in alcoholics: Report of three cases. *J. Clin. Gastroenterol.* **7**, 55–59.

Lesser, P. B., Vietti, M. M., and Clark, W. D. (1986). Lethal enhancement of therapeutic doses of acetaminophen by alcohol. *Dig. Dis. Sci.* **31**, 103–105.

Lew, H., Pyke, S., and Quintanilha, A. (1985). Changes in glutathione status of plasma, liver and muscle following exhaustive exercise in rats. *FEBS Lett.* **185**, 262–266.

MacDonald, C. M. (1973). The effects of ethanol on hepatic lipid peroxidation and on the activities of glutathione reductase and peroxidase. *FEBS Lett.* **35**, 227–230.

MacDonald, C. M., Dow, J., and Moore, M. R. (1977). A possible protective role for sulphydryl compounds in acute alcoholic liver injury. *Biochem. Pharmacol.* **26**, 1529–1531.

McClain, C. J., Krumhout, J. P., and Peterson, F. J. (1980). Potentiation of acetaminophen hepatotoxicity by alcohol. *JAMA-J. Am. Med. Assn.* **244**, 251–253.

Meredith, M. J., and Reed, D. J. (1983). Status of the mitochondrial pool of glutathione in the isolated hepatocyte. *J. Biol. Chem.* **257**, 3747–3753.

Moldeus, P., Andersson, B., Norling, A., and Ormstad, K. (1980). Effect of chronic ethanol administration on drug metabolism in isolated hepatocytes with emphasis on paracetamol activation. *Biochem. Pharmacol.* **29**, 1741–1745.

Morton, S., and Mitchell, M. C. (1985). Effects of chronic ethanol feeding on glutathione turnover in the rat. *Biochem. Pharmacol.* **34**, 1559–1563.

Muller, A., and Sies, H. (1982). Role of alcohol dehydrogenase activity and of acetaldehyde in ethanol-induced ethane and pentane production by isolated perfused rat liver. *Biochem. J.* **206**, 153–156.

Muller, A., and Sies, H. (1983). Ethane release during metabolism of aldehydes and monoamines in perfused rat liver. *Eur. J. Biochem.* **134**, 599–602.

Ookhtens, M., Hobdy, K., Corvasce, M. C., Aw, T. Y., and Kaplowitz, N. (1985). Sinusoidal efflux of glutathione in the perfused rat liver: Evidence for a carrier-mediated process. *J. Clin. Invest.* **75**, 258–265.

Pace-Asciak, C. R., Klein, J., and Spielberg, S. P. (1986). Metabolism of leukotriene $A_4$ into $C_4$ by human platelets. *Biochim. Biophys. Acta* **877**, 68–74.

Perez, H. D., Roll, F. J., Bissell, D. M., and Goldstein, I. M. (1984). Production of chemotactic activity for polymorphonuclear leukocytes by cultured rat hepatocytes exposed to ethanol. *J. Clin. Invest.* **74**, 1350–1357.

Pierson, J. L., and Mitchell, M. C. (1986). Increased hepatic efflux of glutathione after chronic ethanol feeding. *Biochem. Pharmacol.* **35**, 1533–1537.

Pyke, S., Lew, H., and Quintanilha, A. (1986). Severe depletion in liver glutathione during physical exercise. *Biochem. Biophys. Res. Commun.* **139**, 926–931.

Reed, D. J., and Orrenius, S. (1977). The role of methionine in glutathione biosynthesis by isolated hepatocytes. *Biochem. Biophys. Res. Commun.* **77**, 1257–1264.

Reitz, R. C. (1975). A possible mechanism for the peroxidation of lipids due to chronic ethanol ingestion. *Biochim. Biophys. Acta* **380**, 145–154.

Richman, P. G., and Meister, A. (1975). Regulation of gamma-glutamylcysteine synthetase by nonallosteric feedback inhibition by glutathione. *J. Biol. Chem.* **250**, 1422–1426.

Roll, F. J., Bissell, D. M., and Perez, H. D. (1986). Human hepatocytes metabolizing ethanol generate a nonpolar chemotactic factor for human neutrophils. *Biochem. Biophys. Res. Commun.* **137**, 688–694.

Rouach, H., Clement, M., Orfanelli, M.-T., Janvier, B., Nordmann, J., and Nordmann, R. (1983). Hepatic lipid peroxidation and mitochondrial susceptibility to peroxidative attacks during ethanol inhalation and withdrawal. *Biochim. Biophys. Acta* **753**, 439–444.

Sato, C., Matsuda, Y., and Lieber, C. S. (1981). Increased hepatotoxicity of acetaminophen after chronic ethanol consumption in the rat. *Gastroenterology* **80**, 140–148.

Seef, L. B., Cuccherini, B. A., and Zimmerman, H. J. (1986). Acetaminophen hepatotoxicity in alcoholics: A therapeutic misadventure. *Ann. Intern. Med.* **104**, 399–404.

Shaw, S., and Jayatilleke, E. (1987). Acetaldehyde-mediated hepatic lipid peroxidation: Role of superoxide and ferritin. *Biochem. Biophys. Res. Commun.* **143**, 984–990.

Shaw, S., Jayatilleke, E., Ross, W. A., Gordon, E. R., and Lieber, C. S. (1981). Ethanol-induced lipid peroxidation: Potentiation by long term alcohol feeding and attenuation by methionine. *J. Lab. Clin. Med.* **98**, 417–424.

Shaw, S., Rubin, K. P., and Lieber, C. S. (1983). Depressed hepatic glutathione and increased diene conjugates in alcoholic liver disease: Evidence of lipid peroxidation. *Dig. Dis. Sci.* **28**, 585–589.

Sies, H., Koch, O. R., Martino, E., and Boveris, B. (1979). Increased biliary glutathione disulfide release in chronically ethanol-treated rats. *FEBS Lett.* **103**, 287–290.

Smith, M. T., Loveridge, N., Wills, E. D., and Chayen, J. (1979). The distribution of glutathione in the rat liver lobule. *Biochem. J.* **182**, 103–108.

Speisky, H., MacDonald, A., Giles, G., Orrego, H., and Israel, Y. (1985). Increased loss and decreased synthesis of hepatic glutathione after acute ethanol administration: Turnover studies. *Biochem. J.* **225**, 565–572.

Stadtman, T. C. (1980). Selenium-dependent enzymes. *Ann. Rev. Biochem.* **49**, 93–110.

Stege, T. E. (1982). Acetaldehyde-induced lipid peroxidation in isolated hepatocytes. *Res. Commun. Chem. Pathol. Pharmacol.* **36**, 287–297.

Tanner, A. R., Bantock, I., Hinks, L., Lloyd, B., Turner, N. R., and Wright, R. (1986). Depressed selenium and vitamin E levels in an alcoholic population: Possible relationship to hepatic injury through increased lipid peroxidation. *Dig. Dis. Sci.* **31**, 1307–1312.

Vaananen, H. (1986). The distribution of cytochrome *P*-450-mediated drug oxidation and glutathione in periportal and perivenous rat hepatocytes after phenobarbital treatment. *J. Hepatology* **2**, 174–181.

Vendemiale, G., Jayatilleke, E., Shaw, S., and Lieber, C. S. (1984). Depression of biliary glutathione excretion by chronic ethanol feeding in the rat. *Life Sci.* **34**, 1065–1073.

Videla, L. A., Fernandez, V., Ugarte, G., and Valenzuela, A. (1980). Effect of acute ethanol intoxication on the content of reduced glutathione of the liver in relation to its lipoperoxidative capacity in the rat. *FEBS Lett.* **111**, 6–10.

Videla, L. A., Fernandez, V., Valenzuela, A., and Ugarte, G. (1981). Effect of (+)-cyanidanol-3 on the changes in liver glutathione content and lipoperoxidation induced by acute ethanol administration in the rat. *Pharmacology* **22**, 343–348.

Videla, L. A., Fraga, C. G., Koch, O. R., and Boveris, A. (1983). Chemiluminescence of the *in situ* rat liver after acute ethanol intoxication—Effect of (+)-cyanidanol-3. *Biochem. Pharmacol.* **32**, 2822–2825.

Vina, J., Reginald, H., and Krebs, H. A. (1978). Maintenance of glutathione content in isolated hepatocytes. *Biochem. J.* **170**, 627–630.

Vina, J., Estrela, J. M., Guerri, C., and Romero, F. J. (1980). Effect of ethanol on glutathione concentration in isolated hepatocytes. *Biochem. J.* **188**, 549–552.

# 17

# Nutrients in the Pathogenesis and Treatment of Hepatic Encephalopathy


## Steven Schenker and William H. Beer

*Department of Medicine*
*Division of Gastroenterology and Nutrition*
*The University of Texas Health Science Center at San Antonio*
*Audie L. Murphy Veterans' Hospital*
*San Antonio, Texas*

# I. INTRODUCTION

Nutrition plays a key role in the pathogenesis and treatment of hepatic encephalopathy, especially that which occurs in chronic liver disease or cirrhosis and is accompanied by spontaneous and/or surgically induced portal-systemic shunting (PSE). The etiology, clinical presentation, and pathogenesis of encephalopathy with PSE must be clearly distinguished from hepatic coma accompanying acute liver failure, hepatocerebral degeneration (pseudoWilsonian coma), and spastic paraparesis. The present review considers the clinical aspects, pathogenesis, and treatment of hepatic encephalopathy and emphasizes PSE (rather than acute liver failure), controversial issues of pathogenesis, and the role of nutrition.

# II. CLINICAL PICTURE AND DIAGNOSIS

In hepatic encephalopathy, an altered or abnormal mental state is accompanied and caused by impaired liver function and/or increased shunting of blood from portal to systemic circulation. This shunting, which may occur following surgery or spontaneously as a result of disturbed liver architecture, is clearly more important in the encephalopathy that accompanies chronic liver disease or cirrhosis than in the encephalopathy with fulminant hepatic failure that accompanies acute viral or toxic hepatitis.

## A. Events Precipitating Coma

In patients with PSE, a specific event almost always precipitates coma, and identification of this event forms part of the clinical inquiry leading to diagnosis (Table I). The most common precipitating events include azotemia, use of depressant drugs, and gastrointestinal bleeding. In the absence of a precipitating event, the diagnosis should be reevaluated. Exclusion of other causes of coma and the clinical picture outlined below form the basis for diagnosing hepatic encephalopathy.

## B. Mental Changes

The mental changes that are the *sine qua non* in diagnosing hepatic encephalopathy may vary in form and severity and may include impaired intellectual function, nonspecific personality changes, and/or drowsiness. Some changes may be so subtle that sophisticated tests are required to demonstrate and quantify them; others may be as gross as deep coma with no corneal reflexes.

Subtle changes in intellectual function occur frequently in PSE (Rikkers *et al.*, 1978), and significant new ways to assess them have recently emerged. These may require close follow-up, consultation with family members, and confirmation by semiquantitative testing (Gilbertstadt *et al.*, 1978., Elsass *et al.*, 1978., Rikkers *et al.*, 1978). In the past, clinical testing of mental status consisted of evaluating orientation, subtraction of serial sevens, and constructional apraxia (loss of ability to write or form figures, for example). More recently, the numbers connection or ''trailmaking'' test has been seen to be helpful. It has also been suggested that measuring visual evoked potentials—brain-wave responses to flashes of light—may be a sensitive test for incipient encephalopathy (Jones *et al.*, 1984), but we believe the specificity and sensitivity of this approach needs further evaluation. Regardless of how they are assessed, mildly abnormal changes in mental status need to be recognized in order to provide proper treatment of hepatic encephalopathy.

### C. Motor Disturbances

Altered mental state and hepatic dysfunction are but two of the clinical components characterizing hepatic encephalopathy (Schenker and Hoyumpa, 1984). A substantial number of patients may have a flapping asynchronous tremor of the hands, especially at the early stages of disease. This flapping, brought on by sustained hyperextension of the wrists, is mitigated by intentional movements. Lateral tremor of the fingers may precede the flap. A similar disturbance may be seen in other muscle groups as protruding tongue, closed eye muscles or unsustained clonus at the ankle. Metabolic flap or asterixis occurs in many neurological dysfunctions and is not specific for hepatic encephalopathy. The likely cause of these phenomena is abnormal integration of afferent information transmitted at decussating nerve fibers from peripheral muscles to the central nervous system.

### D. Fetor Hepaticus

Many hepatic encephalopathy patients have fetor hepaticus, a pungent, musty odor resembling garlic. This results from exhalation of mercaptans produced through impaired degradation of sulfur-containing amino acids by the diseased liver. However, fetor hepaticus in a comatose patient simply attests to the presence of severe liver disease and not to the nature of the cerebral dysfunction.

### E. Other Bases for Diagnosis

Hyperventilation (sometimes reflected in respiratory alkalosis), mild hypothermia, and fluctuating abnormalities in reflexes are other symptoms

**TABLE I**

**Precipitating Causes of Portal-Systemic Encephalopathy[a]**

| Cause | Incidence | Presumed mechanism(s) | Therapeutic implications |
|---|---|---|---|
| Azotemia (spontaneous or diuretic-induced) | 29% | Increased enterohepatic circulation of urea or nitrogen may increase ammonia production.<br>Uremia exerts a direct sedative effect.<br>Diuretics may induce hypokalemic alkalosis, increase renal vein ammonia output, and enhance ammonia transfer across blood-brain barrier.<br>Excessive diuresis may lead to hypovolemia, prerenal azotemia, and decreased perfusion of vital organs.<br>Hypokalemia may have a separate effect on cerebral function. | Avoid excessive diuresis.<br>Consider prophylactic use of nonabsorbable antibiotics to inhibit bacterial generation of ammonia from urea in the gut. |
| Sedatives, tranquilizers, and analgesics | 24% | These drugs exert a direct depressant effect on the brain.<br>Depression of the respiratory center may lead to hypoxia. | Exercise caution; if use is unavoidable, monitor carefully and reduce dose accordingly.<br>Select an agent with normal metabolism in the presence of liver disease, a short half-life, inactive metabolites, and no cerebral sensitivity. |
| Gastrointestinal bleeding | 18% | Bleeding (100 ml blood = 15–20 g protein) provides substrate for increased production of ammonia and other nitrogenous toxins. | Make prophylactic use of neomycin or lactulose.<br>Evacuate blood from the intestine in bleeding, noncomatose patients with liver disease. |

| | | | |
|---|---|---|---|
| | | Hypovolemic shock and hypoxia may compromise hepatic, cerebral and renal function, the last leading to increases in enterohepatic urea nitrogen cycle activity and ammonia production.<br>Ammonia in stored blood may also be a contributor. | Advise against use of gastrointestinal irritants like alcohol or salicylates.<br>Treat cough or constipation to minimize variceal bleeding from increased portal pressure during coughing or straining. |
| Metabolic alkalosis | 11% | Nonionized ammonia is preferentially diffused across the blood-brain barrier. | Correct defect with intravenous infusion of .5-2 liters of 150 ml hydrochloric acid in 1 liter water over 24 hours.<br>Replace potassium in severe unresponsive cases. |
| Excess dietary protein | 9% | Protein excess provides substrate for production of ammonia and other nitrogenous toxins. | Curtail dietary protein—especially that containing aromatic, sulfuric, or other potentially high ammonia-generating amino acids. |
| Infection | 3% | Increased tissue catabolism leads to a greater endogenous nitrogen load and increased ammonia production.<br>Infection may cause dehydration and prerenal azotemia.<br>Hyposic hyperthermia may potentiate ammonia toxicity. | Search vigorously for infection, and use appropriate antibiotics. |
| Constipation | 3% | Increased contact time between bacteria and nitrogenous substances may increase production and absorption of ammonia and other toxic nitrogen derivatives.<br>Straining at stool may potentially increase portal pressure and cause bleeding. | Make prophylactic use of stool softeners and laxatives. |

[a]Modified from Hoyumpa *et al.*, 1979. Reprinted with permission.

exhibited by patients with hepatic encephalopathy. Convulsions may occur in fulminant hepatic failure, but rarely in cirrhosis. On the other hand, the long-term changes in motor or sensory function that accompany structural neurological changes usually are not found in fulminant hepatic failure. These distinctions are of value in differential diagnosis.

### F. Laboratory Findings

Although not obligatory in every patient, an electroencephalogram (EEG) and measurements of blood ammonia and cerebrospinal fluid glutamine may aid in diagnosis. The EEG usually depicts high amplitude, slow waves (especially bifrontally), and no focal abnormalities, but this pattern is not specific for hepatic encephalopathy. Blood ammonia increases in some but not all patients—a point bearing on pathogenesis. Thus, blood ammonia data may be the most useful when determined serially as an individual patient's mental state changes. The most reliable measurement of blood ammonia requires that arterial blood from a fasted patient be evaluated in a laboratory where the procedure has been carefully validated. Likewise, spinal fluid glutamine, the end product of ammonia detoxification in the brain, is not always elevated. Although less susceptible to laboratory error, spinal fluid evaluation requires a spinal puncture.

### G. Establishing the Diagnosis

The clinical picture is the key to diagnosis. A trial of therapy may be required to establish the diagnosis, especially in the presence of multiple disorders. Fortunately, treatment for PSE is well established, relatively innocuous, and likely to result in improvement, however transient, within 72 hours in about 75% of patients. Such "diagnosis by therapy" is not harmful as long as other possible clues to the origin of the disorder have been vigorously pursued (Hoyumpa *et al.*, 1979).

Although the previously discussed clinical features provide a general picture of hepatic encephalopathy, the disorder spans a wide spectrum of diseases. It is perhaps most important to distinguish between acute and chronic liver failure. In acute liver failure, as in fulminant viral or toxic hepatitis, the onset of encephalopathy is rapid, often with delirium and convulsions; no clear-cut precipitating events can be identified; and response to therapy and prognosis are both poor. In chronic liver disease or cirrhosis, the symptoms and signs of PSE often coexist with subtypes of the disorder, with neurological findings reminiscent of Wilson's disease and demyelinating spinal cord disease. These disorders tend to be progressive, regardless of therapy. Moreover, encephalopathy following liver failure of intermediate duration tends to resemble closely the fulminant failure pattern (Gimson *et al.*, 1986).

## III. PATHOGENESIS

Although much research has been done (Hoyumpa and Schenker, 1982; Schafer and Jones, 1982a), the exact pathogenesis of hepatic encephalopathy remains elusive. Gaps in our knowledge underlie much of the controversy:

1. The neurochemical/neurophysiological basis for normal consciousness remains to be defined, making deviations difficult to assess.
2. The complex functional and biochemical heterogeneity of the brain render studies of the brain difficult and time consuming.
3. Questions remain in developing animal models of the various forms of human hepatic encephalopathy, especially that accompanying cirrhosis: Do studies of acute injury in animal models apply to patients with chronic liver failure? Can we be certain that coma following extensive surgery or administration of a toxin in an experimental animal resulted from liver failure rather than from other, less specific physiological derangements? What should be the gold standard for liver-failure-related experimental hepatic coma? This point deserves greater attention in the development of experimental designs of hepatic coma (Gammal and Geller, 1987). We believe that, until these issues are clarified, findings in each experimental model should not necessarily be extrapolated to others or to humans.
4. The causal relationships and relative importance of associated events such as mental changes and biochemical findings have yet to be determined.
5. The wide clinical spectrum of hepatic encephalopathy raises other questions: Are the mechanisms of coma in patients with fulminant liver failure the same as in patients with cirrhosis and PSE? Do these mechanisms apply to the largely irreversible and progressive neurological syndromes of hepatocerebral degeneration, which include both cerebral abnormalities and spastic paraparesis?

With these concerns in mind, we will consider data available on the pathogenesis of hepatic encephalopathy.

### A. Neurological Factors

Studies in experimental animals, in neurosurgery patients, and in patients with localized brain lesions suggest that consciousness or awareness depends on the normal function of key areas of the brain. These are the reticular-activating substance (RAS) in the brain stem, which controls the on-off aspects of consciousness, and the cortex, which modulates its content, i.e. spectrum of responsiveness. This restricted definition clearly does an injustice to the various interacting circuits and cellular/subcellular biochemical pools in the brain, but it does set forth the known gross cerebral areas most likely to be affected in hepatic encephalopathy and most deserving of careful study.

The potential reversibility of hepatic encephalopathy implies a defect in neurochemical or neurophysiological metabolism rather than a defect in structure. It follows that the astroglial changes and cerebral edema seen in many of these patients are epiphenomena and not determinants of altered mental state. The exact relationships among hepatocerebral dysfunction, paraparesis, and reversibility are uncertain. Moreover, should it turn out that bouts of more conventional hepatic encephalopathy leave subtle residua after treatment (Bernthal *et al.*, 1987), the concept of potential reversibility may need rethinking.

Some have suggested that a deficiency in a key protective substance, more specific than albumin or glucose, may be responsible for hepatic encephalopathy while others have proposed that endogenous brain peptides alter receptor regulation. However, the bulk of current evidence favors an increase in toxins or soporifics or an imbalance between false and true neurotransmitters as the most likely mechanisms of hepatic encephalopathy (Hoyumpa and Schenker, 1982).

## B. Metabolic Factors

PSE is usually induced by a specific clinical event (Table I). Although the mechanisms by which these derangements precipitate PSE are often complex, a common thread is increased nitrogenous load in the intestine. Indeed, despite the high level of controversy about the pathogenesis of PSE, most agree that increased gut nitrogen is a key factor. Although intestinal nitrogen may have various components, the key putative culprit, however, is still ammonia (Schenker and Hoyumpa, 1984). Other components may include sulfur containing or aromatic amino acids and their relative proportions as well as gamma-aminobutyric acid (GABA) and other amines. In addition to the generation of these "toxins" by gut bacteria, ammonia and GABA may be formed enzymatically in small and, to a lesser extent, large gut wall from glutamine and probably other amino acids (Schalm and Van Der Mey, 1979; Sugarbaker *et al.*, 1987; Van Berlo *et al.*, 1987). In fact, most of these amines may be of nonbacterial origin. Thus, nitrogenous substances play a major role in inducing PSE.

Impaired detoxification of nitrogenous products also plays a key role in PSE. Because the liver is the principal site at which ammonia is eliminated by conversion to urea, the nitrogenous load can affect the brain when liver damage interferes with urea synthesis and/or when portal-systemic shunts bypass the liver. Other evidence suggests that skeletal muscle also plays an important role in removing ammonia from the circulation (Lockwood *et al.*, 1979). Thus, decreased muscle mass, often seen in wasted cirrhotic patients, may contribute to high blood ammonia.

*1. Ammonia*

Support for the concept that excess ammonia is a toxin in hepatic encephalopathy is derived from the following data (Schenker and Hoyumpa, 1984):

1. Administration of ammonia or substances that generate it may cause coma.
2. Urea cycle abnormalities result in high blood ammonia and coma.
3. Blood ammonia content is often high in these patients, and therapy to reduce it is frequently beneficial.
4. Ammonia is detoxified in astrocytes, which proliferate in the brain of PSE patients.

On the other hand, elevated blood levels of ammonia do not always occur in patients with hepatic encephalopathy, nor do they always correlate with alterations in mental state. However, single measurements of blood levels may not reflect a prolonged influx of ammonia into the brain, and blood levels may not correlate with brain ammonia pools, which also depend on the pH gradient between blood and brain ammonia levels. Because ammonia is unlikely to be the only relevant toxin, the lack of good correlation is not surprising.

Mechanisms by which ammonia may contribute to PSE are many (Hoyumpa and Schenker, 1982). For example, ammonia may exert a direct depressant effect on the neuronal membrane, thus altering the transfer of chloride and water across this membrane. Another possibility is that ammonia may alter the cytoplasmic NADH/mitochondrial NAD ratio and the malate-aspartate shuttle, thus leading to accumulation of lactate in the cytoplasm and to diminution of the excitatory neurotransmitters aspartate and glutamate. Decreased cerebral energy metabolism has also been detected (Hindfelt *et al.*, 1977; McCandless and Schenker, 1968), Particularly in brainstem RAS (McCandless and Schenker, 1980). A selectively greater use of glucose in brainstem RAS has also been demonstrated in shunted rats given ammonia (Lockwood *et al.*, 1986). The energy deficit, however, may be a later or secondary phenomenon (Hoyumpa and Schenker, 1982). Although these data clearly demonstrate a role of ammonia in the pathogenesis of PSE, we have yet to determine which biochemical/neurophysiological impairments are primary and critical and which are of lesser importance.

*2. False Neurotransmitters*

The concept of false neurotransmitters stipulates an imbalance between plasma branched-chain and aromatic amino acids in cirrhotic patients (Hoyumpa and Schenker, 1982). This imbalance results from poor liver function, with relatively intact muscle metabolism and possibly altered insulin/glucagon homeostasis. The relative deficit in branched chain amino acids in the plasma is believed to bring about decreased competition for transfer of aromatic amino acids into the brain, thus leading to intracerebral generation of false neurotransmitters, displacement of true neurotransmitters, and decreased transmission of synaptic impulses. The net effect would be an increase in octopamine and phenylethylamine at the expense of the normal neurotransmitters serotonin, dopamine, and norepinephrine. Positive and negative aspects of this concept have been extensively discussed, but it remains a hypothesis.

The ammonia and false transmitter concepts have been merged into a unitary hypothesis (James *et al.*, 1979). In this view, brain glutamine and plasma aromatic amino acids share a common carrier at the blood-brain barrier. Greater glutamine efflux is believed to permit greater aromatic amino acid influx, thus further increasing levels of false or weak neurotransmitters in the brain.

The false neurotransmitter concept is disputed, with varying data obtained in different animal models and in patients with hepatic encephalopathy. Perhaps the single, most cited negative study is one in which coma did not result in animals given a large load of false neurotransmitters by intraventricular injection (Zieve and Olsen, 1977). However, the keys to the false neurotransmitter hypothesis may well rest on microregional or synaptic concentrations of these weak neurotransmitters and on the balance between true and false neurotransmitters, which may be critical in the pathogenesis of coma. This hypothesis, although battered, remains viable and deserves further testing.

### 3. *Gamma-Aminobutyric Acid (GABA)*

Gamma-aminobutyric acid (GABA) is the most important inhibitory amino acid in the brain. The most recent hypothesis proposes increased influx of GABA into the brain, or as a variant to this, enhanced cerebral responsiveness to GABA in hepatic encephalopathy (Schafer and Jones, 1982a). The original GABA hypothesis proposed that this substance is generated in the gut by bacterial metabolism, is not metabolized normally by the diseased liver, passes into the brain through a disrupted blood-brain barrier, and inhibits awareness (Ferenci *et al.*, 1981; Fowler and Schafer, 1981; Schafer and Jones, 1982b). The variant theory stipulates increased sensitivity of GABA receptors (Baraldi and Zeneroli, 1982; Zeneroli *et al.*, 1982). Proposed mechanisms for increased sensitivity include decreases in endogenous ligands, altered receptors, or denervation with upregulation of the receptor. However, upregulation would be unusual in the presence of increased amounts of GABA in the brain. Hence, the first and second variants of the GABA concept are somewhat discordant.

The first GABA hypothesis—increased flux of this inhibitor into the brain—suffered a setback when measurement of blood levels of GABA did not confirm a major increase in this amino acid (Ferenci *et al.*, 1986a; Zeneroli *et al.*, 1982; Butterworth *et al.*, 1987). Moreover, studies of alterations in blood-brain permeability have produced varied results depending on the animal model, the method used, and the stage of coma studied (Lo *et al.*, 1987).

The second GABA hypothesis—increased binding to GABA receptors—has also been battered by conflicting results. Many animal models and some human postmortem studies have found no change in binding of GABA to its receptors (Ferenci *et al.*, 1986b; Maddison *et al.*, 1987; Rzepczynski *et al.*, 1986; Thompson *et al.*, 1985). These findings may relate in part to differences in methods for purifying the receptors. Because hepatic encephalopathy is usually rapidly reversible, it is also difficult to conceive how a ''denervated'' receptor could be restored to normal in so brief a time.

In considering the GABA hypotheses, it is especially interesting to note the proximity of cerebral GABA receptors to benzodiazepine receptors. Patients with liver disease, and especially those with the tendency to hepatic encephalopathy, are generally believed to be more sensitive to the sedative effect of benzodiazepines. This pharmacodynamic effect can be distinguished from the pharmacokinetic impairment in elimination of some benzodiazepines in these patients. Thus, enhanced sensitivity to GABA may spill over to enhanced binding of benzodiazepines (Fowler and Schafer, 1981). Indeed, experimental animal studies using positron emission tomography support this view (Samson *et al.*, 1987). Moreover, endogenous benzodiazepine like ligands may participate in inducing coma in PSE patients (Mullen *et al.*, 1987). Reversal of encephalopathy has been attempted using benzodiazepine inhibitors, and anecdotal reports are encouraging (Scollo-Lavizzari and Steinmann, 1985; Bansky *et al.*, 1985).

### 4. *Other Hypotheses*

Both the false neurotransmitter and GABA hypotheses have generated much new research activity, among which has been the study of other excitatory and inhibitory cerebral amino acid neurotransmitters. Some even suggest that hepatic coma may be associated with decreases in excitatory neurotransmitters like aspartate and glutamate and increases in inhibitory neurotransmitters like glycine (Butterworth *et al.*, 1987; Ferenci *et al.*, 1983;

Hindfelt *et al.*, 1977; Hoyumpa and Schenker, 1982). These findings may ultimately be linked to both the ammonia toxicity and the GABA hypotheses.

The lack of a single toxin or concept to explain all aspects of hepatic encephalopathy has brought forth the multifactorial hypothesis (Hoyumpa and Schenker, 1982., Zieve *et al.*, 1974a; Zieve *et al.*, 1974b). In this view, hepatic encephalopathy results from a group of cerebral derangements that together lead to depression and loss of consciousness. In addition to the nitrogenous substances emphasized here, certain fatty acids and mercaptans and perhaps other as yet unknown "toxins," may also contribute to hepatic encephalopathy (Zieve *et al.*, 1974a; Zieve *et al.*, 1974b). At present, a derangement of the normal balance of true neurotransmitters, an influx of weak neurotransmitters, and a secondary impairment of energy metabolism appear to be the mechanisms involved in hepatic encephalopathy. The proposed role for physically altered neuronal membranes is not supported by persuasive data.

## IV. THERAPY

### A. Initial Approaches

Treatment of hepatic encephalopathy involves several approaches. The basic hepatic disorder that led to the development of encephalopathy must be considered first. In alcohol-induced liver disease, for instance, cessation of drinking is the key to treatment. Providing proper nutrition to these often-malnourished patients is essential to enhance hepatic regeneration. Nutritional therapy may be enhanced by appropriate diuresis or by removal of some ascitic fluid to lessen abdominal discomfort and promote improved appetite (Simon *et al.*, 1987). Corticosteroids may be beneficial in patients with certain forms of chronic active hepatitis. In addition to these interventions, general support of the failing liver is critical. In fulminant liver disease, several kinds of support may be required: Glucose must often be administered to prevent or treat hypoglycemia; fresh frozen plasma may be needed to treat hemorrhaging or to prevent the risk of bleeding when clotting factors are depressed; and mannitol may be required to treat cerebral edema.

The events that precipitated encephalopathy should be identified and treated (Table I), especially in patients with PSE. Precipitant causes tend to recur in the same patient but to vary among patients. For instance, the nitrogenous load can be lowered by stopping gut bleeding and by evacuating the blood as nitrogenous substrate, by alleviating azotemia, by decreasing the catabolism caused by sepsis, and by treating constipation.

## B. Approaches to Decreasing the Nitrogenous Load

Many approaches have been used to decrease the nitrogenous load and its impact on the brain; these are most relevant to clinical nutrition.

### 1. *Protein Restriction*

The initial approach to decreasing the nitrogenous load is to stop or lower protein intake. The level of protein restriction depends on the severity of the encephalopathy and the type of follow-up available. If mental status has only changed slightly and the family is adroit in caring for the patient and reporting back, reducing protein intake may be all that is necessary. In contrast, if the encephalopathy is more severe or proper follow-up is impossible, all protein should be withheld, and the patient should be hospitalized for observation. Appropriate use of protein restriction is important because the amino acids essential for hepatic regeneration should not be withheld any longer than necessary.

To spare endogenous nitrogen breakdown while protein is removed, calories should be provided as glucose, supplemented, if necessary, with vitamins and minerals. For example, administering glucose for several days may exacerbate latent thiamine deficiency or may cause marked decreases in serum phosphate levels in patients with alcoholic liver disease. Alert nutritional management requires anticipation of these developments.

After the patient's mental state improves, oral protein should be added in increments of about 10–20 g/day every three days while observing the patient for signs of deterioration. Daily protein increments are inadvisable because it may take a few days for impaired mental status to manifest itself.

### 2. *Lactulose Therapy*

Lactulose has also been used to lower the nitrogen load (Conn *et al.*, 1977; Elkington *et al.*, 1969; Simmons *et al.*, 1970; Zeegan *et al.*, 1970). This synthetic disaccharide, also called galactosidofructose, is not absorbed from the gut but is converted by gut bacteria to organic acids. Lactulose promotes nitrogen excretion in the stool, with a resulting decrease in urea synthesis (Weber, 1979; Weber *et al.*, 1987). Increased excretion of nitrogen occurs primarily via its incorporation into fecal bacteria (Vince *et al.*, 1978), which is believed to result from the action of lactulose or its metabolites on bacterial growth. Lactulose also promotes nitrogen excretion in the soluble stool fraction. Several factors may account for this phenomenon: Bacterial catabolism of dietary nitrogen may be decreased by low gut pH or by carbohydrate-induced inhibition of the synthesis and activity of certain bacterial enzymes. Also, the transit time of nitrogenous substances in the gut may be reduced as a result of the osmotic effect of lactulose products. *In vitro* studies suggest that lactulose, like neomycin, inhibits intestinal glutamine uptake and metabolism to ammonia in tissue harvested from both conventional and germ-free animals (Soeters and Van Leeuwen, 1986).

Lactulose is usually given orally in 30–45 ml doses three to four times per day. The dosage should be adjusted to produce two to three soft stools per day, with the stool pH decreasing from 6.3 to about 5. Although some recommend an hourly schedule until a laxative effect occurs, we prefer to avoid overt diarrhea by using the more conservative regimen. In the presence of ileus, lactulose may be given as an enema. In this form, the initial beneficial effect probably results from the low pH of the solution itself, although organic acids do form within five minutes and an osmotic effect is also present. Lactitol, a lactulose powder, has produced results similar to those obtained with the fluid and may be better tolerated. The benefits of lactulose in patients with PSE are well documented—some 70% improve within 72 hours. Lactose is equally beneficial in patients with PSE and lactose intolerance (Uribe *et al.*, 1981).

Lactulose has no serious side effects, aside from flatulence in some patients and the inconvenience of carrying the bulky fluid form. However, if severe diarrhea is allowed to develop, patients may excrete more water than sodium, and hypernatremia may ensue. These events have been correlated with higher mortality, but the extreme illness of these patients has prevented the establishment of a direct cause-effect relationship.

### 3. *Neomycin Therapy*

Neomycin is not used as frequently today as it was in the past. This antibiotic was presumed to decrease bacterial flora, thereby reducing the formation of ammonia and other potentially toxic amines from nitrogenous substances. It may also affect glutamine conversion to ammonia in the gut wall (Soeters and Van Leeuwen, 1986). The drug was usually given orally in doses of 2–3 g/day or by enema in a 1% solution. About 1 to 3% of the drug appears to be absorbed when given orally or by enema (Breen *et al.*, 1972). The absorbed drug is normally excreted by the kidney, and its concentration in urine may be bactericidal for many organisms. With prolonged use, circulating drug accumulations can cause nephro- and ototoxicity. Hence, its prolonged use in the presence of kidney disease or hearing impairment is dangerous. Moreover, any prolonged use requires monitoring of hearing, renal function, and blood levels. The beneficial effects of neomycin parallel those of lactulose, but lactulose is the preferred treatment because of its relative lack of toxicity. Other antibiotics like metronidazole have also been used (Morgan *et al.*, 1982).

### 4. *Combined Therapies*

Some data suggest that combining neomycin with lactulose may provide incremental benefits in some patients (Weber *et al.*, 1982, Weber *et al.*, 1987). In this instance, neomycin may further reduce urea formation by inhibiting bacterial ureolysis and by preventing recycling of urea nitrogen (Weber *et al.*, 1987). When this combined therapy is used, the stool should be checked to ensure that the pH is low and that the neomycin has not killed the bacterial flora needed to metabolize the lactulose.

More often, lactulose and protein restriction are used together, but protein should be restarted as soon as clinical conditions permit in order to provide optimal nutrition. Some patients with chronic liver disease may need continuous lactulose to permit reasonable protein intake. The benefits of the lactulose/protein restriction regimen have been validated in patients with PSE. In patients with fulminant liver failure, the prognosis is much worse. Although this regimen is used by extrapolation, its validity is unproven.

### 5. *Vegetable-Protein Diet Therapy*

Discussion up to now has centered on reducing the *quantity* of nitrogen ingested or generated, with no attention to the *quality* of the protein. Three studies, each somewhat differently designed, suggest that vegetable protein may be better tolerated than animal protein (De Bruijn *et al.*, 1983; Greenberger *et al.*, 1977; Uribe *et al.*, 1982). In a dissenting report, the combination of lactulose with vegetable or meat protein was compared (Shaw *et al.*, 1983). We use a vegetable-protein-based diet only in the rare patient who is intolerant to lactulose and modest restriction of animal protein. A vegetable-protein diet is less palatable, produces early satiety, and may generate compliance problems (De Bruijn *et al.*, 1983; Weber *et al.*, 1985). Although its benefits are usually modest, they may be substantial in selected patients.

The vegetable-protein diet appears to increase fecal nitrogen excretion, which probably results at least in part from a higher intake of dietary fiber (Weber *et al.*, 1985). This increased excretion lowers nitrogen absorption and urea synthesis (Weber *et al.*, 1985). The lower methionine content in the vegetable diet may also be helpful, but this concept has not been rigorously evaluated. However, plasma methionine levels were comparable in patients on either diet. In diabetic patients, the vegetable-protein diet has an additional effect of lowering blood sugar (Uribe *et al.*, 1982).

### 6. *Amino Acid Therapy*

In patients with chronic liver disease, aromatic amino acids often accumulate because of undermetabolism by the liver, and branched-chain amino acids often decrease because of degradation in muscle. As a result, the aromatic/branched-chain amino acid ratio rises. One proposed mechanism for the pathogenesis of PSE is that this deranged amino acid ratio promotes uptake by the brain of aromatic amino acids that generate false neurotransmitters. Although this theory is far from proven, it was hoped that administration of branched-chain amino acids (BCAA) might benefit PSE patients by improving their amino acid profile. It was further speculated that administering BCAA might improve skeletal muscle protein turnover and function and might enhance ammonia detoxification by these peripheral muscles. The ultimate hope, of course, was to promote positive nitrogen balance while preventing or at least ameliorating hepatic encephalopathy.

Data concerning the possible value of BCAA have been difficult to compare and evaluate. Some studies lacked controls; some used mixed therapeutic protocols; and many had differences in patient groups, amino acid mixtures, or end points for response. It is particularly important to differentiate between attempts to *treat* encephalopathy and attempts to *prevent* overt encephalopathy in susceptible cirrhotic patients by improving their nutrition. Although it is difficult to assign patients to crisp categories, patients with acute encephalopathy and those with chronic recurrent encephalopathy should be evaluated separately. With these caveats, and considering only controlled studies, what is the consensus?

Four studies have evaluated BCAA for treatment of patients with overt or acute encephalopathy (Cerra *et al.*, 1985; Michel *et al.*, 1985; Rossi-Fanelli *et al.*, 1982; Wahren *et al.*, 1983) (Table II). Studies compared 17 to 40 patients receiving BCAA treatment with controls receiving various forms of established treatment. Although variations in study design make comparisons difficult, three studies found no significant differences in encephalopathy grade between patients who received BCAA therapy and those who received other forms of therapy (Michel *et al.*, 1985; Rossi-Fanelli *et al.*, 1982; Wahren *et al.*, 1983), whereas the fourth showed improvement only during the first two days of BCAA therapy (Cerra *et al.*, 1985). One of the studies of acute encephalopathy patients found the benefits of BCAA equalled those of lactulose (Rossi-Fanelli *et al.*, 1982). In a randomized crossover study of chronic PSE with mild encephalopathy, BCAA provided no benefit (Eriksson *et al.*, 1983). Although BCAA therapy appears to provide no benefits over established therapy, it would be interesting to assess the effect of combining BCAA and lactulose therapies. Such studies with adequate numbers of patients are not yet available. As for prevention, two studies have found some evidence that BCAA may lower the risk of encephalopathy by promoting positive nitrogen balance (Egberts *et al.*, 1983; Horst *et al.*, 1984). Silk (1986) has completed an elegant review of this controversial subject.

**TABLE II**

**Controlled Studies of Parental Branched-Chain Amino Acids in Patients With Cirrhosis and Acute Hepatic Encephalopathy[a]**

| | Treatment regimen | | Results | | | |
|---|---|---|---|---|---|---|
| Group | BCAA Formula (% of nitrogen intake) | Control regimen | Encephalopathy grade beginning | Encephalopathy grade end (Days) | Patients showing improvement BCAA/control) | Significance |
| 1 | 100% ($n$ = 17) | Lactulose +glucose ($n$ = 17) | 3–4 | 0 (2–4) | 12/8 | NS |
| 2[b] | 100% ($n$ = 25) | Glucose+ fat ($n$ = 25) | 2–4 | 0–2 (5) | 14/12 (10/11)[c] | NS |
| 3 | 100% ($n$ = 36) | Glucose+ "standard" amino acids ($n$ = 34) | 1–3 | Not stated (5) | 10/12 | NS |
| 4 | 35% ($n$ = 40)[d] | Glucose+ neomycin ($n$ = 35) | 2–4 | Not stated[e] (14) | Not stated | $p < 0.05$ on days 1–2 only |

[a]Adapted from Silk, 1986, and based on studies by Rossi-Fanelli *et al.*, 1982 (Group 1), Wahren *et al.*, 1983 (Group 2), Michel *et al.*, 1985 (Group 3), and Cerra *et al.*, 1985 (Group 4).

[b]Eight patients (5 BCAA, 3 Control) received conventional therapy (lactulose and/or neomycin).

[c]Parenthetical figures for improvement exclude patients receiving BCAA plus conventional therapy.

[d]The other 65% of nitrogen intake consisted of other amino acids.

[e]Only the rate of change was measured for the days in which improvement occurred (days 1–2).

A variation on BCAA therapy is the use of ketoanalogs of amino acids, especially the ornithine salts with endogenous amines (Herlong *et al.*, 1980; Maddrey *et al.*, 1976). These ketoacids have been used to advantage in children with urea cycle abnormalities. Base and associates (1987) reported that ketoacids may promote positive nitrogen balance better than BCAA. However, variable results have been obtained thus far (Chainuvati *et al.*, 1977; Herlong *et al.*, 1980; Walker *et al.*, 1982), and verification of long-term efficacy awaits further studies. At the moment, these ketoanalogs are not commercially available.

### 7. *Other Therapeutic Approaches*

Many other drugs and procedures have been used to treat PSE. Urease-inhibiting drugs have been used to decrease the generation of ammonia. Colon removal has occasionally been employed to decrease bacterial generation of amines, but the realization that much ammonia is produced in the small bowel has all but eliminated this relatively rare procedure. One procedure that may become more widely used is attempting to occlude the portal-systemic shunts thought to be responsible for PSE. Another is hepatic transplant, especially in patients with the acute, progressive coma associated with fulminant liver disease; transplants have already been found to offer some benefits (Bismuth *et al.*, 1987).

## V. FUTURE RESEARCH NEEDS

Research is the key to progress in this field, and future needs are many. In the experimental setting, these include:

1. better and more diverse animal models, especially for chronic liver disease,
2. greater emphasis on brain microheterogeneity,
3. additional studies of neurophysiology including more studies of the astroglial cells that mobilize ammonia in the brain,
4. more precise definition of the blood-brain barrier in experimental models of liver failure, and
5. *in vivo* studies involving administration of potential toxins and agonists/antagonists to determine their effects on functional impairment or recovery.

In the clinical setting, several thoughts come to mind:

1. The use of adrenal transplant techniques in Parkinsonism raises the question of whether such techniques might be used to provide key brain areas with specific neurotransmitters such as dopamine.

2. Better definition of minimal encephalopathy and better ways to assess the potential for full recovery are needed. Newer techniques like nuclear magnetic resonance should be used to define brain metabolism.

3. A critical assessment of the various therapeutic modalities, such as the use of antagonists of putative endogenous soporifics and combination therapy, would also be useful.

Above all, in this controversial field, is the need for an open mind as new data emerge.

## ACKNOWLEDGMENTS

Supported by funds from the Veterans Administration (Research Service, Audie L. Murphy Memorial Veterans Hospital).

## REFERENCES

Bansky, G., Meier, P. J., Ziefler, W. H., Walser, H., Schmid, M., and Huber, M. (1985). Reversal of hepatic coma by benzodiazepine antagonist (Ro 15-1788) [Letter to Editor]. *Lancet* **1**, 1324–1325.

Baraldi, M., and Zeneroli, M. L. (1982). Experimental hepatic encephalopathy: Changes in the binding of gamma-aminobutyric acid. *Science* **216**, 427–429.

Base, W., Barsigian, C., Schaeffer, A., Shaw, E., Martinez, J., and Maddrey, W. C. (1987). Influence of branched chain amino acids and branched chain keto acids on protein synthesis in isolated hepatocytes. *Hepatology* **7**, 324–329.

Basile, A. E., Gammal, S. H., Mullen, K. D., Jones, E. A., and Skolnick, P. (1988). Hepatic encephalopathy: Evidence for the involvement of an endogenous benzodiazepine receptor ligand. *Hepatology*. (In press.)

Bernthal, P., Hays. A., Tarter, R. E., Van Thiel, D., Lecky, J., and Hegedus, A. (1987). Cerebral CT scan abnormalities in cholestatic and hepatocellular disease and their relationship to neuropsychologic test performance. *Hepatology* **7**, 107–114.

Bismuth, H., Samuel, D., Gugenheim, J., Castaing, D., Bernuau, J., Rueff, B., and Benhamou, J.-P. (1987). Emergency liver transplantation for fulminant hepatitis. *Ann. Intern. Med.* **107**, 337–341.

Breen, K. J., Bryant, R. E., Levinson, J. D., and Schenker, S. (1972). Neomycin absorption in man. Studies of oral and enema administration and effect of intestinal ulceration. *Ann. Intern. Med.* **76**, 211–218.

Butterworth, R. F., Lavoie, J., Giguere, J-F., Layrargues, G. P., and Bergeron, M. (1987). Cerebral GABA-ergic and glutamatergic function in hepatic encephalopathy. *Neurochem. Pathol.* **6**, 131–144.

Cerra, F. B., Cheung, N. K., Fischer, J. E., Kaplowitz, N., Schiff, E. R., Dienstag, J. L., Bower, R. H., Mabry, C. D., Leevy, C. M., and Kiernan, T. (1985). Disease specific amino acid infusion (F080) in hepatic encephalopathy: A prospective, randomized, double-blind, controlled trial. *JPEN* **9**, 288–295.

Chainuvati, T., Plengvanit, U., and Viranuvatti, V. (1977). Effect of ornicetil (ornithine alpha-ketoglutarate) on encephalopathy in patients with acute and chronic liver disease. *Acta Hepatogastroenterol* **24**, 434–439.

Conn, H. O., Leevy, C. M., Vlahcevic, Z. R., Rodgers, J. B., Maddrey, W. C., Seef, L., and Levy, L. L. (1977). Comparison of lactulose and neomycin in the treatment of chronic portal systemic encephalopathy. *Gastroenterology* **72**, 573–583.

De Bruijn, K. M., Blendis, L. M., Zilm, D. H., Carlen, P. L., and Anderson, G. H. (1983). Effect of dietary protein manipulations in subclinical portal-systemic encephalopathy. *Gut* **24**, 53–60.

Egberts, E. H., Schomerus, H., Hamster, W., and Jurgens, P. (1983). Branched-chain amino acids in the treatment of latent portal systemic encephalopathy. A double blind placebo-controlled crossover study. *Gastroenterology* **88**, 887–895.

Elkington, S. G., Floch, M. H., and Conn, H. O. (1969). Lactulose in the treatment of chronic portal-systemic encephalopathy. *N. Engl. J. Med.* **281**, 408–412.

Elsass, P., Lund, Y., and Ranek, L. (1978). Encephalopathy in patients with cirrhosis of the liver: A neurophysiological study. *Scand. J. Gastroenterol.* **13**, 241–247.

Eriksson, L. S., Person, A., and Wahren, J. (1983). Branched chain amino acids in the treatment of chronic hepatic encephalopathy. *Gut* **23**, 801–806.

Ferenci, P., Schafer, D. F., Shrager, R., and Jones, E. A. (1981). Metabolism of the inhibitory neurotransmitter gamma-aminobutyric acid in a rabbit model of acute hepatic failure [Abstract]. *Hepatology* **1**, 509.

Ferenci, P., Schafer, D. F., Pappas, S. C., and Jones, E. A. (1983). Inhibitory and excitatory amino acid neurotransmitters in hepatic coma. *In* "New Aspects of Clinical Nutrition" (G. Kleinberger and E. Deutsch, eds.), pp. 485–504. S. Karger, New York.

Ferenci, P., Ebner, J., Zimmerman, C. H., Roth, E., and Haussinger, D. (1986a) Is blood gamma-aminobutyric acid (GABA) increased in hepatic encephalopathy? [Abstract]. *Hepatology* **6**, 1157.

Ferenci, P., Zieve, L., Ebner, J., Zimmerman, C. H., and Rzepczynski, D. (1986b). Postsynaptic neural membrane affinity for GABA and receptor density are unaltered in hepatic coma following portacaval shunt (PCS) and hepatic artery ligation (HAL) [Abstract]. *Hepatology* **6**, 1143.

Fowler, J. M., and Schafer, D. F. (1981). A mechanism for the increased sensitivity to benzodiazepines in hepatocellular failure: Evidence from an animal model [Abstract]. *Gastroenterology* **80**, 1359.

Gammal, S., and Geller, D. (1987). Correspondence to the editor. *Hepatology* **7**, 617–618.

Gilbertstadt, S., Gilbertstadt, H., Beugel, B., Collier, R., McClain, C. J., and Zieve, L. (1978). Defective intellectual function in alcoholic cirrhotics and non-cirrhotic alcoholics: Relationship to severity of liver disease [Abstract]. *Gastroenterology* **74**, 1037.

Gimson, A. E. S., O'Grady, J., Ede, R. J., Portmann, B., and Williams, R. (1986). Late onset hepatic failure: Clinical, serological, and histological features. *Hepatology* **6**, 288–294.

Greenberger, N. J., Carley, J., Schenker, S., Bettinger, I., Stamnes, C., and Beyer, P. (1977). Effect of vegetable and animal protein diets in chronic hepatic encephalopathy. *Dig. Dis. Sci.* **22**, 845–855.

Herlong, H. F., Maddrey, W. C., and Walser, M. (1980). The use ornithine salts of branched-chain ketoacids in portal-systemic encephalopathy. *Ann. Intern. Med.* **95**, 545–550.

Hindfelt, B., Plum, F., and Duffy, T. E. (1977). Effect of acute ammonia intoxication on cerebral metabolism in rats with portacaval shunts. *J. Clin. Invest.* **59**, 386–396.

Horst, D., Grace, N. D., Conn, H. O., Schiff, E., Schenker, S., Viteri, A., Low, D., and Atterbury, C. E. (1984). Comparison of dietary protein with an oral, branched chain-enriched amino acid supplement in chronic portal-systemic encephalopathy. A randomized controlled trial. *Hepatology* **4**, 279–287.

Hoyumpa, A. M., Jr., and Schenker, S. (1982). Perspectives in hepatic encephalopathy. *J. Lab. Clin. Med.* **100**, 477–487.

Hoyumpa, A. M., Desmond, P. V., Avant, G. R., Roberts, R. K., and Schenker, S. (1979). Clinical conference: hepatic encephalopathy. *Gastroenterology* **76**, 184–195.

James, J. H., Jeppson, B., Ziparo, V., and Fischer, H. E. (1979). Hyperammonaemia, plasma amino acid imbalance, and blood-brain amino acid transport: A unified theory of portal systemic encephalopathy. *Lancet* **2**, 772–775.

Jones, E. A., Schafer, D. F., Ferenci, P., and Pappas, C. S. (1984). The neurobiology of hepatic encephalopathy. *Hepatology* **4**, 1235–1242.

Lo, W. D., Ennis, S. R., Goldstein, G. W., McNeely, D. L., and Betz, A. L. (1987). The effects of galactosamine-induced hepatic failure upon blood-brain barrier permeability. *Hepatology* **7**, 452–456.

Lockwood, A. H., McDonald, J. M., Reiman, R. E., Gelbard, A. S., Laughlin, D. S., Duffy, T. E., and Plum, F. (1979). The dynamics of ammonia metabolism in man: effects of liver disease and hyperammonemia. *J. Clin. Invest.* **63**, 449–460.

Lockwood, A. H., Ginsberg, M. D., Rhoades, H. M., and Gutierez, M. T. (1986). Cerebral glucose metabolism after portacaval shunting in the rat. Patterns of metabolism and implications for the pathogenesis of hepatic encephalopathy. *J. Clin. Invest.* **78**, 86–95.

Maddison, J. E., Dodd, P. R., Morrison, M., Johnston, G. A. R., and Farrell, G. E. (1987). Plasma GABA, GABA-like activity and the brain GABA-benzodiazepine receptor complex in rats with chronic hepatic encephalopathy. *Hepatology* **7**, 621–628.

Maddrey, W. C., Weber, F. A., Coulter, A. W., Chura, C. M., Champanis, N. P., and Walser, M. (1976). Effects of keto analogues of essential amino acids in portal-systemic encephalopathy. *Gastroenterology* **71**, 190–195.

McCandless, D. W., and Schenker, S. (1968). Encephalopathy of thiamine deficiency: Studies of intracerebral mechanisms. *J. Clin. Invest.* **47**, 2268–2280.

McCandless, D. W., and Schenker, S. (1980). Effect of acute ammonia intoxication on energy stores in the cerebral reticular activating system. *Exp. Brain Res.* **44**, 325–330.

Michel, H., Bories, P., Aubin, J. P., Pomier-Layrargues, G., Bauret, P., and Bellet-Herman, H. (1985). Treatment of acute hepatic encephalopathy in cirrhotics with a branched chain amino acid enriched versus a conventional amino acid mixture. *Liver* **5**, 282–289.

Morgan, W. H., Read, A. E., and Speeller, D. C. E. (1982). Treatment of hepatic encephalopathy with metronidazole. *Gut* **23**, 1–7.

Mullen, K. D., Szauter, K. M., Galloway, P. G., and Kaminsky, K. (1987). CSF of patients with hepatic encephalopathy (HE) contains significant benzodiazepine (BZ) binding activity. Correlation with post mortem cortical BZ binding studies [Abstract]. *Hepatology* **7**, 1103.

Rikkers, L., Jenko, P., Rudman, D., and Freides, D. (1978). Subclinical hepatic encephalopathy: Detection, prevalence, and relationship to nitrogen metabolism. *Gastroenterology* **75**, 462–469.

Rossi-Fanelli, F., Riggio, D., and Cangiano, C., Cascino, A., DeConcilis, D., Merli, M., Stortoni, M., Giunchi, G., and Capocaccia, L. (1982). Branched chain amino acids vs. lactulose in the treatment of hepatic coma. A controlled study. *Dig. Dis. Sci.* **27**, 929–935.

Rzepczynski, D., Zieve, L., Lindblod, S., and LaFontaine, D. (1986). *In vivo* studies of GABAergic effects in experimental hepatic encephalopathy. *Hepatology* **6**, 902–905.

Samson, Y., Bernuau, J., Pappata, S., Chavoix, P., Baron, J. C., and Maziere, M. A. (1987). Cerebral uptake of benzodiazepine measured by positron emission tomography in hepatic encephalopathy. *N. Engl. J. Med.* **316**, 414–415.

Schafer, D. F., and Jones, E. A. (1982a). Potential neural mechanisms in the pathogenesis of hepatic encephalopathy. *In* "Progress in Liver Diseases" (H. Popper and F. Schaffner, eds.), pp. 615–628. Grune & Stratton, New York.

Schafer, D. F., and Jones, E. A. (1982b). Hepatic encephalopathy and the gamma-aminobutyric acid neurotransmitter system. *Lancet* **1**, 18–20.

Schalm, S. W., and Van Der Mey, T. (1979). Hyperammonemic coma after hepatectomy in germ-free rats. *Gastroenterology* **77**, 231–234.

Schenker, S., and Hoyumpa, A. M., Jr. (1984). Pathophysiology of hepatic encephalopathy. *Hospital Practice* **19**, 99–121.

Scollo-Lavizzari, G., and Steinmann, E. (1985). Reversal of hepatic coma by benzodiazepine antagonist (Ro 15-1788). *Lancet* **1**, 1324–1325.

Shaw, S., Worner, T. M., and Lieber, C. S. (1983). Comparison of animal and vegetable protein sources in the dietary management of hepatic encephalopathy. *Amer. J. Clin. Nutr.* **38**, 59–63.

Silk, D. B. A. (1986). Branched chain amino acids in liver disease: Fact or fantasy? *Gut* **27**, S1, 103–110.

Simmons, F., Goldstein, H., and Boyle, J. D. (1970). A controlled clinical trial of lactulose in hepatic encephalopathy. *Gastroenterology* **59**, 827–832.

Simon, D. M., McCain, J. R., Bonkovsky, M. L., Wells, J. O., Hartle, D. K., and Galambos, J. T. (1987). Effects of therapeutic paracentesis on systemic and hepatic hemodynamics and on renal and hormonal function. *Hepatology* **7**, 423–429.

Soeters, P. B., and Van Leeuwen, M. (1986). Laktulose, neomyzin und ammoniakstoffwechsel. *Infusion Therapie und Klinische Ernahrung* **13**, 186–190.

Sugarbaker, S. P., Revhaug, A., and Wilmore, D. W. (1987). The role of the small intestine in ammonia production after gastric blood administration. *Ann. Surg.* **206**, 5–17.

Thompson, J. S., Schafer D. F., Schafer, G. S., and Hodgson, P. E. (1985). Gamma-aminobutyric acid plasma levels and brain binding in Eck-fistula dogs. *J. Surg. Res.* **38**, 143–148.

Uribe, M., Berthier, J. M., Lewis, H., Mata, J. M., Sierra J. G., Garcia-Ramos, G., Acosta, J. R., and Dehesa, M. (1981). Lactose enemas plus placebo tablets vs. neomycin tablets plus starch enemas in acute portal systemic encephalopathy. *Gastroenterology* **81**, 101–106.

Uribe, M., Marquez, M. A., Ramos, G. G., Ramos-Uribe, M. H., Vargas, F., Villalobos, A., and Ramos, C. (1982). Treatment of chronic portalsystemic encephalopathy with vegetable and animal protein diets: A controlled crossover study. *Dig. Dis. Sci.* **27**, 1109–1116.

Van Berlo, C. L. H., De Jonge, H. R., Van Den Bogaard, A. E. J. M., Van Eijk, H. M. H., Janssen, M. A., and Soeters, P. B. (1987). Gamma-aminobutyric acid production in small and large intestine of normal and germ-free Wistar rats. Influence of food intake and intestinal flora. *Gastroenterology* **93**, 472–479.

Vince, A., Killingley, M., and Wrong, O. M. (1978). Effect of lactulose on ammonia production in a fecal incubation system. *Gastroenterology* **74**, 544–549.

Wahren, J., Denis, J., Desurmont, P., Eriksson, L. S., Escoffier, J. M., Gauthier, A. P., Hagenfeldt, L., Michel, H., Opolon, P., Paris, J-C., Veyrac, M. (1983). Is the intravenous administration of branched chain amino acids effective in the treatment of hepatic encephalopathy? A multicenter study. *Hepatology* **3**, 475–480.

Walker, S., Gotz, R., Czygan, P., Stiehl, A., Lanziger, G., Sieg, A., Raedsch, R., and Komerell, B. (1982). Oral ketoanalogs of branched chain amino acids in hyperammonemia in patients with cirrhosis of the liver. A double-blind crossover study. *Digestion* **24**, 105–111.

Weber, F. L., Jr. (1979). The effect of lactulose on urea metabolism and nitrogen excretion in cirrhotic patients. *Gastroenterology* **77**, 518–523.

Weber, F. L., Jr., Fresard, K. M., and Lally, B. R. (1982). Effects of lactulose and neomycin on urea metabolism in cirrhotic subjects. *Gastroenterology* **82**, 213–217.

Weber, F. L., Jr., Minco, D., Fresard, K. M., and Banwell, J. G. (1985). Effects of vegetable diets on nitrogen metabolism in cirrhotic subjects. *Gastroenterology* **89**, 538–544.

Weber, F. L., Jr., Banwell, J. G., Fresard, K. M., and Cummings, J. H. (1987). Nitrogen in fecal bacterial, fiber and soluble fractions of patients with cirrhosis: Effects of lactulose and lactulose plus neomycin. *J. Lab. Clin. Med.* **110**, 259–263.

Zeegen, R., Drinkwater, J. E., Fenton, J. C. B., Vince, A., and Dawson, A. M. (1970). Some observations on the effects of treatment with lactulose on patients with chronic hepatic encephalopathy. *Q. J. Med.* **39**, 245–263.

Zeneroli, M. L., Iuliano, E., Racagni, G., and Baraldi, M. (1982). Metabolism and brain uptake of gamma-aminobutyric acid in galactosamine-induced hepatic encephalopathy in rats. *J. Neurochem.* **38**, 1219.

Zieve, L., and Olsen, E. L. (1977). Can hepatic coma be caused by a reduction of brain noradrenaline or dopamine? *Gut* **18**, 688–691.

Zieve, F. J., Zieve, L., Doizaki, W. M., and Gilsdorf, R. B. (1974a). Synergism between ammonia and fatty acids in the production of coma. Implications for hepatic coma. *J. Pharmacol. Exo. Ther.* **191**, 10–16.

Zieve, L., Doizaki, W. M., and Zieve, F. J. (1974b). Synergism between mercaptans and ammonia or fatty acids in the production of coma. A possible role for mercaptans in the pathogenesis of hepatic coma. *J. Lab. Clin. Med.* **83**, 16–28.

# 18

# Nitrogen Metabolism in the Intestine

## Norman Kretchmer

*Department of Nutritional Sciences*
*College of Natural Resources*
*University of California, Berkeley*
*Berkeley, California*
*Department of Pediatrics*
*University of California, San Francisco*
*San Francisco, California*

## Ruth Hurwitz

*Department of Nutritional Sciences*
*College of Natural Resources*
*University of California, Berkeley*
*Berkeley, California*

# I. INTRODUCTION

Many assign the intestine a minor physiologic role in the total metabolic economy of the organism because they only consider its functions as in the absorption of fluid and nutrients and as an inert barrier to prevent offensive elements in food from entering the body. However, the intestine is actually highly complex and is an active, integrated participant in total body metabolism. This discussion will be limited to nitrogen metabolism in the intestine, which has ramifications both within the intestine and throughout the body.

# II. INTESTINAL STRUCTURE AND FUNCTION

The primary functional unit of the intestine includes two cell systems, the crypt and the villus (Fig. 1), whose biologies are very different. The crypt consists of stem cells, proliferating cells, and motile cells. These cells differentiate as they move out of the crypt toward the junctional zone.

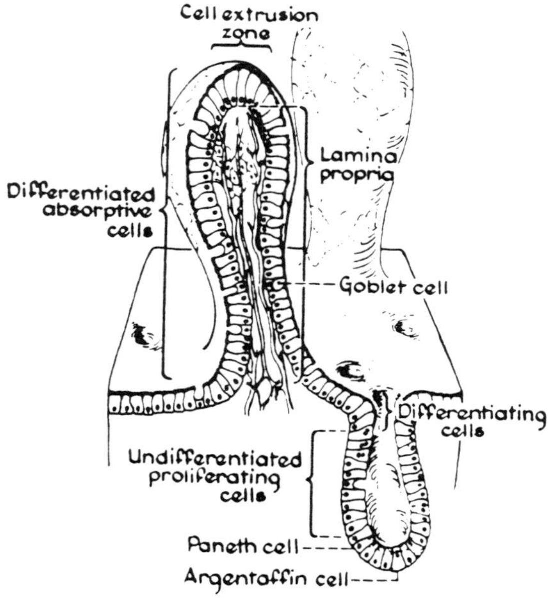


**Fig. 1.** Diagram of the functional unit of the small intestine, illustrating the proliferating cells in the crypt, the differentiating cells, and the matured differentiated cells on the villus. (From Herbst *et al.*, 1969. Reprinted with permission.)

The maturing, differentiated cells move up to occupy the villus, where they take on the biochemical characteristics of fully mature enterocytes with a highly specialized brush border. Characteristic enzymes, such as sucrase and lactase, can be identified in mature enterocytes. Intracellular nitrogen metabolism occurs throughout the crypt-villus unit, and as cells mature, they take part in the nitrogen metabolism of the entire organism.

## III. INTESTINAL NITROGEN METABOLISM AND AMINO ACID SYNTHESIS

Ammonia is of primary importance in nitrogen metabolism. It is derived from several nitrogenous compounds, including glutamine. As indicated in Fig. 2, glutamine also functions as a source of energy by providing a

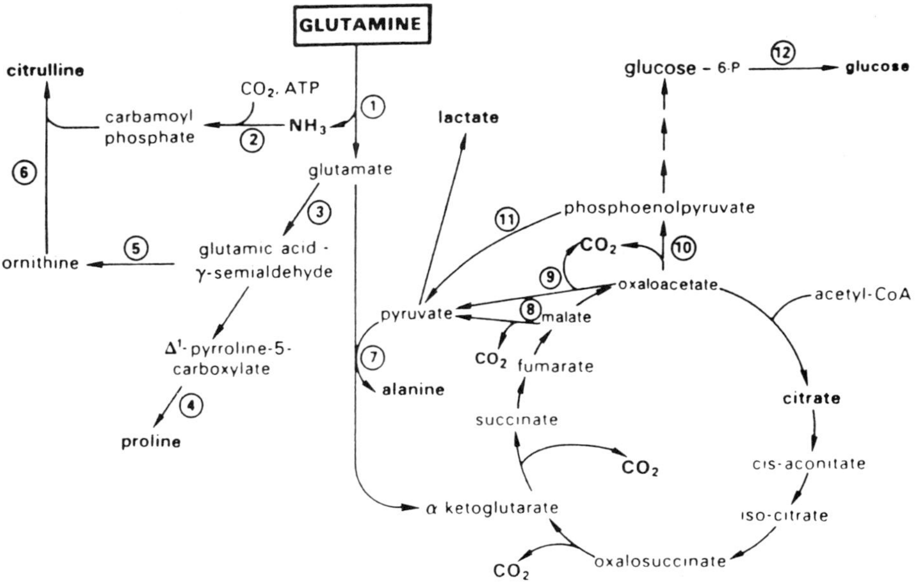


**Fig. 2.** Several pathways of glutamine metabolism are operative in rat intestinal mucosa. Boldface type indicates metabolic products released into intestinal venous blood. Numbered reactions have all been individually demonstrated *in vitro* with mucosal preparations from rat small intestine. Circled numbers refer to the enzyme responsible for the metabolic reaction: (1) glutaminase, (2) carbamoyl-phosphate synthase, (3) pyrroline-5-carboxylate synthase, (4) pyrroline-5-carboxylate reductase, (5) ornithine-oxo-acid aminotransferase, (6) ornithine carbamoyltransferase, (7) alanine aminotransferase, (8) malate dehydrogenase, (9) oxaloacetate decarboxylase, (10) phosphoenolpyruvate carboxykinase, (11) pyruvate kinase, (12) glucose-6-phosphatase. (From Windmueller, 1980. Reprinted with permission.)

carbon skeleton to be used in the Krebs cycle. When glutamine enters the Krebs cycle, another ammonia molecule is released. In each instance, ammonia is used by the carbamyl phosphate synthetases. Carbamyl phosphate synthetase I (CPS I) is a mitochondrial enzyme, and carbamyl phosphate synthetase II (CPS II) is a cytosolic enzyme.

### A. Pyrimidine and Purine Synthesis

Ammonia from glutamine can be used for *de novo* pyrimidine or purine synthesis. These pathways predominate in crypt cells. CPS II participates in *de novo* formation of pyrimidine, and the nitrogen required for its synthesis is derived directly from glutamine. From all indications, the most active pyrimidine synthesis occurs in proliferating enterocytes, which have an increased need to synthesize nucleic acids. This contention was confirmed in a study that showed much greater incorporation of tritiated cytidine into RNA in crypts than in villi (Herbst *et al.*, 1970) (Fig. 3).

At times, the carbamyl phosphate formed in mitochondria overflows into the cytoplasm and is metabolized in the pathway of pyrimidine synthesis to form orotic acid. Excess orotic acid that cannot be further metabolized in the liver can be found in body fluids. Other enzymes

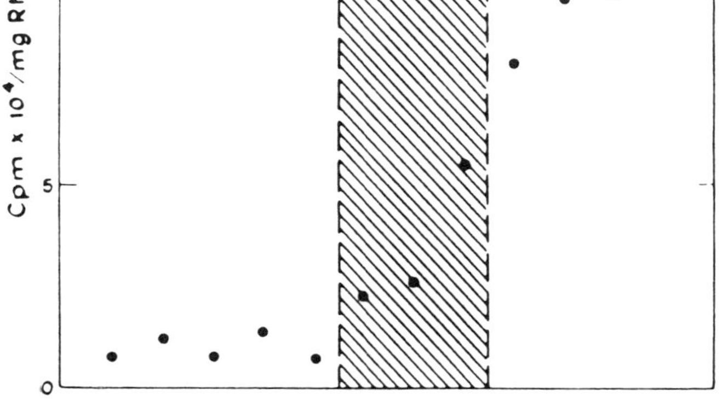


**Fig. 3.** Incorporation of tritiated cytidine into RNA was measured in crypts, junctional zone, and villi of jejunal mucosa. Each point represents an average of results obtained with mucosa from 6 animals. (From Herbst *et al.*, 1970. Reprinted with permission.)

involved in pyrimidine synthesis, such as aspartic transcarbamase and dihydroorotase, are elevated in crypt cells (Herbst *et al.*, 1970; Fortin-Magana *et al.*, 1970) (Fig. 4).

## B. Arginine and Citrulline Synthesis

Ammonia participates in arginine synthesis in hepatic mitochondria. The important intermediates in this pathway are citrulline, ornithine, and argininosuccinate. The first step in this pathway is activated by *N*-acetylglutamate, a compound synthesized via acetylglutamate synthetase. Arginine activates this enzyme. When arginase is present in the cell,

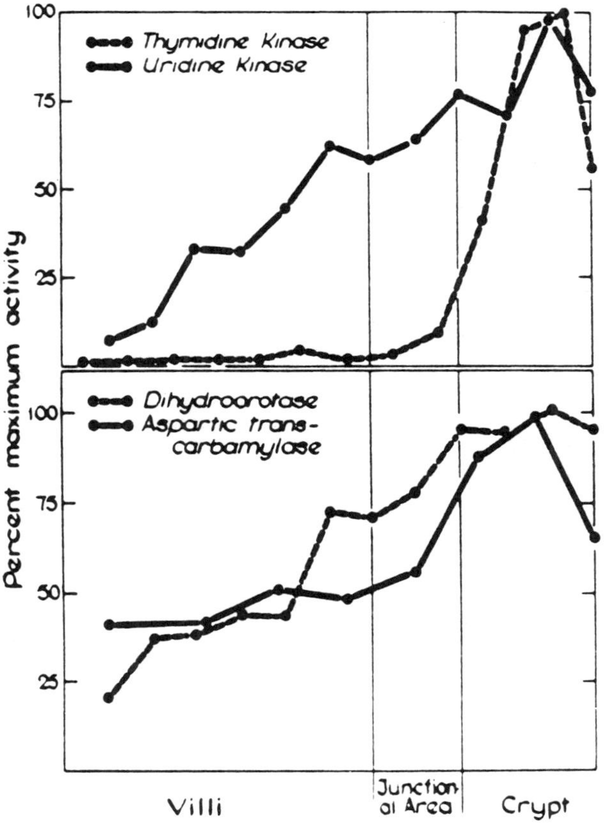


**Fig. 4.** Activities of thymidine kinase and uridine kinase (above) and dihydroorotase and aspartate transcarbamylase (below) were measured in various layers of jejunal mucosa. At least three animals were used in each study. (From Herbst *et al.*, 1970. Reprinted with permission.)

arginine is hydrolyzed, forming ornithine and urea. Ornithine is an important intermediate in this and other pathways to be discussed.

### 1. *Studies in Adult Rats*

The adult rat enterocyte has been shown to contain ornithine transcarbamylase, thus giving it the potential to synthesize citrulline (Jones *et al.*, 1961). The critical physiologic studies were carried out in the rat (Windmueller and Spaeth, 1974). Using perfusion techniques, these authors showed that glutamine is the main energy source for the intestine (Windmueller and Spaeth, 1980). In their studies, 30% of labeled glutamine in blood was removed in one passage through the intestine (Windmueller and Spaeth, 1975), and the major products of intestinal glutamine metabolism were carbon dioxide, citrulline, proline and lactate. Because they did not find labeled arginine, the authors concluded that citrulline must be the end-product of nitrogen metabolism in the rat (Windmueller and Spaeth, 1980). Similar conclusions were reached for sheep (Wolff *et al.*, 1972) and for humans (Felig and Wahren, 1971). Windmueller and Spaeth (1981) demonstrated that citrulline is not taken up by the liver, whereas the kidney removes citrulline from blood and converts it to arginine (Featherston *et al.*, 1973; Windmueller and Spaeth, 1981). The ability of the kidney to convert citrulline to arginine was first shown by Borsook and Dubnoff (1941). This finding is interesting in view of the fact that arginase, although present in the kidney of the adult animal, is sequestered distal to the site of arginine synthesis (Szepesi *et al.*, 1970). Thus, arginine metabolism takes place in a different locus in the kidney than arginine synthesis.

Studies by Windmueller and Spaeth further indicate that the intestine is not the sole source of citrulline because removal of the entire splanchnic contents lowers the circulating citrulline concentration by only 25%. The source of the remaining citrulline is unknown. These authors also showed that the kidney is not the sole site at which citrulline is used; the brain and other organs may also participate in synthesizing arginine from citrulline.

### 2. *Studies in Neonatal and Weanling Rats and Mice*

All enzymes necessary for arginine synthesis are present in the intestine of the neonatal $C_{57}B1$ mouse, but not in the neonatal rat (Hurwitz and Kretchmer, 1986). These enzymes include CPS I, ornithine transcarbamylase (OTC), argininosuccinate synthetase (ASS) and argininosuccinate lyase (ASL). The developmental curves for the activities of CPS I and ASL are the most elevated at birth (Fig. 5), when ASL activity is six to seven times that found in the adult intestine. At birth, ASL activity in the mouse

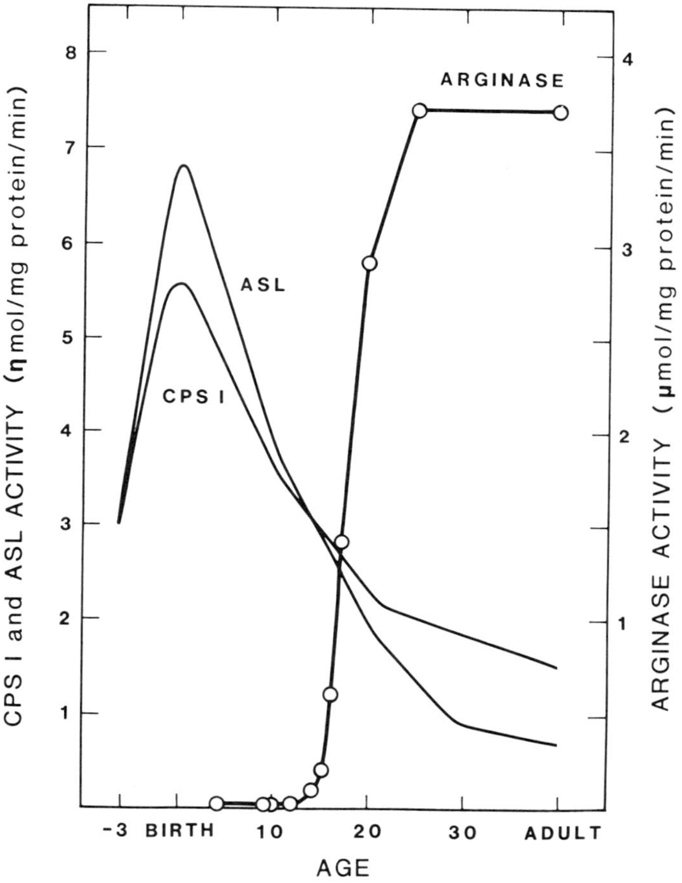


**Fig. 5.** The activity of arginase in mouse jejunum during development was measured. Each open circle represents value of a single jejunum. Developmental curves for argininosuccinate lyase (ASL) and carbamyl phosphate synthetase I (CPS I) are also included to show contrast in pattern. (From Hurwitz and Kretchmer, 1986. Reprinted with permission.)

kidney is five times less than in the adult kidney, but ten times less than in the weanling kidney (Fig. 6). Theoretically, all citrulline produced in the intestine of the neonatal mouse would be used for local synthesis of arginine and would thus be unavailable to kidney. If citrulline availability exceeded intestinal needs, then the slight synthesizing power of the neonatal mouse kidney might be able to utilize the small amount of circulating citrulline.

To demonstrate the function of this system, free arginine was measured after a reaction of $NH_3$ + [$^{14}C$]$NaHC0_3$ with slices of neonatal and adult

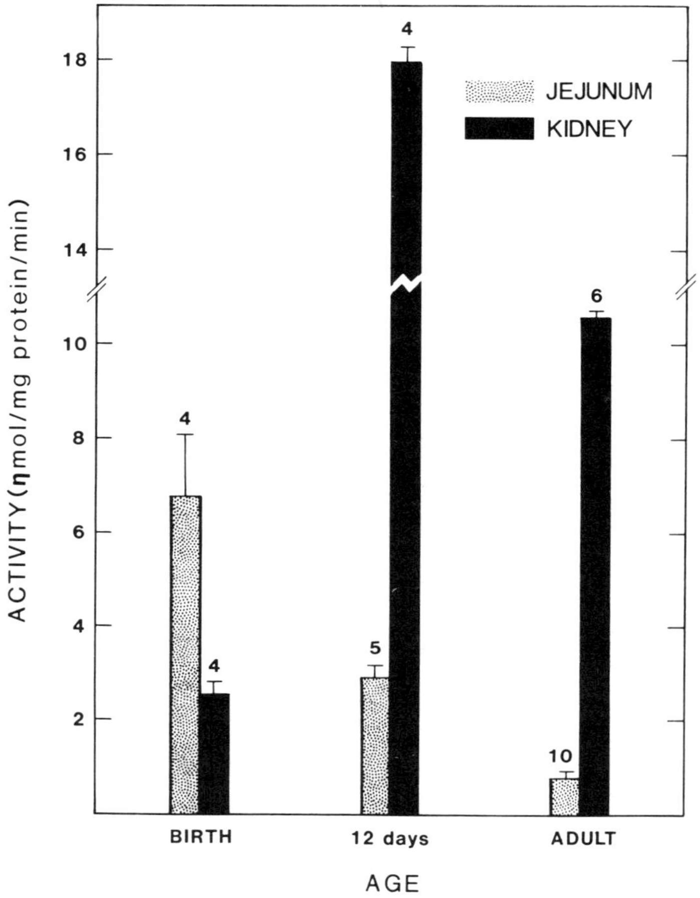


**Fig. 6.** Specific activity of argininosuccinate lyase (ASL) was compared in mouse jejunum and kidney at various ages. Each bar represents mean ± SD. Numbers above bars indicate numbers of animals in each group. (From Hurwitz and Kretchmer, 1986. Reprinted with permission.)

mouse intestine (Table I). Neonatal tissue formed three times more free arginine than adult tissue. With citrulline as the substrate, neonatal intestinal enzymes formed 150 times more free arginine, and 75 times more arginine was incorporated into protein.

Maternal milk of the rat contains more arginine during the first day after parturition than maternal milk of the mouse (unpublished observations). In both the rat and the mouse, the combination of synthesized arginine and arginine in maternal milk is sufficient for growth until weaning. At weaning, arginase activity first appears in the intestine and increases

TABLE I

**Synthesis of Arginine from $NH_3$ + $CO_2$ and from Citrulline By Intestine of Newborn and Adult Mouse[a]**

| | $NH_3 + CO_2$ | Citrulline | |
|---|---|---|---|
| Group | Free arginine | Free arginine | Free arginine incorporated into protein |
| Newborn | 163 ± 20 (5) | 165.0 ± 15.0 (4) | 7.5 ± 1.00 (4) |
| Adult | 68 ± 31 (5) | 1.0 ± 0.5 (4) | 0.1 ± 0.08 (4) |
| | $p < 0.025$ | $p < 0.001$ | $p < 0.001$ |

[a]Values are expressed as means ± SD of picomoles of arginine formed in 30 min/mg intestinal protein. Parenthetical number is number of assays. Each assay was performed on three combined minced jejunums from newborn mice or 2- to 3-mm slices of 2 cm of adult jejunum. Substrates were either $NH_3$ and [$^{14}$C]$NaHCO_3$ or [carbamyl-$C^{14}$]citrulline. After acid precipitation of the protein in the incubated mixture, free arginine in the soluble portion was enzymatically converted to $CO_2$ to measure arginine content. The precipitate was washed, solubilized, and counted to measure arginine incorporated into protein. (Data from unpublished observations.)

rapidly (Fig. 5). At the same time, arginase increases in the mammary gland (Folley, 1947). These findings support the contention that arginine fulfills the role of an essential amino acid during rapid growth periods.

Arginine, or its substitute, citrulline, is necessary for adequate growth. In an elegant series of experiments, Hoogenraad and associates (1976) showed that severe growth retardation occurred in six-week-old rats fed a glycine-glycine derivative of *N*-(phosphonacetyl-L-ornithine)(Gly-Gly-PALO), an inhibitor of the OTC enzyme. Gly-Gly-PALO penetrated enterocytes, but not hepatocytes. In enterocytes, the peptide was removed enzymatically, leaving PALO free to inhibit OTC. Growth retardation was prevented by administering citrulline or, to a lesser degree, arginine, at the same time as Gly-Gly-PALO. Administration of Gly-Gly-PALO lowered serum arginine and citrulline content and produced a corresponding increase in ornithine.

Although the rat intestine cannot synthesize arginine, the enterocyte of the $C_{57}$B1 mouse has an intact pathway for arginine synthesis (unpublished observations). Mice of the $C_{57}$B1 and $C_3$H strains show very high ASL and CPS I activity during the perinatal period. ASL activity can be detected in the mouse kidney at birth. This activity, on the basis of mg protein, is about one third of that found in the intestine. However, if total activity in both organs is compared, activity in the intestine is about

245 (7 × 35 mg) nmols/whole intestine/min, whereas activity in the kidney is about 24 (2.2 × 11 mg) nmols/both kidneys/min. Thus ASL activity in the total intestine is approximately 10 times that in both kidneys (unpublished observations).

At 10 to 12 days after birth, the activity of arginine-synthesizing enzymes increases in the kidney and decreases in the intestine. By that time, OTC activity in the intestine has increased twofold (unpublished observations). At natural weaning 12 to 15 days after birth, the activity of the ASL and CPS I enzymes in the intestine decreases to one-third to one-half of that seen in the perinatal period (Fig. 5). Arginase also appears in the intestine at weaning and may function in producing ornithine, which is essential in polyamine formation. Arginase appears at weaning simultaneously in the rat intestine (Herzfeld and Raper, 1976) and in the mammary gland (Folley, 1947). It has been postulated that the organism can use endogenously synthesized arginine and that the high arginase content allows for metabolism of exogenous arginine to produce ornithine in the intestine and liver (Hoogenraad *et al.*, 1976).

## IV. FUTURE RESEARCH DIRECTIONS

A number of metabolic pathways require arginine. Thus, it is important to understand how the neonatal intestine uses arginine. Because arginase is not present in the neonatal intestine, the intestine cannot produce ornithine. Preliminary results show that ornithine cannot be produced in the neonatal intestine via the action of transamidinase (glycine–arginine amidinotransferase) (unpublished observations).

Another pathway that remains to be investigated in the neonatal mouse is the formation of ornithine from glutamate via L-glutamyl-semialdehyde. The activity of the intestinal enzyme pyrroline-5-carboxylate-synthetase (Wakabayashi and Jones, 1983) in the cat (Rogers and Phang, 1985) is about one-fifth of that in the rat. The low activity of this enzyme, which is necessary for the formation of ornithine and eventually citrulline, undoubtedly explains why the cat is extremely dependent on dietary arginine (Morris and Rogers, 1978). An ornithine source must exist in the neonatal mouse because the intestine cannot regenerate ornithine from arginine until 12 days after birth and because ornithine is necessary for synthesis of arginine and polyamines (Luk *et al.*, 1980). Hydrolysis of arginine in the liver does produce ornithine, but this ornithine is needed for recycling in urea synthesis in liver cells and probably does not enter circulation.

## V. SUMMARY

All organs use metabolically derived nitrogen for synthesis of intracellular proteins, nucleic acids, and other nitrogenous substances. The intestine has several unique characteristics: its cells are in a constant state of proliferation and differentiation, the enterocyte has a highly specialized brush border that functions in both digestion and absorption, and glutamine is the major source of energy for this organ. Nitrogen derived from glutamine is used for the formation of purines and pyrimidines and for synthesis of citrulline. In certain animals, the intestine can utilize glutamine–nitrogen for the synthesis of arginine.

Differences in the developmental aspects of arginine metabolism have been demonstrated in three species of animals, the mouse, the rat and the cat. Neonatal mice of certain strains synthesize arginine in the intestine, but this capability disappears at about 12 days after birth. At weaning, the activities of argininosuccinate synthetase (ASS) and argininosuccinate (ASL) enzymes disappear in the intestine while they simultaneously develop maximal activity in the kidney. Unlike the mouse, carnivores such as the cat are dependent on dietary arginine. Intraspecies differences in activity of ASL have been found in rats and mice.

## REFERENCES

Borsook, J., and Dubnoff, J. W. (1941). The conversion of citrulline to arginine in kidney. *J. Biol. Chem.* **141**, 717–738.

Featherston, W. R., Rogers, Q. R., and Freedland, R. A. (1973). Relative importance of kidney and liver in synthesis of arginine by the rat. *Biochem. J.* **224**, 127–129.

Felig, P., and Wahren, J. (1971). Amino acid metabolism in exercising man. *J. Clin. Invest.* **50**, 2703–2714.

Folley, S. J. (1947). Changes in the arginase and alkaline phosphatase contents of the mammary gland and liver of the rat during pregnancy, lactation and mammary involution. *Biochem. J.* **41**, 261–269.

Fortin-Magana, R., Hurwitz, R., Herbst, J. J., and Kretchmer, N. (1970). Intestinal enzymes: Indicators of proliferation and differentiation in the jejunum. *Science* **167**, 1627–1628.

Herbst, J. J., Sunshine, P., and Kretchmer, N. (1969). Intestinal malabsorption in infancy and childhood. *Adv. in Pediatr.* **16**, 16.

Herbst, J. J., Fortin-Magana, R., and Sunshine P. (1970). Relationship of pyrimidine biosynthetic enzymes to cellular proliferation in rat intestine during development. *Gastroenterology* **59**, 240–246.

Herzfeld, A., and Raper, S. M. (1976). Enzymes of ornithine metabolism in adult and developing rat intestine. *Biochim. Biophys. Acta* **428**, 600–610.

Hoogenraad, N., Totino, N., Elmer H., Wraight, C., Alewood, P., and Jones, R. B. (1976). Inhibition of intestinal citrulline synthesis causes severe growth retardation in rats. *Amer. J. Physiol.* **249**, G792–G799.

Hurwitz, R., and Kretchmer, N. (1986). Development of arginine synthesizing enzymes in mouse intestine. *Amer. J. Physiol.* **251**, G103–G110.

Jones, M. E., Anderson, A. D., Anderson, C., and Hodes, S. (1961). Citrulline synthesis in rat tissues. *Arch. Biochem. Biophys.* **95**, 499–507.

Luk, G. D., Marton, L. J., and Baylin, S. B. (1980). Ornithine decarboxylase is important in intestinal mucosal maturation and recovery from injury in rats. *Science* **210**, 195–198.

Morris, J. G., and Rogers, Q. R. (1978). Ammonia intoxication in the near-adult cat as a result of dietary deficiency of arginine. *Science* **199**, 431–432.

Rogers, Q. R., and Phang, J. M. (1985). Deficiency of pyrroline-5-carboxylate synthase in the intestinal mucosa of the cat. *J. Nutr.* **115**, 146–150.

Szepesi, B., Avery, H., and Freedland, R. A. (1970). Role of kidney gluconeogenesis and amino acid catabolism. *Amer. J. Physiol,* **219**, 1627–1631.

Wakabayashi, Y., and Jones, M. E. (1983). Pyrroline-5-carboxylate synthesis from glutamate by rat intestinal mucosa. *J. Biol. Chem.* **258**, 3865–3872.

Windmueller, H. G. (1980). *In* "Glutamine: Metabolism, Enzymology, and Regulation" (J. Mora and R. Palacios, eds.), p. 235. Academic Press, New York.

Windmueller, H. G., and Spaeth, A. E. (1974). Uptake and metabolism of plasma glutamine by the small intestine. *J. Biol. Chem.* **249**, 5070–5079.

Windmueller, H. G., and Spaeth, A. E. (1975). Intestinal metabolism of glutamine and glutamate from the lumen as compared to glutamine from blood. *Arch. Biochem. Biophys.* **171**, 662–672.

Windmueller, H. G., and Spaeth, A. E. (1980). Respiratory fuels and nitrogen metabolism *in vivo* in small intestine of fed rats. *J. Biol. Chem.* **255**, 107–112.

Windmueller, H. G., and Spaeth, A. E. (1981). Source and fate of circulating citrulline. *Amer. J. Physiol.* **241**, E473–E480.

Wolff, J. E., Bergman, E. N., and Williams, H. H. (1972). Net metabolism of plasma amino acids by liver and portal-drained viscera of fed sheep. *Amer. J. Physiol.* **223**, 438–446.

# 19

## Role of Gastrointestinal Hormones in Adaptation

Vay Liang W. Go

*Division of Digestive Diseases and Nutrition*
*National Institute of Diabetes and Digestive and Kidney Diseases*
*Bethesda, Maryland*
*Mayo Medical School*
*Rochester, Minnesota*



### I. INTRODUCTION

Nutritional adaptation takes place from the prenatal stage of development, which is characterized by continuous transfer of nutrients from maternal to fetal circulation, to the postnatal stage, which is characterized by oral ingestion of nutrients on a feed-fast cycle. The gastrointestinal neuroendocrine system plays an important role in this adaptive process.

The focus of research into intestinal adaptation has recently swung from direct localized nutritional effects to gastrointestinal hormones and growth factors (Johnson, 1987). The endocrine and paracrine actions of hormones and peptides in the gastrointestinal mucosa and intrinsic nerves appear to be important regulators of trophic responses to such local stimuli as food ingestion and digestion and gastrointestinal secretions (Fig. 1).

The gastrointestinal tract is believed to have the largest mass of endocrine cells and the greatest diversity of endocrine products of any organ in the body. The ultrastructure of gastrointestinal endocrine cells resembles that of other endocrine cells—the base of each cell contains secretory granules that discharge peptides into adjacent capillaries. Each endocrine cell secretes a specific peptide hormone (Thompson *et al.*, 1987; Walsh, 1987). Oral nutrients are potent stimuli for release of hormones from the endocrine cells, which are scattered throughout the gastrointestinal mucosa and dispersed among ordinary epithelial absorptive cells. The release of gastrointestinal hormones in response to nutrients and the trophic effect of gut hormones on gut mucosal and parenchymal tissues may influence human postnatal adaptation (Lucas *et al.*, 1983).

This chapter reviews the role of nutrients in the release of gastrointestinal hormones and regulatory peptides and describes the resulting alterations in gut function. The synthesis, structure, biology, and metabolism of these hormones and peptides are described elsewhere (Thompson *et al.*, 1987; Walsh, 1987).

## II. DISTRIBUTION OF GUT HORMONES AND REGULATORY PEPTIDES

The gastrointestinal tract is an endocrine organ that releases a variety of hormones, each of which is predominantly found at one location (Fig. 2). Gastrin is primarily a gastric hormone. Cholecystokinin (CCK), secretin, gastric inhibitory polypeptide (GIP), and motilin are found mainly in the upper small intestine. Neurotensin and enteroglucagon (GLI) are lower small bowel hormones, and peptide YY (PYY) is a colon hormone. Insulin, glucagon, human pancreatic polypeptide (HPP), and pancreostatin and are present in the pancreatic islets (Go and Koch, 1988; Koch *et al.*, 1987). Nonhormonal regulatory peptides are found in the neurons, ganglia, and nerve fibers of the gut intrinsic plexus. These include vasoactive intestinal polypeptide (VIP), substance P, bombesin-like peptide, somatostatin, the enkephalins, peptide histidine-isoleucine (PHI), calcitonin, gene-related peptide (peptide G), and galanin.

The embryological origin of the gut neuroendocrine system, derived from the ectoderm and neural crest, is similar to that of the cerebral cortex,

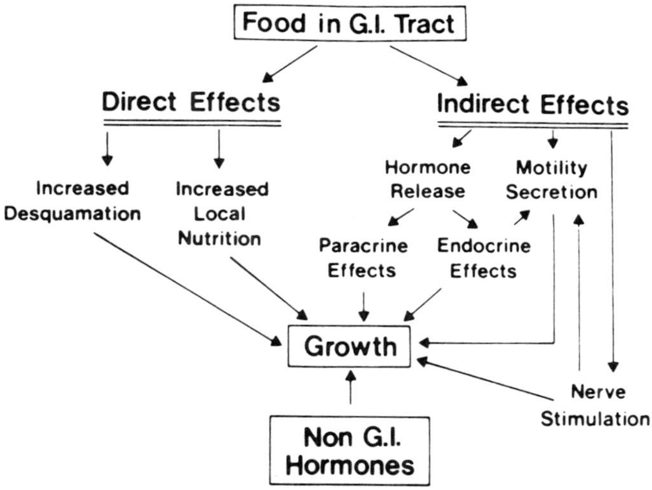


**Fig. 1.** Ingestion and digestion and food has both direct and indirect effects on the growth of gastrointestinal mucosa. (From Johnson, 1987. Reprinted with permission.)

hypothalamus, pituitary, and sympathetic nervous system. Gut regulatory peptides and hormones, with the exception of secretin, GIP, and GLI, are also found in nervous tissue. Regional differences in distribution of these substances have been demonstrated in the gut, spinal cord, and brain (Go and Koch, 1988; Yaksh *et al.*, 1988). Regulatory peptides and hormones influence the release of gut hormones and directly affect the functions of gut muscle as well as epithelial, vascular, and immune cells.

## III. ROLE OF INTRALUMINAL NUTRIENTS IN THE RELEASE OF GASTROINTESTINAL HORMONES

The substances that bathe the microvilli in the gastrointestinal lumen provide the most important stimuli for release of gastrointestinal hormones. Release of these hormones is stimulated by products of protein, fat, and carbohydrate digestion, by adjacent nerves, and by other hormones and ions in the circulation. Each nutrient has a different specificity for each peptide hormone as well as a different and dose-dependent ability to stimulate its release (Table I).

### A. Carbohydrate Digestion

Glucose is a potent stimulator of GIP release. Studies in humans have shown that perfusion of glucose into the upper gut increased GIP release

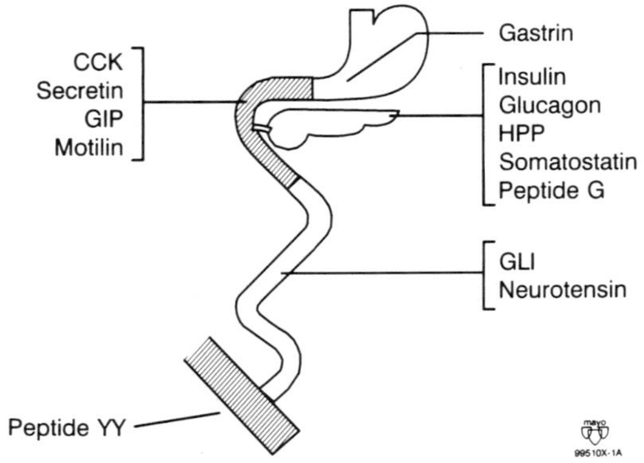


**Fig. 2.** Gastrointestinal hormones and regulatory peptides are regionally distributed in the gastrointestinal mucosa and in the pancreatic islets. Distinct regional differences are found in the concentrations of these substances. Gastrin is primarily a gastric hormone. Cholecystokinin (CCK), secretin, gastric inhibitory polypeptide (GIP), and motilin are found mainly in the upper small intestine. Neurotensin and enteroglucagon (GLI) are lower small bowel hormones, and peptide YY is a colon hormone. Insulin, glucagon, human pancreatic polypeptide (HPP), somatostatin and peptide G are present in the pancreatic islets (Go and Koch, 1988. Reprinted with permission.)

(McCullough *et al.*, 1983), whereas inhibition of carbohydrate digestion by purified amylase inhibitor or by acarbose, a mucosal disaccharidase inhibitor, diminished GIP release (Boivin *et al.*, 1987; Dimitriadis *et al.*, 1982). Glucose does not stimulate the release of gastrin, CCK, or secretin and only weakly stimulates release of the distal gut hormones GLI, neurotensin, and PYY. GIP is the leading candidate as the gut hormone responsible for augmenting insulin release. This insulinotrophic effect, which occurs only after plasma glucose reaches 17–20 mg/dl, is linearly related to plasma glucose levels (McCullough *et al.*, 1983). The autonomic nervous system does not directly affect glucose-stimulated GIP secretion in humans (Nelson *et al.*, 1986).

## B. Protein Digestion

Peptides and amino acids have a potent effect on release of proximal gut hormones, particularly gastrin, CCK, and GIP, and a lesser effect on release of HPP.

### 1. *Gastrin*

Gastrin was the first gastrointestinal hormone proposed to have trophic effects on gastrointestinal mucosa and on growth of the oxyntic gland

**TABLE I**

**Specificity and Potency of Intraluminal Nutrients In the Release of Gut Hormones**

| | Stimuli | | |
|---|---|---|---|
| Hormone | Protein | Carbohydrate | Fat |
| Gastrin | + + + + | | |
| CCK | + + + | | + + + + |
| Secretin | | | + |
| GIP | + + + | + + + + | + + |
| Motilin | | | + + |
| HPP | + + + | + | + + |
| GLI | | + | + + + + |
| Neurotensin | + | + | + + + + |
| PYY | | | + + + + |

(Johnson, 1987). In a study of duodenal ulcer patients, intragastric concentrations of 1 to 8% peptone solutions produced linear increases in plasma gastrin (Lam *et al.*, 1980). Although a gastric luminal pH below 3 inhibited gastrin release in the presence of amino acids or protein, the magnitude and duration of gastrin release were increased by maintaining the pH above 3. This feedback inhibition modulated the amount of gastrin normally released after a meal (Walsh, 1987). The amino acids phenylalanine and tryptophan stimulated gastrin release when perfused intraluminally but had no effect on gastrin release when administered intravenously, although intravenous administration did stimulate acid secretion (Taylor *et al.*, 1982).

### 2. *Cholecystokinin (CCK)*

CCK stimulates pancreatic enzyme secretion and gallbladder contraction, both of which require intraluminal protein digestion. In addition, CCK has recently been found to regulate pancreatic acinar and ductal cell replication (Beglinger and Gyr, 1987). In bioassays of human subjects, phenylalanine and tryptophan had a potent effect on CCK release when perfused intraduodenally (Go *et al.*, 1970). Long-term infusion of CCK can lead to progressive reduction of pancreatic enzyme content and to increased DNA synthesis; it can also contribute to hormone-dependent pancreatic growth (Beglinger and Gyr, 1987). These findings have led to speculation that CCK may mediate pancreatic enzyme adaptation following prolonged intake of a high-protein diet.

### 3. *Gastric Inhibitory Polypeptide (GIP)*

A mixed amino acid solution stimulated GIP release in humans when perfused intraduodenally but not when perfused intravenously (Thomas *et al.*, 1978). Intraduodenal infusion of a mixture containing arginine, histidine–isoleucine, leucine, lysine, and threonine caused significant GIP release, whereas a mixture of phenylalanine, tryptophan, methionine, and valine produced no response. These findings suggest that GIP release is stimulated by a different group of amino acids than those causing pronounced release of CCK and gastrin.

### 4. *Human Pancreatic Polypeptide (HPP)*

Ingestion of a protein meal and cholinergic reflexes cause release of HPP into the circulation, whereas anticholinergic agents markedly inhibit its release (Floyd *et al.*, 1977). On the other hand, intravenous infusion of amino acids produced an even smaller release of HPP than ingestion of fat.

## C. Fat Digestion

### 1. *Distal Gut Hormones*

Fat hydrolysates are potent stimuli for release of the distal gut hormones neurotensin, GLI, and PYY (Walsh, 1977). The effect of fatty acids on the release of these hormones is both dose- and carbon-chain-length-dependent. For example, oleic acid is a more powerful stimulator of hormone release than short- or medium-chain fatty acids. In humans, the inhibition of gastric emptying and intestinal transit in response to ileal fat has been called the "ileal brake" (MacFarlane *et al.*, 1983). This phenomenon may be mediated by ileal and colonic hormones. All three distal gut hormones may function as enterogastrones—hormones that mediate the inhibition of gastric acid secretion after fat ingestion. However, only GLI has been suggested as a physiological regulator of intestinal cell turnover. An association has been reported between intestinal crypt cell production and GLI. Intestinal resection, colonic glucose perfusion, and bombesin injection have all been shown to stimulate intestinal mitotic activity and to increase GLI cell degeneration and plasma GLI content in rats (Buchan *et al.*, 1985; Miazza *et al.*, 1985). The physiological significance of these findings remains unclear.

### 2. *Proximal Gut Hormones*

Fat hydrolysates are also potent stimuli for the proximal gut hormones CCK and GIP (Walsh, 1987). We have investigated the effects of intraduodenal glycerol perfusion, fatty acid chain length, and fatty acid load on pancreatic and gallbladder function, which are thought to be related to CCK release (Malagelada *et al.*, 1976). Although glycerol had no effect, pancreatic and gallbladder responses were augmented by increasing fatty acid chain length and fatty acid load until the maximum capacity for pancreatic secretion and gallbladder emptying were attained. In later investigations using a glucose-insulin clamp technique, we found that oral fat increased GIP release in humans and that insulin did not inhibit fat-stimulated GIP secretion under normal glycemic conditions (Verdonk *et al.*, 1980). We observed a higher GIP response to oral fat in the hypoglycemic clamp and a lower GIP response in the hyperglycemic clamp. These results suggest a glycemic effect on GIP secretion in the presence of hyperinsulinemia.

### D. The Enteroinsular Axis

The interrelationship between gut hormones and pancreatic islets has been referred to as the ''enteroinsular axis'' (Creutzfeldt and Ebert, 1986). An exciting new hypothesis suggests that different gut hormones may function as incretins for different foodstuffs. Thus, CCK released by oral amino acids might potentiate their action on pancreatic islet insulin release, or GIP released by oral glucose might potentiate the action of glucose on insulin release. Recent findings indicate that GIP may potentiate CCK-stimulated secretion of pancreatic exocrine enzymes (Mueller *et al.*, 1987) and that gut hormones may potentiate maturation of both endocrine and exocrine pancreatic cells (Williams, 1987).

### E. Trace Minerals

Certain trace minerals appear to have a role in the synthesis and release of gut hormones and regulatory peptides. Intraduodenal perfusion or intravenous infusion of calcium, magnesium, and zinc caused significant stimulation of plasma CCK in the dog (Inoue *et al.*, 1985), and intraduodenal perfusion of calcium and magnesium in humans produced similar results (Malagelada *et al.*, 1978).

## IV. ACTIONS OF GUT HORMONES AND REGULATORY PEPTIDES

Each gastrointestinal hormone has characteristic and distinct effects on various gastrointestinal target organs as well as on other endocrine secretions. The release of gut hormones subjects each target organ to many simultaneous agonistic and antagonistic influences. Thus, the activity of the gastrointestinal hormones differs significantly from that of the classical endocrine hormones released by the pituitary, thyroid, and adrenal glands (Go and Miller, 1983). All gastrointestinal hormones alter gut secretion and absorption as well as motor, immunological, and metabolic functions. Some gastrointestinal hormones also have trophic effects on gastrointestinal tissue that may affect adaptation in the gut. Receptors on cell membranes allow these hormones to enter gut cells, where they may affect the regulation of gene products such as digestive enzymes or the synthesis of endocrine products such as insulin. The biological actions of each hormone are reviewed elsewhere (Walsh, 1987).

Because each gastrointestinal hormone and regulatory peptide has multiple actions in many target tissues, it is difficult to determine the physiological actions specific to any single hormone or peptide. For example, the interpretation of a radioimmunoassay measurement of a circulating gut hormone is frustrated by the need for simultaneous quantification of all intraluminal digestive events. The recent availability of synthetic hormones for intravenous use has led to a better understanding of the physiological and pharmacological functions of gastrointestinal hormones. Table II lists the commonly accepted physiological activities of the gastrointestinal hormones. Gastrin, CCK, and GLI all have specific trophic actions in gastrointestinal tissue; the possible trophic activities of other gut hormones have not been evaluated.

Little is known about the activities of gut hormones and regulatory peptides in neural tissues such as the brain and spinal cord, and much remains to be learned about the role of nutrients in the synthesis and release of gut hormones and peptides in neural tissues. However, one widely accepted concept is that some of these regulatory substances may serve as neurotransmitters in regulating physiological functions within autonomic nervous system tissues (Dockray, 1987). Several gut peptides, such as CCK and neuropeptide Y, may be involved in regulating centrally mediated functions such as food intake in health and disease. We recently quantitated the release of hypothalamic CCK after feeding in primates and showed that its release could be interrupted by vagotomy (Schick *et al.*, 1987). We also found that intracerebroventricular injections of CCK suppressed feeding in rats (Schick *et al.*, 1986). Whether these effects on the satiety center are physiological or pharmacological is unknown.

## V. SUMMARY

The gastrointestinal neuroendocrine system plays an important role in the nutritional adaptation that takes place from the prenatal to the postnatal stages of development. We now know that nutrients can regulate the secretion of gastrointestinal hormones and regulatory peptides, each of which has a unique regional distribution in both gut and neural tissues.

TABLE II

**Currently Accepted Physiological Activities of Gastrointestinal Hormones**

| Hormone | Primary positive effects on gastrointestinal function |
|---|---|
| Gastrin | Stimulates gastric acid and pepsin secretion<br>Stimulates gastric motility<br>Exerts trophic action on growth |
| Secretin | Stimulates pancreatic and hepatic bicarbonate secretion<br>Augments CCK action on pancreatic secretion<br>Stimulates Brunner's gland and intestinal bicarbonate secretion |
| CCK | Stimulates gallbladder contraction and pancreatic enzyme secretion<br>Augments secretin action on pancreatic secretion<br>Decreases tone of body of stomach<br>Exerts trophic action on growth of the pancreas |
| GIP | Stimulates release of insulin<br>Inhibits gastric acid secretion |
| Motilin | Initiates interdigestive motor complex |
| HPP | Inhibits pancreatic enzyme secretion<br>Inhibits gallbladder contraction |
| Enteroglucagon | Stimulates release of insulin<br>Exerts trophic action on mucosal growth |
| Neurotensin | Stimulates release of glucagon<br>Inhibits gastric acid secretion |
| PYY | Inhibits gastric secretion and emptying<br>Inhibits pancreatic exocrine secretion |

These hormones and peptides control the gut functions that are essential in converting food into absorbable nutrients and in the metabolic processes required for growth, development, and survival. Carbohydrates, proteins, and fats have different specificities and potencies in regulating secretion of different gut hormones and peptides, some of which exhibit trophic effects. The chronic release of a gut hormone or peptide in response to stimulation by a particular nutrient could lead to adaptation in organ function. The cellular mechanisms involved in these processes remain to be elucidated.

## REFERENCES

Beglinger, C., and Gyr, K. (1987). Frontiers in pancreatic physiology. *Pancreas* **2**, 120–125.

Boivin, M. Zinsmeister, A. R., Go, V. L. W., and DiMagno, E. P. (1987). Effect of a purified amylase inhibitor on carbohydrate metabolism after a mixed meal in healthy humans. *Mayo Clinic Proceedings* **62**, 249–255.

Buchan, A., Griffiths, C., Morris, J., and Polak, J. (1985). Enteroglucagon cell hyperfunction in rat small intestine after gut resection. *Gastroenterology* **88**, 8–12.

Creutzfeldt, W., and Ebert, R. (1986). The enteroinsular axis. *In* "The Exocrine Pancreas" (V. L. W. Go, J. D. Gardner, F. P. Brooks, E. Lebenthal, E. P. DiMagno, and G. A. Scheele, eds.), pp. 333–342. Raven Press, New York.

Dimitriadis, G., Tessari, P., Go, V., and Gerich, J. (1982). Effects of acarbose on metabolic and hormonal responses to meal ingestion and intravenous glucose in normal man. *In* "Proceedings of the First International Symposium on Acarbose" (W. Creutzfeldt, ed.), pp. 216–222. Excerpta Medica, Amsterdam.

Dockray, G. J. (1987). Physiology of enteric neuropeptides. *In* "Physiology of the Gastrointestinal Tract" (L. R. Johnson, J. Christensen, M. J. Jackson, E. D. Jacobson, and J. H. Walsh, eds.), 2nd edition, pp. 41–66. Raven Press, New York.

Floyd, J., Fajan, S., Pek, S., and Chance, R.-E. (1977). A newly recognized pancreatic polypeptide: Plasma levels in health and disease. *Recent Prog. Horm. Res.* **33**, 519–570.

Go, V. L. W., and Koch, T. R. (1988). Distribution of gut peptides. *In* "Handbook of Physiology: Neuroendocrinology of the Gut" (G. M. Makhlouf, ed.), Vol. 1. American Physiological Society, Bethesda. (In press.)

Go, V. L. W., and Miller, L. J. (1983). The role of gastrointestinal hormones in the control of postprandial and interdigestive gastrointestinal function. *Scand. J. Gastroenterol.* **18**, 135–142.

Go, V. L. W., Hofmann, A. F., and Summerskill, W. H. J. (1970). Pancreozymin bioassay in man based on pancreatic enzyme secretion: Potency of specific amino acids and other digestive products. *J. Clin. Invest.* **49**, 1558–1564.

Inoue, K., Fried, G., Wilner, I., Sakamoto, T., Lilja, P., Greeley, G., Jr., Watson, L., and Thompson, J. (1985). Effect of divalent cations on gastrointestinal hormone release and exocrine pancreatic secretion in dogs. *Amer. J. Physiol.* **248**, G28–G34.

Johnson, L. R. (1987). Regulation of gastrointestinal growth. *In* "Physiology of the Gastrointestinal Tract" (L. R. Johnson, J. Christensen, M. J. Jackson, E. D. Jacobson, and J. H. Walsh, eds.), 2nd edition, pp. 301–333. Raven Press, New York.

Koch, T. R., Carney, J. A., and Go, V. L. W. (1987). Distribution and quantitation of gut neuropeptides in normal intestine and inflammatory bowel diseases. *Dig. Dis. Sci.* **32**, 369–376.

Lam, S. K., Isenberg, J. I., Grossman, M. I., Lane, W. H., and Walsh, J. H. (1980). Gastric acid secretion is abnormally sensitive to endogenous gastrin released after peptone test meals in duodenal ulcer patients. *J. Clin. Invest.* **65**, 555–562.

Lucas, A., Bloom, S. R., and Aynsley-Green, A. (1983). Metabolic and endocrine consequences of depriving preterm infants of enteral nutrition. *Acta Paediatr. Scand.* **72**, 245–249.

MacFarlane, A., Kinsman, R., Read, N. W., and Bloom, S. R. (1983). The ileal brake: Ileal fat slows bowel transit and gastric emptying in man. *Gut* **24**, A471–A472.

Malagelada, J.-R., DiMagno, E. P., Summerskill, W. H. J., and Go, V. L. W. (1976). Regulation of pancreatic and gallbladder functions by intraluminal fatty acids and bile acids in man. *J. Clin. Invest.* **58**, 493–499.

Malagelada, J.-R., Holtermuller, K. H., McCall, J. T., and Go, V. L. W. (1978). Pancreatic, gallbladder and intestinal responses to intraluminal magnesium salts in man. *Amer. J. Dig. Dis.* **23**, 481–485.

McCullough, A. J., Miller, L. J., Service, F. J., and Go, V. L. W. (1983). Effect of graded intraduodenal glucose infusions on the release and physiological action of gastric inhibitory polypeptide. *J. Clin. Endocrinol. Metab.* **56**, 234–241.

Miazza, B. M., Al-Mukhtar, M. Y. T., Salmeron, M., Ghatei, M. A., Felce-Dachez, M., Filali, A., Villet, R., Wright, N. A., Bloom, S. R., and Rambaud, J.-C. (1985). Hyperenteroglucagonaemia and small intestinal mucosal growth after colonic perfusion of glucose in rats. *Gut* **26**, 518–524.

Mueller, M. K., Scheck, T., Dressman, V., Miodonski, A., and Goebell, H. (1987). GIP potentiates CCK stimulated pancreatic enzyme secretion: Correlation of anatomical structures with the effect of GIP and CCK on amylase secretion. *Pancreas* **2**, 106–113.

Nelson, R. L., Go, V. L. W., McCullough, A. J., Ilstrup, D. M., and Service, F. J. (1986). Lack of a direct effect of the autonomic nervous system on glucose-stimulated gastric inhibitory polypeptide (GIP) secretion in man. *Dig. Dis. Sci.* **31**, 929–935.

Schick, R. R., Reilly, W. M., Roddy, D. R., Yaksh, T. L., and Go, V. L. W. (1987). Neuronal cholecystokinin-like immunoreactivity is postprandially released from primate hypothalamus. *Brain Res.* **418**, 20–26.

Schick, R. R., Yaksh, T. L., and Go, V. L. W. (1986). Intracerebroventricular injections of cholecystokinin octapeptide suppress feeding in rats—pharmacological characterization of this action. *Regul. Peptides* **14**, 277–291.

Taylor, I., Byrne, W., Christie, D., Ament, M., and Walsh, J. (1982). Effect of individual L-amino acids on gastric acid secretion and serum gastrin and pancreatic polypeptide release in humans. *Gastroenterology* **83**, 273–278.

Thomas, F., Sinar, D., Mazzaferri, E., Cataland, S., Mekhjian, H., Caldwell, J., and Fromkes, J. (1978). Selective release of gastric inhibitory polypeptide by intraduodenal amino acid perfusion in man. *Gastroenterology* **74**, 1261–1265.

Thompson, J. C., Greeley, G. H., Jr., Rayford, P. L., and Townsend, C.M., eds. (1987). "Gastrointestinal Endocrinology." McGraw-Hill, New York.

Verdonk, C. A., Rizza, R. A., Nelson, R. L., Go, V. L. W., Gerich, J. E., and Service, F. J. (1980). Interaction of fat-stimulated gastric inhibitory polypeptide on pancreatic alpha and beta cell function. *J. Clin. Invest.* **65**, 1119–1125.

Walsh, J. H. (1987). Gastrointestinal hormones. *In* "Physiology of the Gastrointestinal Tract" (L. R. Johnson, J. Christensen, M. J. Jackson, E. D. Jacobson, and J. H. Walsh, eds.), pp. 181–253. Raven Press, New York.

Williams, J. A. (1987). Gut–islet–pancreatic acinar interaction. *Pancreas* **2**, 240–241.

Yaksh, T. L., Michener, S. R., Bailey, J. E., Harty, G. J., Lucas, D. L., Nelson, D. K., Roddy, D. R., and Go, V. L. W. (1988). Survey of distribution of substance P, vasoactive intestinal polypeptide, cholecystokinin, neurotensin, met-enkephalin, bombesin and PHI in the spinal cord of cat, dog, sloth and monkey. *Peptides*. (In press.)

# 20

# Nutrient Regulation of Intestinal Surface Membrane Hydrolases

Gary M. Gray

*Division of Gastroenterology and the Digestive Disease Center*
*Stanford University School of Medicine*
*Stanford, California*

Ann M. Reisenauer

*Division of Clinical Nutrition*
*University of California, Davis*
*School of Medicine*
*Davis, California*

Richard Quan

*Department of Pediatric Gastroenterology-Nutrition*
*University of Texas Southwestern Medical Center at Dallas*
*Dallas, Texas*

# I. INTRODUCTION

The enterocyte, by virtue of its specialized membrane at the intestinal surface, is essential in the interfacial digestion of polar oligomeric nutrients that must first be reduced to dimers or monomers before they can be absorbed by specific transporters. These digestive activities tend to decrease when the required substrate is excluded from the diet. Many of the molecular mechanisms responsible for maintaining intestinal hydrolases at levels appropriate for efficient nutrient digestion at the intestinal surface remain undefined. We have identified two distinctly different mechanisms of dietary regulation of intestinal surface-membrane hydrolases (Reisenauer and Gray, 1985; Quan and Gray, 1987).

# II. ACUTE INDUCTION OF AMINOOLIGOPEPTIDASE (AOP) BY ITS INTRAINTESTINAL TETRAPEPTIDE SUBSTRATE

The aminooligopeptidase (AOP), often called aminopeptidase N, is essential for the hydrolysis of the oligopeptide products of luminal pancreatic proteases (Smithson and Gray, 1977). In intact rats, rapid synthesis of the immature AOP protein occurred within 15 minutes in the endoplasmic reticulum (ER). This protein then increased in molecular size within 30 to 45 minutes after assembly and modification of its carbohydrate chains in the intracellular ER-Golgi compartment. Transport to the brush-border surface membrane occurred 3 to 6 hours later (Ahnen *et al.*, 1982; Ahnen *et al.*, 1983). Although AOP activity in the brush border decreased after starvation and increased after a high-protein diet (Kim *et al.*, 1973; Nicholson *et al.*, 1974), the mechanism of this regulation is unknown. Our *in vivo* studies in rats examined the role of high-affinity substrates in regulating intracellular synthesis and assembly of AOP and its transport to the brush-border surface.

## A. AOP Synthesis

Male Sprague-Dawley rats were fed a protein-deficient diet for 12 days (Reisenauer and Gray, 1985). After the rats were anesthetized, a 25-cm jejunal loop was isolated, and catheters were installed into its proximal and distal ends. Two rats were perfused intraintestinally in each experiment: One received 2m*M* of L-glycyl-leucyl-glycyl-glycine (Gly-Leu-Gly-Gly), a high-affinity tetrapeptide substrate for AOP, and the control received an equivalent amino acid solution of 6 m*M* glycine and 2 m*M* L-leucine (Gly + Leu). Each solution was made isotonic with 150 m*M* NaCl and perfused into the intestinal loop at 0.5 ml/minute. After perfusion of the test peptide or the control amino-acid mixture for 30 minutes, the solutions were removed, and 2.5 mCi of L-[$^3$H]leucine was placed in the loop for a 5-minute pulse. This was followed by a 30-, 60-, or 180-minute perfusion with the solution originally administered to each animal. Animals were then killed, the intestine was recovered, and subcellular fractions of brush border and ER-Golgi membranes were prepared (Ahnen *et al.*, 1982). We then assayed the activities of AOP, using the high-affinity substrate leucyl-beta-naphthylamide (LeuNA); sucrase, a marker for the brush-border membranes; aryl esterase, a marker for the ER-Golgi membranes; and protein (Ahnen *et al.*, 1983). Brush-border and ER-Golgi membranes were solubilized with 0.5% Triton X-100. AOP and sucrase were immunoprecipitated with monospecific rabbit antibodies.

Figure 1 compares the incorporation of [$^3$H]leucine into AOP in ER-Golgi and brush-border membranes in paired rats receiving intraintestinal Gly-Leu-Gly-Gly or its constituent amino acids, Gly + Leu. More radiolabel was incorporated into newly synthesized AOP in the ER-Golgi fraction in rats perfused with Gly-Leu-Gly-Gly than in rats perfused with the amino acid solution; the difference was 89 $\pm$ 17% ($p < 0.025$) at 30 minutes and 124 $\pm$ 14% ($p < 0.01$) at 60 minutes (Reisenauer and Gray, 1985). In two of three experiments, 200% more labeled AOP was incorporated in the brush border from tetrapeptide-perfused rats than in brush border from amino acid-perfused rats after 180 minutes, even though newly synthesized AOP does not reach its maximum at the intestinal surface membrane until after about 6 hours (Ahnen *et al.*, 1982). Labeled AOP in the brush border at 180 minutes was significantly increased in the tetrapeptide-perfused rats as compared to the amino-acid perfused animals (178 $\pm$ 32 disintegrations per minute (dpm)/mU AOP vs. 128 $\pm$ 23 dpm/mU AOP; $p < 0.05$). However, the total brush-border AOP activity was similar in both groups in these short-term studies. This finding suggests that the surface membrane contains a relatively large, stable pool of this enzyme. The synthesis of sucrase, an unrelated brush-border hydrolase, was no different in Gly-Leu-Gly-Gly-perfused and amino-acid-perfused animals (Reisenauer and Gray, 1985).

Another paired pulse-chase experiment involved perfusion of jejunal loops with 150 m*M* NaCl plus 1.5 m*M* LeuNA, a high-affinity substrate for AOP, or with 150 m*M* NaCl alone (Reisenauer and Gray, 1985). Again, significant differences between groups were observed in the amount of newly synthesized AOP in the ER-Golgi fraction. In rats perfused with LeuNA plus saline, the total incorporation of the label into AOP was 1.8-fold greater at 30 minutes and 3.7-fold greater at 60 minutes than in rats perfused with saline alone.

These studies demonstrate that rapid and specific AOP synthesis is induced by high-affinity substrates such as Gly-Leu-Gly-Gly or LeuNA.

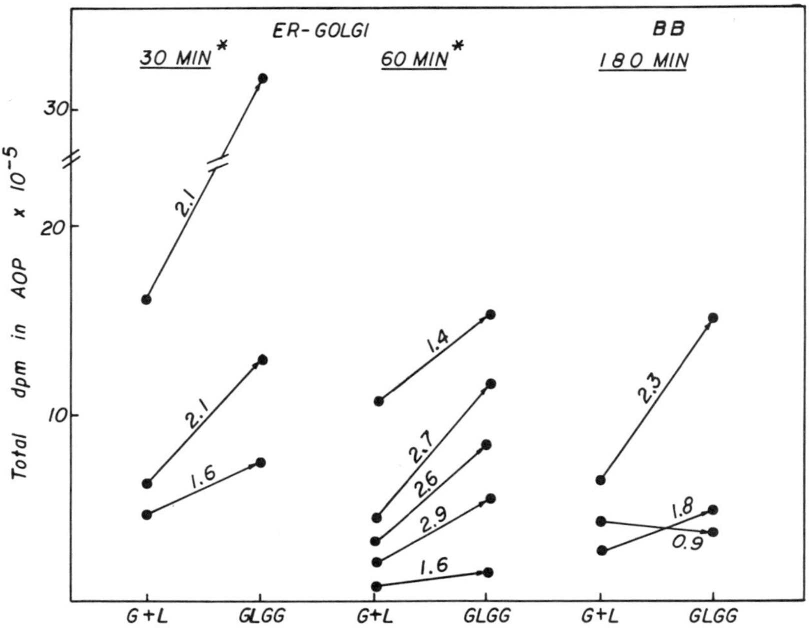


**Fig. 1.** Total incorporation of [$^3$H]leucine into aminooligopeptidase (AOP) was compared in endoplasmic reticulum-Golgi (ER-Golgi) and brush-border (BB) fractions from paired rats receiving intraintestinal 2 m*M* Gly-Leu-Gly-Gly (GLGG) or its constituent amino acids (G+L). Arrows connect paired animals, which were perfused with tetrapeptide or amino acid solution for 30 minutes, pulse-labeled with [$^3$H]leucine, and then chased with the peptide or amino-acid solution for 30, 60, or 180 minutes. Values are reported in disintegrations per minute (dpm) in AOP. Numbers above arrows denote the ratios of the amount of label in AOP from the GLGG-perfused rats to that from the G + L-perfused control rats. The increase in synthesis in ER-Golgi was significant at 30 minutes ($p < 0.025$) and at 60 minutes ($p < 0.001$) by paired t-test. Data are reported as means ± SEM. (From Reisenauer and Gray, 1985. Reprinted with permission.)

These substrates appear to promote intracellular AOP synthesis by interacting with this hydrolase at the lumen-membrane interface.

In other studies, we analyzed the possibility that Gly-Gly, the C-terminal dipeptide product released during hydrolysis of Gly-Leu-Gly-Gly (Smithson and Gray, 1977), can induce AOP synthesis. When rats were perfused with a solution containing 2 m*M* each of glycine, leucine, and Gly-Gly, the amount of newly synthesized AOP was identical to that found with the mixture of amino acids only (Reisenauer and Gray, 1985). Thus, the hydrolytic products of Gly-Leu-Gly-Gly, whether amino acids or the terminal dipeptide, do not appear to induce AOP synthesis. From these experiments, we concluded that induction of AOP synthesis requires an intact oligopeptide substrate.

### B. Postsynthesis Assembly and Modification of AOP

To determine whether acute induction of AOP synthesis involved structural alteration of the AOP glycoprotein and/or enhancement of shuttling from intracellular to brush-border membranes, we examined the kinetics of *in vivo* assembly by sodium dodecyl sulfate (SDS) electrophoresis and autoradiography after intraintestinal pulse-chase with [$^3$H]leucine (Reisenauer and Gray, 1985). Maximal incorporation of the label in ER-Golgi occurred at 30 minutes after the pulse in both the tetrapeptide-perfused rats and the amino-acid-perfused controls. The newly synthesized, labeled AOP was assembled in the intracellular ER-Golgi compartment and transferred to the brush border at comparable rates. The final result was a doubling of the number of new AOP molecules, which were then processed and transported to the brush border at normal rates.

To assess possible differences in AOP assembly between tetrapeptide- and amino-acid-perfused rats, we examined immunoprecipitates from the ER-Golgi and brush-border fractions (Reisenauer and Gray, 1985). Both immature and mature molecules of the enzyme were indistinguishable from those found in normal rats (Ahnen *et al.*, 1983). In essence, AOP synthesis increased, while the subsequent carbohydrate chain processing and membrane-associated shuttling to the luminal surface remained unchanged. The final result was a two- to threefold increase in the number of AOP molecules that were synthesized, processed, and transported to the brush-border surface.

These experiments clearly demonstrate that luminal exposure of a high-affinity tetrapeptide substrate to protein-depleted rats abruptly and specifically induces AOP synthesis in the enterocyte. Because the amino-acid and dipeptide products of the tetrapeptide substrate did not induce synthesis, we believe that the acute induction of synthesis requires the interaction of the intact substrate with this enzyme at the enterocyte surface. This abrupt enhancement of the synthesis of a digestive peptide by its luminal substrate constitutes a discrete, immediate, and local mechanism for the regulation of digestion at the intestinal surface. These provocative results prompted us to explore the mechanism of regulation of another important digestive hydrolase, sucrase-$\alpha$-dextrinase.

## III. RESPONSE OF SUCRASE-$\alpha$-DEXTRINASE (S-D) TO CARBOHYDRATE WITHDRAWAL

Sucrase-$\alpha$-dextrinase (S-D) is a hybrid glycoprotein digestive hydrolase, initially synthesized as a single-chain macromolecule of $>200$ kDa in the ER-Golgi and subsequently transferred to the brush-border membrane. There S-D is cleaved by luminal pancreatic proteases to a hybrid dimer, one component of which hydrolyzes dietary sucrose to transportable monosaccharides and the other of which digests the α-dextrin products of starch to glucose (Gray, 1982). Although this hydrolase is essential for the intestinal surface-membrane digestion of luminal carbohydrate nutrients, little is known of the molecular details of its regulation by its intraluminal substrates. Studies have shown that markedly decreased dietary carbohydrate reduced sucrase activity by at least 50% (Deren *et al.*, 1967; Goda *et al.*, 1985). On the other hand, a carbohydrate-rich diet increased sucrase activity within a few days in animals (Goda *et al.*, 1985) as well as humans (Rosensweig and Herman, 1968).

## A. Effect on S-D Activity

We examined S-D structure and function in rats fed a carbohydrate-free diet (Quan and Gray, 1987). Male Wistar rats weighing 250–350 g were maintained on regular rat chow with 70% carbohydrate for 5 days. Control rats were then continued on regular chow, while another group of animals was fed a carbohydrate-free diet for 7 days. Weights for the two groups did not differ significantly throughout the experiment. Removal of dietary carbohydrate for 7 days produced the expected marked reduction in sucrase activity to about one-half of normal (Quan and Gray, 1987). This reduction was observed in whole intestinal homogenate and in brush-border membranes. However, the specific activity of sucrase in purified ER-Golgi membranes remained unchanged in animals on the carbohydrate-free diet and in controls. The sucrase-to-dextrinase ratio of activity was about 1.2:1 in both the control and carbohydrate-free diet groups. Hence, both sucrase and dextrinase activities decreased proportionally in response to carbohydrate withdrawal.

We then explored the possibility that loss of S-D molecules may have caused the reduction in hydrolytic activities in response to carbohydrate withdrawal (Quan and Gray, 1987). If this were the explanation, then kinetic analysis should reveal no alteration in the $K_m$ because the affinity of the remaining active sites would be expected to be normal, but reduction in $V_{max}$ would be expected because of the loss of enzyme molecules. When brush borders from rats fed a carbohydrate-free diet for 7 days were incubated with sucrose in a range of concentrations from 1 to 100mM, the $K_m$ did not differ from the 20 m*M* found in normal rats, but the maximal hydrolytic rate or $V_{max}$ was reduced to 50% of normal (Quan and Gray, 1987).

## B. Effect on S-D Synthesis Rate

Experiments were then carried out to determine whether the reduction in S-D activity resulted from a decrease in the synthetic rate of the enzyme (Quan and Gray, 1987). After being allowed water for the 18 hours preceding the experiment, rats were anesthetized, and a 25-cm jejunal segment was prepared as in the AOP studies described above (Smithson and Gray, 1977; Ahnen *et al.*, 1982; Ahnen *et al.*, 1983). After preperfusion with 150 m*M* NaCl at 0.5 ml/minute for one hour, 1 mCi of [$^{35}$S]methionine was instilled in the loop and allowed to remain for 5 minutes as a pulse. The isotope was then flushed out, and the loop was filled and perfused with 1 m*M* unlabeled methionine for the remainder of the experiment, which involved a 30- to 180-minute chase period. Quantitation of radioactivity and analysis by SDS electrophoresis were carried out as in the AOP experiments detailed above. S-D was isolated by immunoprecipitation with the specific polyclonal antibody raised in rabbits, and SDS electrophoresis was carried out as previously described (Ahnen *et al.*, 1983), except that immune pellets were heated at 100° for 2 minutes, and a 6.5% total acrylamide–2% crosslinked gel was used as the separation gel. Bands were cut from the dried gel and quantified for specific total radioactivity for the particular membrane organelles.

Administration of nonradioactive methionine in chase periods of 30 to 180 minutes promoted label incorporation into the ER-Golgi compartment and subsequently into the brush-border surface membrane. However, total label incorporated into ER-Golgi was not altered in carbohydrate-deprived animals compared to the control group. Hence, the synthesis of sucrase appears to continue at normal rates during substrate deprivation (Quan and Gray, 1987). This suggested that a mechanism other than decreased synthesis of S-D protein may be responsible for the marked reduction in sucrase catalytic activity in carbohydrate deprivation. Thus, we were prompted to consider whether a change in the relationship of S-D glycoprotein structure and function occurs in response to carbohydrate withdrawal. Because preliminary studies revealed a normal pattern for the S and D subunits on SDS electrophoresis (Quan and Gray, 1987), another approach was used to identify a possible structural change.

## C. Effect on Total S-D Protein in Brush Border Membrane

Because polyvalent antiserum contains several species of antibodies that identify various domains of the S-D protein, specific immunoassays can provide an estimate of total sucrase protein. The active S-D can be determined by sucrase activity and total S-D protein by immunoassay; thus the following equation can be assumed to pertain:

$$S_t = S_a + S_i \qquad \text{(Reaction 1)}$$

In this equation, $S_t$ equals total S-D by immunoassay, $S_a$ equals catalytically active S-D by sucrase assay, and $S_i$ equals inactive S-D protein. This equation can be rearranged to allow determination of inactive S-D:

$$S_i = S_t - S_a \qquad \text{(Reaction 2)}$$

Immunoassay specific for S-D was carried out by two different methods after solubilizing samples from ER-Golgi and brush-border membranes with 50 pulses in a Bronson cell sonicator. Samples were centrifuged at 100,000 × g for 1 hour, and the supernatant was applied to 1 × 1 cm squares of nitrocellulose that were prewashed in distilled water and dried. The solubilized sucrase, diluted at least 100-fold, was applied to the nitrocellulose and exposed to 2% fetal bovine serum to block any residual binding sites. The immobilized sucrase antigen was then incubated with 100 ml of monospecific rabbit anti-sucrase at 1:1,000 dilution for 3 hours and exposed to goat anti-rabbit gamma-globulin that had been covalently bound to horseradish peroxidase. The nitrocellulose squares were transferred to 12 × 75 mm tubes, and the chromogen product of the horseradish peroxidase reaction was determined (Hawkes *et al.*, 1982). In other analyses (Quan and Gray, 1987), S-D was quantified by rocket immunoelectrophoresis (Laurell, 1972). Highly purified rat intestinal S-D, with an activity of 20 μmol/min/mg protein, served as the standard, and the height of the rocket arc was a linear function of the quantity of antigen added.

By both immunoassays, the total S-D protein was the same in carbohydrate-deprived and control rats, but only about 50% of the sucrase activity was required to produce the same level of immunoassay signal in enterocyte surface membranes from carbohydrate-deprived rats, reflecting the presence of appreciable amounts of sucrase protein devoid of catalytic sites. As can be seen from the equation above, this indicates that a marked shift of active to inactive sucrase occurs in response to removal of dietary carbohydrate. The S-D protein remains intact, but a conversion of the catalytic site causes the majority of the hydrolase to be in the inactive form (Quan and Gray, 1987).

This regulatory mechanism may preserve S-D protein in an inactive and possibly more stable form until carbohydrate is returned to the diet; then the reserve of S-D molecules would presumably be available for conversion to the catalytically active form. The mechanism for reduction in sucrose digestive capacity, which involves conversion of an active to an inactive enzyme, is very different than that seen for the augmentation of AOP in response to dietary substrate, which is achieved by production of new enzyme molecules rather than by any conversion of a preexisting inactive moiety. Other studies are needed to ascertain the mechanism of recovery of intestinal carbohydrate digestive capacity in response to carbohydrate feeding.

## IV. SUMMARY

The mechanisms regulating two intestinal brush-border hydrolases were examined in intact rats. Our first studies determined the effects of 12-day dietary protein restriction, followed by short-term substrate induction, on synthesis and assembly of AOP. Paired animals were intraintestinally perfused with Gly-Leu-Gly-Gly, a high-affinity substrate for AOP, or with its hydrolytic products, Gly + Leu, for 30 minutes. They were then pulse-labeled with [$^3$H]L-leucine and chased for 30 to 180 minutes with the tetrapeptide or the control amino-acid solution. In the tetrapeptide-perfused animals, incorporation of the label into immunoprecipitated AOP was 200% higher than in controls at 30 and 60 minutes in the ER-Golgi and at 180 minutes in the brush-border. The post-synthesis movement from ER-Golgi to the brush border was maintained at normal rates. Thus, acute induction of synthesis appears to require the interaction of intact oligopeptide substrate with AOP at the intestinal surface.

By contrast, we demonstrated in other studies that substrate withdrawal does not alter the synthesis rate of sucrase-$\alpha$-dextrinase, a hydrolase essential for digestion of several dietary carbohydrates. In rats fed a carbohydrate-free diet for 7 days, catalytic activity decreased 50% while *in vivo* synthesis of S-D, measured by specific quantitative immunoassay, remained normal. We therefore concluded that loss of catalytic sites caused the decrease in S-D activity. We have hypothesized that the inactivated S-D protein may become reactivated when carbohydrate is returned to the diet.

These two complementary mechanisms of dietary regulation of intestinal hydrolases allow local modulation of the hydrolytic capacity of the enterocyte in response to changes in nutrients present at the luminal surface.

## ACKNOWLEDGMENTS

This work was supported by research grants DK 11270, DK 15802, and training grants AM 07056, and GM 07026 from the National Institutes of Health.

## REFERENCES

Ahnen, D. J., Santiago, N. A., Cezard, J. P., and Gray, G. M. (1982). Intestinal aminooligopeptidase: *In vivo* synthesis on intracellular membranes of the rat jejunum. *J. Biol. Chem.* **257**, 12129–12135.

Ahnen, D. J., Mircheff, A. K., Santiago, N. A., Yoshioka, C., and Gray, G. M. (1983). Intestinal surface aminooligopeptidase: Distinct molecular forms during assembly on intracellular membranes *in vivo*. *J. Biol. Chem. 258*, 5960–5966.

Deren, J. J., Broitman, S. A., and Zamcheck, N. (1967). Effect of diet upon intestinal disaccharidases and disaccharide absorption. *J. Clin. Invest.* **46**, 186–195.

Goda, T., Bustamante, S., and Koldovsky, O. (1985). Dietary regulation of intestinal lactase and sucrase in adult rats: Quantitative comparison of effect of lactose and sucrose. *J. Pediatr. Gastroenterol. Nutr.* **4**, 998–1008.

Gray, G. M. (1982). Intestinal disaccharidase deficiencies and glucose-galactose malabsorption. *In*: "Metabolic Basis of Inherited Disease" (J. B. Stanbury, J. B. Wyngaarden,

D. S. Fredrickson, J. L. Goldstein, and M. S. Brown, eds.), 5th ed., pp. 1719–1742. McGraw-Hill, New York.

Hawkes, R., Niday, E., and Gordon, J. (1982). A dot immunobinding assay for monoclonal and other antibodies. *Anal. Biochem.* **119**, 142–147.

Kim, Y. S., McCarthy, D. M., Lane, W., and Fong, W. (1973). Alterations in the levels of peptide hydrolases and other enzymes in brush border and soluble fractions of rat small intestinal mucosa during starvation and refeeding. *Biochim. Biophys. Acta* **321**, 262–273.

Laurell, C. B. (1972). Electroimmunoassay. *Scand. J. Clin. Lab. Invest.* **29** (P Suppl. 124), 21–37.

Nicholson, J. A., McCarthy, D. M., and Kim, Y. S. (1974). The responses of rat intestinal brush border and cytosol peptide hydrolase activities to variation in dietary protein content: Dietary regulation of intestinal peptide hydrolases. *J. Clin. Invest.* **54**, 890–898.

Quan, R., and Gray, G. M. (1987). Sucrase-α-dextrinase reduction by carbohydrate-free (CF) diet: Conversion of active to inactive enzyme [Abstract]. *Gastroenterology* **92**, 1585.

Reisenauer, A. M., and Gray, G. M. (1985). Abrupt induction of a membrane digestive enzyme by its intraintestinal substrate. *Science* **227**, 70–72.

Rosensweig, N. S., and Herman, R. H. (1968). Control of jejunal sucrase and maltase activity by dietary sucrose or fructose in man. A model for the study of enzyme regulation in man. *J. Clin. Invest.* **47**, 2253–2262.

Smithson, K. W., and Gray, G. M. (1977). Intestinal assimilation of a tetrapeptide in the rat. Obligate function of brush border aminopeptidase. *J. Clin. Invest.* **60**, 665–674.

# 21

# Intestinal Adaptation to Parenteral Nutrition

Elliot Weser

*Medicine Service*
*Audie L. Murphy Memorial Veterans Hospital*
*University of Texas Health Science Center*
*San Antonio, Texas*



## I. INTRODUCTION

Small bowel mucosal mass and function depend on the efficiency of nutrient absorption and the ability to compensate for injured or partially resected small intestine. In animals receiving enteral nutrition after small bowel resection, mucosal hyperplasia was apparent in the remaining intestine and was particularly prominent in the residual ileum after jejunectomy (Nygaard, 1967; Dowling and Booth, 1967; Tilson and Wright,

1970; Weser and Hernandez, 1971). Adaptive growth responses also occur in the jejunum after ileal resection, but these responses, partly related to adaptive increases in caloric consumption, are usually less extensive and variable than those in the ileum (Young and Weser, 1974). Mucosal hyperplasia is associated with an increased rate of crypt cell production and migration to the villus tip (Hanson and Osborne, 1971; McDermott and Roudnew, 1976). This adaptive increase in cell renewal begins as early as two days following surgical resection and may occur in proportion to the amount of intestine resected (Obertop *et al.*, 1977; Hanson *et al.*, 1977a; Hanson *et al.*, 1977b). A peak increase in ileal mucosal ornithine decarboxylase (ODC) activity also occurs two days after jejunectomy (Luk and Baylin, 1982). This enzyme catalyzes the decarboxylation of ornithine to putrescine, which is the rate-limiting step in polyamine synthesis. Polyamine synthesis is required to facilitate the adaptive response of DNA and protein synthesis following intestinal resection (Luk and Baylin, 1983). Inhibition of ODC by difluormethyl ornithine suppresses polyamine synthesis and prevents adaptive hyperplasia after jejunal resection (Luk and Baylin, 1984).

Several studies have demonstrated that the mucosal morphology of a transposed segment within the small intestine conforms to that of the local region. For example, mucosal weight and villous height increased in an ileal segment transposed to the jejunum, whereas, conversely, villous height decreased in a jejunal segment transposed to the ileum (Altmann and Leblond, 1970; Gronqvist *et al.*, 1975; Philipson, 1975). However, mucosal hypoplasia was observed in segments of bypassed intestine that were out of contact with chyme (Gleeson *et al.*, 1972; Keren *et al.*, 1975; Rijke *et al.*, 1977). Therefore, significant adaptive mucosal hyperplasia after resection requires that the remaining small intestine be exposed to intraluminal chyme. These findings suggest that the intraluminal environment exercises an important influence on intestinal adaptation.

Other studies showed that the presence of nutrients in the enteric lumen is essential for the adaptive mucosal hyperplasia of residual small bowel (Feldman *et al.*, 1976; Levine *et al.*, 1976). Animals with intestinal resection that are nourished isocalorically by total parenteral nutrition (TPN) gain weight but do not develop mucosal hyperplasia in the remaining intestine. In TPN-maintained animals with intact intestine, the duodenojejunal mucosa underwent hypoplasia and loss of the proximal to distal gradient of mucosal mass (Levine *et al.*, 1974; Eastwood, 1977). Mucosal alterations that follow the absence of nutrients from the intestinal lumen may increase susceptibility to mucosal injury.

The effects of single-nutrient enteral infusions on intestinal mucosal mass have been studied in animals otherwise maintained on TPN. Small quantities of intraluminal long-chain fats and fatty acids prevented TPN-induced mucosal hypoplasia or stimulated adaptive hyperplasia after resection (Morin *et al.*, 1982; Grey *et al.*, 1984). These effects were equivalent to those produced by complete mixtures of macromolecular nutrients. Other single substrates that produced similar effects include amino acids, amines, and a variety of carbohydrates (Spector *et al.*, 1977; Spector *et al.*, 1981; Tabata and Johnson, 1986; Weser *et al.*, 1982a; Weser *et al.*, 1982b; Weser *et al.*, 1982c; Weser *et al.*, 1985; Weser *et al.*, 1986). These substrates, which may be absorbed by active or diffusion mechanisms, have been shown to stimulate adaptive mucosal growth, independent of their metabolism by the mucosa. Several of our studies of the regulation of intestinal adaptation are described below.

## II. EFFECTS OF ENTERAL AND PARENTERAL NUTRITION ON INTESTINAL ADAPTATION

### A. Experimental Methods

Male Sprague-Dawley rats weighing about 240 g were fasted overnight and anesthetized with intraperitoneal sodium pentobarbital (40 mg/kg). A sterile silastic catheter was placed into the superior vena cava via the right jugular vein. The entire small bowel length was measured *in situ*, and a second catheter was placed in the mid-small intestinal lumen for distal small bowel infusion. After being tunneled subcutaneously, both the intravenous and intestinal catheters exited from the rat dorsally between the scapulae and were connected to their respective infusion solutions via a Holter infusion pump. All rats were then maintained in individual metabolic cages designed to minimize coprophagy and permit urine collection. A harness attachment with swivel arrangement for the two catheters permitted each animal unrestrained movement in its cage.

For the entire experimental period, an intravenous nutrient solution was continuously infused at the rate of 2 ml/hr, and an experimental single-nutrient solution or saline control was continuously infused at the rate of 2 ml/h via the enteral catheter. At the end of this experimental period, rats were killed by decapitation. The entire small bowel was rapidly removed, rinsed, blotted, and divided into 8 equal segments, beginning with the duodenojejunum and ending with the terminal ileum. Segments of 2 cm proximal and distal to the catheter site were discarded. Segments were weighed and their length determined using a 5 g weight suspended from the segment. After mucosa were scraped with a glass slide and weighed, a 1:20 homogenate was prepared in cold 0.9% saline. Mucosal DNA and protein were measured in all studies, and mucosal ODC was also measured in some studies. Statistical analyses were verified by analysis of variance and, where appropriate, by the unpaired Student's t-test.

## B. Adaptive Hyperplasia Following Enteral Carbohydrate Infusion in Rats Maintained on Total Parenteral Nutrition (TPN)

### 1. *Monosaccharide Infusions*

The midgut infusion of 15% glucose or 15% fructose increased segment and mucosal weight, DNA, and protein concentration/cm gut adjacent to and downstream from the enteral infusion site in TPN-maintained rats (Weser *et al.*, 1982c) (Fig. 1). Fructose appeared to produce greater changes than glucose. In addition, both sugars stimulated mucosal hyperplasia in the proximal small bowel segments. This hyperplasia was greatest in segment 1, even though it was far from the infusion site. The finding that nutrients absorbed from the ileal lumen stimulate mucosal adaptation locally and in the proximal small bowel suggested that a humoral or

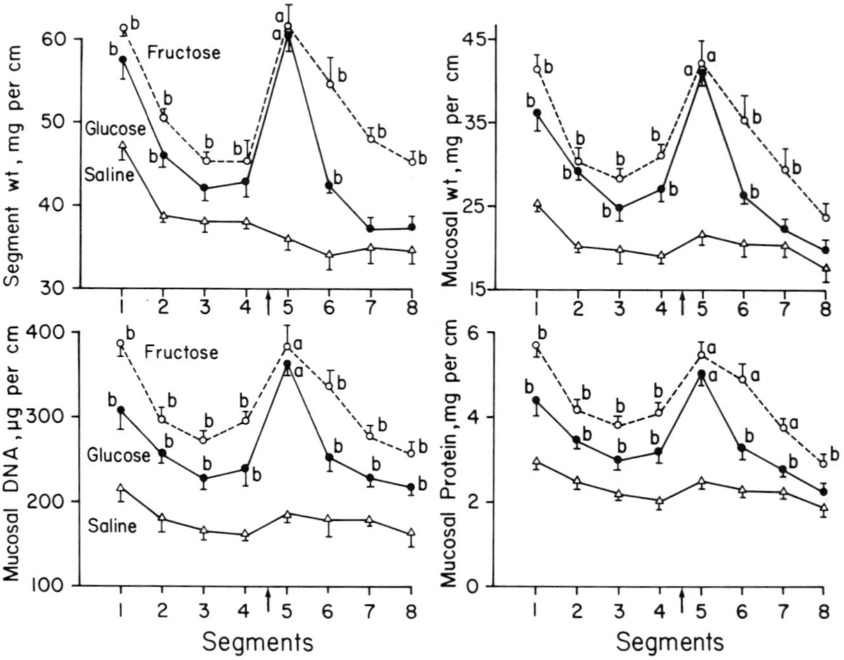


**Fig. 1.** TPN-maintained rats receiving midgut infusion of glucose or fructose were compared with saline controls to determine effects of a single enteral nutrient on stimulation of mucosal growth. Solid circles represent 15% glucose ($n$ = 7); open circles, 15% fructose ($n$ = 6); open triangles, 0.9% saline ($n$ = 5); arrow indicates infusion site. Values represent mean ± SEM. For measurements marked "a," $p < 0.01$; "b," $p < 0.05$. (From Weser *et al.*, 1982c. Reprinted with permission.)

hormonal mechanism was involved. Reflux of the infused substrate did not reach the proximal bowel segments (unpublished observations).

### 2. *Effect of Phlorizin on Monosaccharide-Induced Mucosal Hyperplasia*

Phlorizin was added to the glucose solution to determine whether mucosal growth could be altered by inhibiting glucose transport in the TPN-maintained rats. Midgut infusion of the glucose plus phlorizin solution significantly increased mucosal weight in segments distal to the infusion site (Fig. 2), shifting the peak effect on mucosal growth to segment 6 (Weser *et al.*, 1982c). Similar findings were noted for the other parameters of mucosal mass. This suggests that phlorizin partially decreased glucose uptake in the midgut segments, allowing unabsorbed glucose to reach the more distal segments of the lumen where it exerted its growth effect. The addition of phlorizin to fructose or saline control solutions did not affect mucosal adaptive responses nor did it alter the remote proximal growth effects of the sugars.

### 3. *Dose Response of Glucose-Induced Mucosal Adaptation*

Midgut infusion of increasing concentrations of glucose resulted in progressive increases in mucosal adaptation in TPN-maintained rats (Weser *et al.*, 1985) (Fig. 3). The 20% glucose solution produced the greatest increase in mucosal mass versus saline controls, whereas 5% glucose produced no increase versus controls. A similar progression of mucosal mass

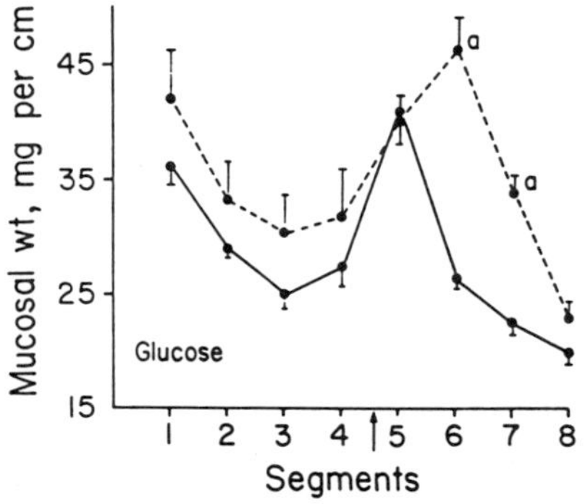


**Fig. 2.** The effect of phlorizin on mucosal growth stimulated by midgut infusion of glucose was studied in TPN-maintained rats. Solid line represents 15% glucose ($n$ = 5); broken line, 15% glucose plus 200 mg phlorizin/ml ($n$ = 5); arrow indicates infusion site. Values represent mean ± SEM ($p < 0.001$). (From Weser *et al.*, 1982c. Reprinted with permission.)

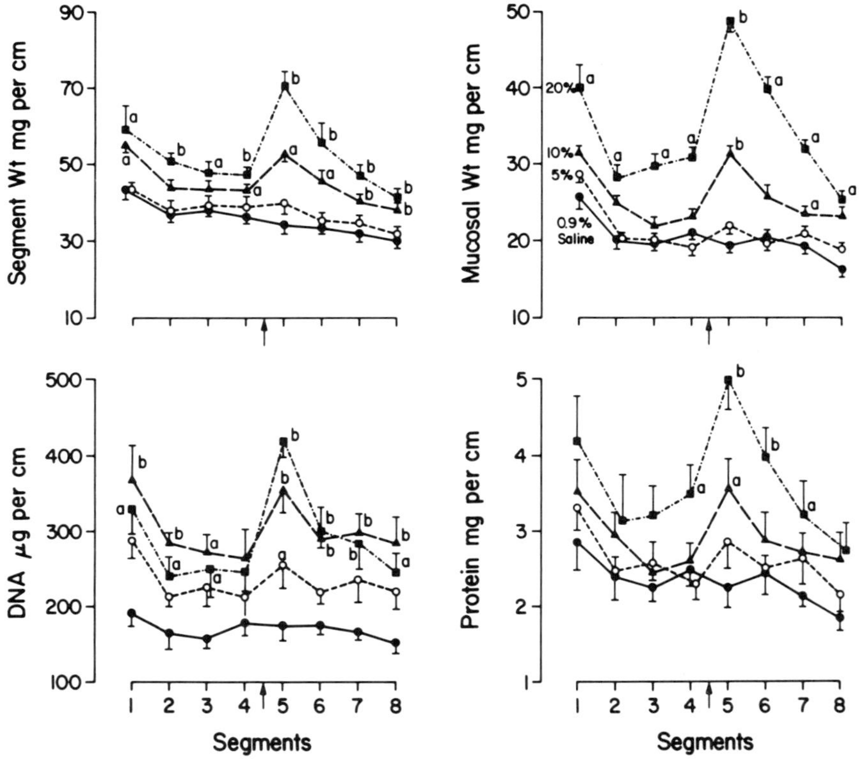


**Fig. 3.** The increase in mucosal mass after 2 days of 2 ml/hr midgut infusion of varied concentrations of glucose was compared with normal saline infusion in TPN-maintained rats. Open circles represent 5% glucose; solid triangles, 10% glucose; solid squares, 20% glucose; solid circles, normal saline; arrow indicates infusion site. Values represent mean ± SEM of 5 rats. For measurements marked "a," $p < 0.05$; "b," $p < 0.01$. (From Weser *et al.*, 1985. Reprinted with permission.)

appeared to occur in the proximal segments, but this was clearly significant only for 20% glucose. Midgut infusions of saline solutions with osmolarity equal to that of the glucose solutions produced no significant changes in mucosal mass compared with normal saline infusion. This finding suggests that the proportional growth changes observed with increasing glucose concentrations were not related to the osmolarity of the solutions but rather to the amount of glucose in the intestinal lumen.

### 4. *Dose Response of Sucrose-Induced Mucosal Adaptation*

Infusion of increasing concentrations of sucrose was also associated with a progressive increase in mucosal mass adjacent to and downstream from the infusion site in TPN-maintained rats (Weser *et al.*, 1986) (Fig. 4). In segment 5, mucosal mass generally increased in proportion to the amount of sucrose delivered into the lumen. Progressive increases in mucosal mass also occurred in proximal segments far removed from the infusion site, particularly with 20% sucrose.

### 5. *Dose Response of Disaccharide Versus Monosaccharide-Induced Adaptation*

The growth effects on mucosal mass associated with infusion of 5% sucrose and other disaccharides were compared with 5% glucose and normal saline in TPN-maintained rats (Weser *et al.*, 1986) (Fig. 5). Increases in mucosal mass similar to those for sucrose occurred following infusion of maltose and lactose, but no significant differences were seen between glucose and saline. In other studies involving infusions of higher

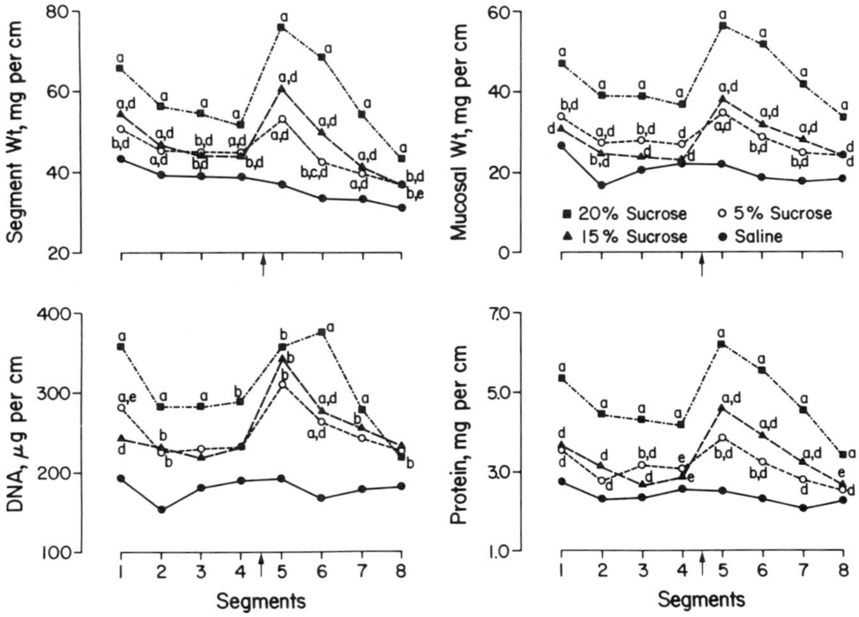


**Fig. 4.** The increase in mucosal mass after 7 days of 2 ml/hr midgut infusion of varied concentrations of sucrose was compared with saline infusion in TPN-maintained rats. Open circles represent 5% sucrose; solid triangles, 15% sucrose; solid squares, 20% sucrose; solid circles, 0.9% saline; arrow indicates infusion site. Values represent mean ± SEM of 5 rats. For measurements marked "a," $p < 0.01$; "b," $p < 0.01$ vs. saline; "c," $p < 0.05$ vs. 15% sucrose; "d," $p < 0.01$ vs. 20% sucrose; "e," $p < 0.05$ vs. 20% sucrose. (From Weser *et al.*, 1986. Reprinted with permission.)

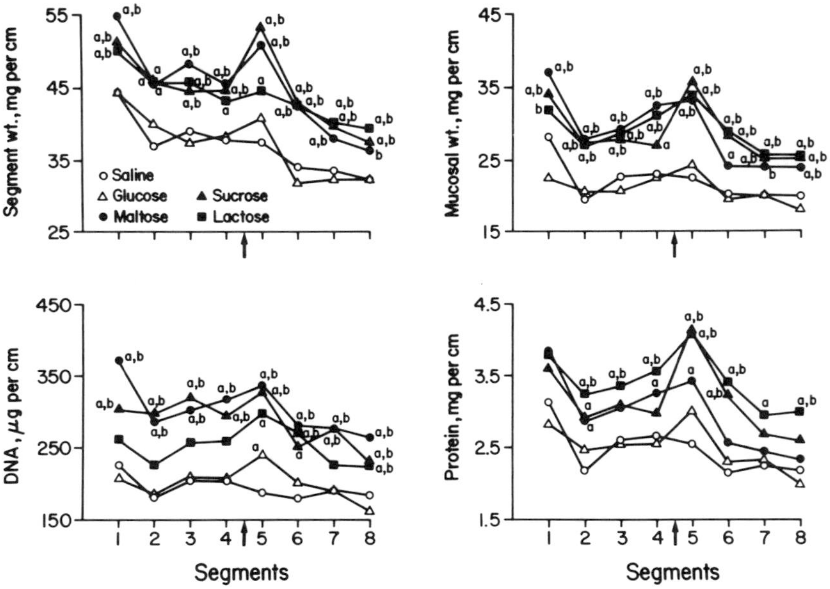


**Fig. 5.** The effect on mucosal mass of midgut infusions of 5% disaccharide was compared with 5% glucose and 0.09% saline in TPN-maintained rats. Open circles represent 0.09% saline; open triangles, 5% glucose; solid circles, 5% maltose; solid triangles, 5% sucrose; solid squares, 5% lactose; arrow indicates infusion site. Values represent mean ± SEM of 5 rats. For measurements marked "a," $p < 0.05$ vs. saline; "b," $p < 0.05$ vs. glucose. (From Weser *et al.*, 1986. Reprinted with permission.)

concentrations of saccharides, sucrose consistently induced greater mucosal adaptive growth than equal concentrations of glucose or other monosaccharides. Thus, enteral disaccharides appear to produce greater increases in mucosal growth than equivalent loads of monosaccharides by weight.

### 6. *Disaccharide Hydrolysis and Mucosal Adaptation*

The advantage of disaccharides over monosaccharides in promoting mucosal growth appeared to be significant only with disaccharides capable of being hydrolyzed by intestinal disaccharidases. To determine whether inhibition of sucrose hydrolysis would impair its absorption and destroy its growth effect on small bowel mucosa, we added acarbose, an alpha-glucosidase inhibitor, to a midgut infusion of 10% sucrose in TPN-maintained rats (Weser *et al.*, 1986) (Fig. 6). This maneuver significantly inhibited sucrose-induced mucosal growth downstream from the infusion site. In other experiments, we found that lactulose, a nonhydrolyzable

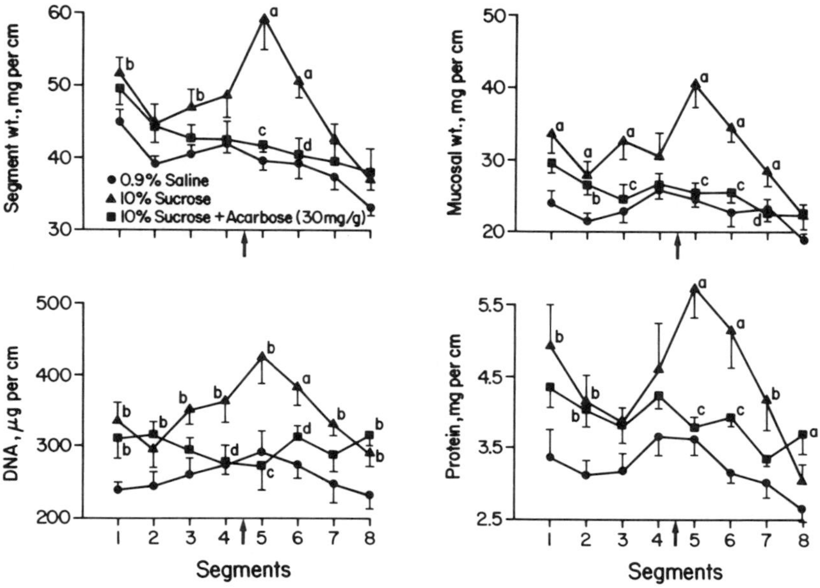


**Fig. 6.** The effect of 30 mg acarbose/g sucrose on sucrose-induced intestinal adaptation was studied in TPN-maintained rats. Solid circles represent 0.9% saline; solid triangles, 10% sucrose; solid squares, 10% sucrose plus acarbose; arrow indicates infusion site. Values represent mean ± SEM of 5 rats. For measurements marked "a," $p < 0.01$ vs. saline; "b," $p < 0.05$ vs. saline; "c," $p < 0.01$ vs. sucrose; "d," $p < 0.05$ vs. sucrose. (From Weser *et al.*, 1986. Reprinted with permission.)

disaccharide, did not induce mucosal adaptation; its effects were similar to those of saline or 5% glucose. Thus, disaccharides affect mucosal adaptation only after hydrolysis releases their component monosaccharides for absorption.

The finding that hydrolyzed disaccharides trigger greater mucosal growth than free monosaccharides suggests that the mechanisms involved in absorption and transport of a nutrient substrate may also influence mucosal growth. This also supports the theory that absorption, secretion and other aspects of the "functional work load" have a greater influence on the rate of crypt cell production than mucosal metabolism (Clark, 1977).

## C. Relationship between Total Parenteral Nutrition (TPN) and Small Bowel Mucosal Mass

The absence of intestinal nutrients results in hypoplasia in intestinal mucosa (Feldman *et al.*, 1976; Levine *et al.*, 1976). To study some of the mechanisms involved in this hypoplasia, we measured the effects of TPN on DNA concentration, ODC activity, and small bowel mucosal mass in TPN-maintained rats. We also examined the effects of enteral infusion of a single nutrient, with and without addition of an ODC inhibitor, in these animals.

### 1. *Effect of TPN on ODC Activity and DNA Concentration*

In chow-fed control rats, ODC activity was highest in the distal ileum, even though mucosal mass was lowest in this part of the small bowel (unpublished observations) (Table I). It is unclear whether luminal bacteria or other factors specific to this region of the bowel cause this high level of ODC activity. Within two days after initiating TPN, ODC activity decreased significantly in all regions, and low ODC concentrations persisted after seven days. Thus, the hypoplasia of small bowel mucosa induced by the absence of enteral nutrients is associated with a marked decrease in intestinal ODC activity.

In chow-fed controls, mucosal DNA concentration/cm of bowel segment decreased progressively from duodenojejunum to proximal ileum to distal ileum (unpublished observations) (Table II). This proximal to distal gradient of DNA concentration and mucosal mass is typically found in animals fed orally. Within two days after initiating TPN, mucosal DNA concentration decreased significantly in the proximal duodenojejunum, accompanied by lesser decreases in the proximal and distal ileum. These decreases persisted throughout the seven-day experimental period.

The data showed that the absence of nutrient absorption from the lumen rapidly and markedly reduced ODC activity, DNA concentration and mucosal mass.

### 2. *Effect of Enteral Infusion of a Single Nutrient on ODC Activity and DNA Concentration in TPN-Maintained Rats*

Solutions of 20% sucrose or saline were infused into the midgut of rats otherwise maintained on TPN. Within two days, ODC activity increased

**TABLE I**

**Effect of TPN on Rat Small Bowel Mucosal Ornithine Decarboxylase (ODC) Activity[a]**

| Group | Duodeno–jejunum | Proximal ileum | Distal ileum |
|---|---|---|---|
| Chow-fed ($n$ = 5) | 12.1 ± 4.5 | 12.4 ± 6.8 | 30.2 ± 7.4 |
| TPN 2 d ($n$ = 5) | 3.6 ± 1.3 | 0.4 ± 0.2 | 1.2 ± 0.5 |
| TPN 7 d ($n$ = 5) | 3.6 ± 1.2 | 2.5 ± 1.6 | 2.2 ± 1.0 |

[a]Data are given in pmol [$^{14}CO_2$]ODC/hr/mg protein ± SEM ($p < 0.05$ vs. chow). (Data from unpublished observations.)

**TABLE II**

**Effect of TPN on Rat Small Bowel Mucosal DNA Concentration[a]**

| Group | Duodeno-jejunum | Proximal ileum | Distal ileum |
|---|---|---|---|
| Chow-fed ($n$ = 5) | 327 ± 26 | 264 ± 24 | 205 ± 18 |
| TPN 2 d ($n$ = 5) | 205 ± 15[b] | 227 ± 11 | 209 ± 15 |
| TPN 7 d ($n$ = 5) | 198 ± 22[b] | 190 ± 23[b] | 151 ± 19[b,c] |

[a]Data are given in mcg DNA/cm of intestine ± SEM. (Data from unpublished observations.)

[b]$p < 0.05$ vs. chow.

[c]$p < 0.05$ vs. TPN 2 d.

significantly in the proximal and distal ileum of sucrose-infused rats but not in controls (unpublished observations) (Table III). The enteral infusion of 20% sucrose also stimulated ODC activity in the duodenojejunum, which was far removed from the midgut infusion site. At seven days, however, no significant differences in ODC activity were observed between sucrose) and saline-infused rats. When 1.5 mg% difluormethyl ornithine (DFMO), a known inhibitor of ODC activity and intestinal adaptation, was added to the sucrose solution, sucrose-induced stimulation of ODC activity was blocked not only in the downstream proximal and distal ileal segments but in the proximal duodenojejunum as well (Table III).

As anticipated, midgut infusion of 20% sucrose increased mucosal DNA concentration in the downstream proximal and distal ileum as well as in the proximal duodenojejunum, whereas infusion of saline did not

**TABLE III**

**Effect of Midgut 20% Sucrose Infusion for 2 Days on Small Bowel Mucosal Ornithine Decarboxylase (ODC) Activity in TPN-Maintained Rats[a]**

| Group | Duodeno-jejunum | Proximal ileum | Distal ileum |
|---|---|---|---|
| Saline ($n$ = 8) | 3.6 ±1.3 | 0.4 ± 0.2 | 1.2 ± 0.5 |
| Sucrose ($n$ = 8) | 11.2 ± 3.8[b] | 17.0 ± 6.7[b] | 8.9 ± 3.8[b] |
| Sucrose + DFMO ($n$ = 5) | 1.9 ± 0.5[c] | 0.0 ± 0.0[c] | 0.1 ± 0.0[c] |

[a]Data are given in pmol [$^{14}CO_2$]ODC/hr/mg protein ± SEM. (Data from unpublished observations.)

[b]$p < 0.05$ vs. saline.

[c]$p < 0.05$ vs. sucrose alone.

(unpublished observations) (Table IV). The addition of DFMO to the sucrose solution significantly inhibited this adaptive response (Table IV).

Thus, in these experiments, stimulation or inhibition of mucosal growth in the ileum appeared to influence the adaptive response in the duodenojejunum, suggesting that an ileal-enteric feedback mechanism contributes to overall adaptation in the small intestine. The adaptive mucosal growth response is mediated through the activities of mucosal ODC. The effects on mucosal mass of a single nutrient delivered into the proximal ileum in TPN-maintained animals are similar to those observed following exposure of the ileum to enteral nutrients after jejunectomy.

## III. SUMMARY

Small bowel mucosal mass and function depend on the efficiency of nutrient absorption and the ability to compensate for injured or partially resected small intestine. Our laboratory and others have defined several mechanisms by which enteral nutrients stimulate adaptive mucosal growth or prevent or reverse TPN-induced mucosal hypoplasia in the ileum.

In enterally fed animals, mucosal hyperplasia and a peak increase in ornithine decarboxylase activity occurred in ileal mucosa within two days after partial small bowel resection. Because ODC is the rate-limiting enzyme in polyamine synthesis, its inhibition suppresses polyamine synthesis and prevents adaptive hyperplasia. Animals nourished exclusively by TPN gain weight but do not develop mucosal hyperplasia, in part because TPN markedly and rapidly reduces mucosal ODC activity and DNA concentration.

**TABLE IV**

**Effect of Midgut 20% Sucrose Infusion for 7 Days on Small Bowel Mucosal DNA Concentration in TPN-Maintained Rats[a]**

| Group | Duodeno-jejunum | Proximal ileum | Distal ileum |
|---|---|---|---|
| Saline ($n$ = 10) | 196 ± 13 | 191 ± 11 | 166 ± 11 |
| Sucrose ($n$ = 10) | 301 ± 37[b] | 449 ± 65[b] | 253 ± 43 |
| Sucrose + DFMO ($n$ = 5) | 195 ± 20[c] | 170 ± 19[c] | 144 ± 32[c] |

[a]Data are given in mcg DNA/cm of intestine ± SEM. (Data from unpublished observations.)

[b]$p < 0.05$ vs. saline.

[c]$p < 0.05$ vs. sucrose alone.

Single substrates that prevent TPN-induced mucosal hypoplasia include long-chain fats and fatty acids, amino acids, amines, and a variety of carbohydrates. A proportional relationship appears to exist between the concentration of an intraluminal nutrient and the level of mucosal growth. In TPN-fed rats, the stimulation or inhibition of mucosal growth in the ileum appears to influence the adaptive response in the duodenojejunum, suggesting that an ileal-enteric feedback mechanism contributes to overall adaptation in the small intestine. Further studies of entero-enteric regulation of mucosal growth are needed to delineate other mechanisms involved in intestinal adaptation.

## REFERENCES


Altmann, G. C., and Leblond, C. F. (1970). Factors influencing villus size in the small intestine of adult rats as revealed by transposition of intestinal segments. *Amer. J. Anat.* **127**, 15–36.

Clark, R. M. (1977). "Luminal nutrition" versus "functional work load" as controllers of mucosal morphology and epithelial replacement in rat small intestine. *Digestion* **15**, 411–424.

Dowling, R. H., and Booth, C. C. (1967). Structural and functional changes following small intestinal resection in the rat. *Clin. Sci.* **32**, 139–149.

Eastwood, C. L. (1977). Small bowel morphology and epithelial proliferation in intravenously alimented rabbits. *Surgery* **82**, 613–620.

Feldman, E. J., Dowling, R. H., McNaughton, J., and Peters, T. J. (1976). Effects of oral vs intravenous nutrition on intestinal adaptation after small bowel resection. *Gastroenterology* **70**, 712–719.

Gleeson, M. H., Cullen, J., and Dowling, R. H. (1972). Intestinal structure and function after small bowel bypass in the rat. *Clin. Sci.* **43**, 731–742.

Grey, V. L., Garofalo, C., Greenberg, G. R., and Morin, C. L. (1984). The adaptation of the small intestine after resection in response to free fatty acids. *Amer. J. Clin. Nutr.* **40**, 1235–1242.

Gronqvist, B., Engstrom, B., and Grimelius, L. (1975). Morphological studies of the rat small intestine after jejuno-ileal transposition. *Acta Chir. Scand.* **141**, 208–217.

Hanson, W. R., and Osborne, J. W. (1971). Epithelial cell kinetics in the small intestine of the rat 60 days after resection of 70 per cent of the ileum and jejunum. *Gastroenterology* **60**, 1087–1097.

Hanson, W. R., Osborne, J. W., and Sharp, J. G. (1977a). Compensation by the residual intestine after intestinal resection in the rat. I. Influence of the amount of tissue removed. *Gastroenterology* **72**, 692–700.

Hanson, W. R., Osborne, J. W., and Sharp, J. G. (1977b). Compensation by the residual intestine after intestinal resection in the rat. II. Influence of postoperative time interval. *Gastroenterology* **72**, 701–705.

Keren, D. F., Elliott, H. L., Brown, G. D., and Yardley, J. H. (1975). Atrophy of villi with hypertrophy and hyperplasia of paneth cells in isolated (Thiry-Vella) ileal loops in rabbits. *Gastroenterology* **68**, 83–93.

Levine, G. M., Deren, J. J., Steiger, E., and Zinno, R. (1974). Role of oral intake in maintenance of gut mass and disaccharidase activity. *Gastroenterology* **67**, 975–982.

Levine, G. M., Deren, J. J., and Yezdimir, E. (1976). Small bowel resection. Oral intake is the stimulus for hyperplasia. *Amer. J. Dig. Dis.* **21**, 542–546.

Luk, G. D., and Baylin, S. B. (1982). Ornithine decarboxylase in intestinal maturation, recovery, and adaptation. *In* "Mechanisms of Intestinal Adaptation. Falk Symposium 30" (J. W. L. Robinson, R. H. Dowling, and E. O. Riecken, eds.), pp. 65–78. MTP Press, Lancaster, England.

Luk, G. D., and Baylin, S. B. (1983). Polyamines and intestinal growth-increased polyamine biosynthesis after jejunectomy. *Amer. J. Physiol.* **245**, G656–G660.

Luk, G. D., and Baylin, S. B. (1984). Inhibition of intestinal epithelial DNA synthesis and adaptive hyperplasia after jejunectomy in the rat by suppression of polyamine biosynthesis. *J. Clin. Invest.* **74**, 698–704.

McDermott, F. T., and Roudnew, B. (1976). Ileal crypt cell population kinetics after 40 per cent small bowel resection. *Gastroenterology* **70**, 707–711.

Morin, C. L., Grey, V. L., and Garofalo, C. (1982). Influence of lipids on intestinal adaptation after resection. *In* "Mechanisms of Intestinal Adaptation. Falk Symposium 30" (J. W. L. Robinson, R. H. Dowling, and E. O. Riecken, eds.), pp. 175–184. MTP Press, Lancaster, England.

Nygaard, K. (1967). Resection of the small intestine in rats. III. Morphological changes in the intestinal tract. *Acta Chir. Scand.* **133**, 233–248.

Obertop, H., Nundy, S., Malamud, D., and Malt, R. A. (1977). Onset of cell proliferation in the shortened gut. Rapid hyperplasia after jejunal resection. *Gastroenterology* **72**, 267–270.

Philipson, B. (1975). Morphology in the cat ileal mucosa following construction of an ileal reservoir or transposition of patches to different locations. *Scand. J. Gastroenterol.* **10**, 369–377.

Rijke, R. P. C., Plaisier, H. M., deRuiter, H., and Galjaard, M. D. (1977). Influence of experimental bypass on cellular kinetics and maturation of small intestinal epithelium in the rat. *Gastroenterology* **72**, 896–901.

Spector, M. H., Levine, G. M., and Deren, J. J. (1977). Direct and indirect effects of dextrose and amino acids on gut mass. *Gastroenterology* **72**, 706–710.

Spector, M. H., Traylor, J. B., Young, E. A., and Weser, E. (1981). Stimulation of mucosal growth by gastric and ileal infusion of single amino acids in parenterally nourished rats. *Digestion* **21**, 33–40.

Tabata, K., and Johnson, L. R. (1986). Ornithine decarboxylase and mucosal growth in response to feeding. *Amer. J. Physiol.* **251**, G270–G274.

Tilson, M. D., and Wright, H. K. (1970). Adaptation of functioning and bypassed segments of ileum during compensatory hypertrophy of the gut. *Surgery* **64**, 687–693.

Weser, E., and Hernandez, M. H. (1971). Studies of small bowel adaptation after intestinal resection in the rat. *Gastroenterology* **60**, 69–75.

Weser, E., Tawil, T., and Fletcher, J. T. (1982a). Stimulation of small bowel mucosal growth by gastric infusion of different sugars in rats maintained on total parenteral nutrition. *In* "Mechanisms of Intestinal Adaptation. Falk Symposium 30" (J. W. L. Robinson, R. H. Dowling, and E. O. Riecken, eds.), pp. 141–149. MTP Press, Lancaster, England.

Weser, E., Vandeventer, A., and Tawil, T. (1982b). Non-hormonal regulation of intestinal adaptation. *Scand. J. Gastroenterol.* **17** (Suppl. 74), 105–113.

Weser, E., Vandeventer, A., and Tawil, T. (1982c). Stimulation of small bowel mucosal growth by mid-gut infusion of different sugars in rats. *J. Pediatr. Gastroenterol. Nutr.* **1**, 411–416.

Weser, E., Babbitt, J., and Vandeventer, A. (1985). Relationship between enteral glucose load and adaptative mucosal growth in the small bowel. *Dig. Dis. Sci.* **30**, 675–681.

Weser, E., Babbitt, J., Hoban, M., and Vandeventer, A. (1986). Intestinal adaptation. Different growth responses to disaccharides compared with monosaccharides in rat small bowel. *Gastroenterology* **91**, 1521–1527.

Young, E. A., and Weser, E. (1974). Nutritional adaptation after small bowel resection in rats. *J. Nutr.* **104**, 994–1001.

# 22

# Immunoregulation in the Mucosal Immune System and the Pathogenesis of Immunologic Diseases of the Gastrointestinal Tract

Warren Strober, Marjorie E. Kanof, Martin Zeitz, and Stephen P. James

*Mucosal Immunity Section*
*Laboratory of Clinical Investigation*
*National Institute of Allergy and Infectious Diseases*
*Bethesda, Maryland*

# I. INTRODUCTION

The mucosal immune system is that part of the lymphoid system that is in immediate contact with the antigenic environment of the gastrointestinal tract. As a first line of defense against infection, the mucosal immune system responds to potential oral pathogens by producing reactive immune effector products. This response is only part of the story, however, because the mucosal immune system does not respond to the vast majority of innocuous substances in food or in resident microbial flora (Strober *et al.*, 1981; Mowat, 1987).

The mucosal immune system is anatomically and functionally subdivided into two major areas: the inductive area, in which lymphocytes undergo the initial interactions with mucosal antigens that lead to lymphocyte proliferation and differentiation, and the effector area, in which the primed lymphocytes again interact with antigens via antibody- and cell-mediated processes (Strober and Brown, 1987). The inductive area is centered in gut-associated lymphoid tissues (GALT) such as Peyer's patches, and the effector area is located in the lamina propria underlying the mucosal epithelium. The pattern of cellular migration linking these two areas favors the movement of GALT-derived cells to the lamina propria. This migration moves lymphocytes induced by mucosal antigens to sites enriched for these antigens.

The following discussion examines the cellular processes underlying the differential responsiveness of the mucosal immune system and focuses on immune responses in the GALT and the lamina propria. The role of abnormalities of the mucosal immune response in the pathogenesis of gastrointestinal diseases is also discussed.

# II. STIMULATION OF THE GUT-ASSOCIATED LYMPHOID TISSUES (GALT) BY ORAL ANTIGENS

## A. Proposed Mechanisms Regulating Unresponsiveness

Three mechanisms have been proposed to explain the unresponsiveness of the mucosal immune system to oral stimulation by diet-derived antigens. These mechanisms have been best described for events occurring in the Peyer's patches.

### 1. *Generation of Suppressor T Cells*

The mucosal immune system most often responds to antigenic stimulation by generating suppressor T cells. In animal studies, the transfer of

Peyer's patch or spleen cells from an orally immunized donor suppressed the recipient's subsequent response to the immunizing antigen, even when the antigen was introduced by a normally immunogenic route (Strober *et al.*, 1981; Mowat, 1987; Richman *et al.*, 1978). This response was mediated by suppressor T cells that developed in Peyer's patches as a result of antigen-specific cellular cascades similar to those found elsewhere in the lymphoid system. Ultimately, these suppressor T cells were disseminated to distant parts of the lymphoid system (Mowat, 1987; Gautam and Battisto, 1985). The suppressor T cell-dominated responses that follow mucosal immunization have been elicited by oral administration of many different protein antigens and nonliving particulates such as killed viruses, bacteria, and heterologous red cells (Mowat, 1987; Strober and Brown, 1987). However, such responses were not elicited by antigens that react directly with B cells nor by oral challenge with live replicating organisms or cells, perhaps because antigens within these organisms react directly with B cells (Mowat, 1987; Strober and Brown, 1987).

To some extent, the T cell responsiveness to oral antigens is immunoglobulin (Ig) class specific. The oral administration of antigen substances may be followed by concurrent suppression of IgG and enhancement of IgA antibody responses (Challacombe and Tomasi, 1980) as well as by simultaneous development of IgA-specific helper cells and IgG-specific suppressor cells (Richman, 1981). After prolonged oral administration of an antigen, IgA antibody levels increased steadily until a plateau was reached while IgM and IgG antibody levels steadily declined (Emancipator *et al.*, 1987). These seemingly antagonistic IgA and IgM/IgG responses may synergistically prevent potentially detrimental systemic reactions to environmental antigens. Thus, mucosal helper T-cells may upregulate IgA responses causing decreased absorption of potentially pathogenic antigens at the mucosal surface, whereas mucosal suppressor T cells may downregulate systemic IgM/IgG responses to innocuous antigens that breach the mucosal barrier.

### 2. *Clonal Inhibition or Deletion*

Clonal inhibition or deletion, most commonly associated with immature cells, may also explain mucosal unresponsiveness to stimulation by oral antigens. Evidence for this mechanism came from the demonstration that unresponsiveness to orally administered antigens continued long after the demonstration of transferred suppressor T cells (Richman, 1979). In sheep, Peyer's patches are sites of massive cell turnover and death, as might be expected in a lymphoid area undergoing simultaneous cell elaboration and deletion following encounters with antigens (Reynolds, 1986). However, studies in rodents and humans have failed to demonstrate that the many relatively immature cells in Peyer's patches are susceptible to interactions that result in antigen tolerance. This evidence suggests the alternate possibility that clonal inhibition or deletion affects more mature cells as a result of special conditions of antigen presentation in Peyer's patches. Schwartz's laboratory has defined conditions of antigen presentation that produce signals causing cell inactivation (Jenkins *et al.*, 1987).

### 3. *Activity of Mucosal Mitogens*

This hypothesis stipulates that certain mucosal mitogens, most notably lipopolysaccharide (LPS), may condition responses to mucosal antigens by downregulating antigen-nonspecific suppressor T cells. In contrast to the first hypothesis, which proposes that mucosal system suppression results from antigen-specific cell interactions, this theory suggests that suppression results from antigen-nonspecific stimulation of cells by a polyclonal activator. Evidence for the mucosal mitogen hypothesis comes from several observations: First, oral administration of antigens from the surface of sheep erythrocytes produced a greater response in LPS-unresponsive mice than in normal LPS-responsive mice (Kiyono *et al.*, 1982). Second, the LPS-responsive mice developed antigen-specific suppressor and helper T cells, whereas the LPS-unresponsive mice developed only helper T cells (Michalek, 1982). These findings suggest that the absence of LPS responsiveness probably accounted for the development of contrasuppressor T cells rather than suppressor T cells in the LPS-unresponsive mice. Recent studies demonstrated that induction of contrasuppressor T cells is a normal part of mucosal immune response and that this response is exaggerated in LPS-unresponsive mice (Kitamura *et al.*, 1987). The absence of LPS responsiveness may also reduce the activation of B cells and macrophages, thus reducing stimulation of the autoreactive suppressor T cells that recognize the autologous major histocompatibility complex (MHC) on activated cells (Kotani *et al.*, 1986). Although autoreactive suppressor T cells are normally involved in antigen-specific cell interactions throughout the immune system, they may have a heightened role in the LPS-enriched environment of the mucosa.

## B. Predominance of Unresponsiveness

Although the mechanisms regulating mucosal immune response to oral antigens could theoretically affect the systemic immune response, their predominance in mucosal immune response has yet to be explained. One study supports the hypothesis that the breakdown of antigens in the gastrointestinal tract produces antigen fragments that preferentially activate suppressor T cells (Bruce and Ferguson, 1986). In this study, serum of animals recently fed ovalbumin (OVA) contained antigen fragments that activated OVA-specific suppressor T cells, whereas serum of animals injected with OVA did not contain such fragments. Another, perhaps related, explanation is that antigen processing by antigen-presenting cells preferentially induces suppressor rather than helper T cells in the mucosal immune system but not in the systemic immune system. Evidence for this theory, which is scanty at best, rests primarily on the recent demonstration that antigen-presenting intestinal epithelial cells preferentially stimulated T cells with suppressor-cell-associated markers and function (Mayer and Shlein, 1987). A third possibility is that antigen concentration in the mucosal immune system is far higher than in the systemic immune system, leading to high dose tolerance via the previously described mechanism of clonal inhibition or deletion.

### C. Reversal of Unresponsiveness

Despite the above evidence, the responses of the mucosal immune system are not always negative. Recent work has shown that antigen-presenting cells can be activated by administering muramyl peptide, by inducing graft-versus-host reactions, or by feeding cholera toxin, a substance with direct but unexplained biochemical effects on lymphoid cells (Mowat, 1987; Elson and Ealding, 1984). Therefore, the tendency of the mucosal system to be immunologically unresponsive is at least partially reversible. Transient and localized changes in mucosal immune response may be important in the appropriately positive reactions to potential pathogens that lead to host defense as well as in the inappropriately positive reactions that lead to disease.

## III. PHENOTYPE AND FUNCTION OF LAMINA PROPRIA T CELLS

New extraction methods now make it possible to define the phenotype, function, and immunoregulatory potential of lamina propria T cells in the effector area of the mucosal immune system.

### A. Phenotype Studies

Studies of peripheral blood T cells have identified various surface markers and the immunoregulatory characteristics of T cells bearing these markers. With these data, our laboratory determined the proportions of extracted lamina propria T cells bearing each marker (James *et al.*, 1986). The distribution of T-cells bearing fluorochrome-labeled monoclonal antibodies specific for each marker was analyzed using dual channel flow cytometry, which allowed us to identify cells with two markers. Lamina propria contained equal proportions of T cells bearing CD4 and CD8 antigens, but markedly fewer T cells bearing CD4 or CD8 and the Leu-8 or 2H4 antigen. For example, only 10% of CD4 T cells were Leu-8 positive in the lamina propria, whereas 60% of CD4 T cells were Leu-8 positive in peripheral blood. These differences, which were not attributable to cell extraction methods, were corroborated in studies of intact lamina propria stained with immunoperoxidase-labeled antibodies. These findings seem compatible with the observation that stimulation by various mitogens led to rapid disappearance of Leu-8 and 2H4 markers from the surface of lamina propria T cells (Kanof and James, 1987). The more activated state of lamina propria T cells, described below, may explain their lower expression of Leu-8.

## B. Function Studies

### 1. *State of Activation of Lamina Propria T Cells*

The following data from our laboratory support the hypothesis that lamina propria T cells are in a more activated state than peripheral blood T cells (Zeitz *et al.*, 1988a):

1. A very low proportion of T cells from peripheral blood and other nonmucosal sites and a high proportion of T cells from lamina propria expressed interleukin-2 (IL-2) receptors.
2. In the absence of other stimulants, T cells from lamina propria proliferated more actively when cultured with IL-2 than T cells from other sites.
3. Resting T cells from lamina propria contained detectable IL-2-specific mRNA, whereas other T cells did not.
4. Compared with T cells at other sites, lamina propria T cells expressed more MHC class II antigen, another surface marker associated with cell activation.
5. Freshly isolated lamina propria T cells, in common with other T cells, did not produce IL-2. After stimulation by mitogens, however, they produced far more of this lymphokine than other T cells.

Thus, T cells from lamina propria are in a more activated state than T cells from peripheral blood or other lymphoid areas, probably because they receive greater exposure to environmental antigens and mitogens and thus more frequent stimulation.

### 2. *Immunoregulatory Potential of Lamina Propria T Cells*

In studies of T cells in peripheral blood, CD4/Leu-8+ T cells had a relatively low response to antigens, but autoreactive T cells responded to autologous MHC antigens (Kansas *et al.*, 1985). Peripheral blood T cells also induced CD8+ T cells to mediate increased suppressor activity. In contrast, CD4/Leu-8− T cells, which act as helper T cells, had a high response to antigens and a low response to autologous MHC antigens. In more recent studies, CD4/Leu-8+ T cells functioned as direct suppressor T cells in the absence of CD8+ T cells (Kanof *et al.*, 1987a). This activity was most evident when the Leu-8 antigen was crosslinked with anti-Leu-8 antibody.

In the lamina propria, the low levels of Leu-8 T cells significantly affect its immunoregulatory potential. The low proportion of CD4/Leu-8+ cells results in low suppressor capability. In pokeweek mitogen-induced *in vitro* assay systems, suppressor activity in lamina propria CD4+ T cells was lower than in peripheral blood CD4+ T cells. This low suppressor activity was attributable to low levels of CD4+/Leu-8+ T cells rather than to qualitative defects in these cells (unpublished observations). Because the proportion of CD8+/Leu-8+ T cells in the lamina propria is also low, we compared the suppressor capacity of CD8+ T cells in isolated lamina propria and in peripheral blood; the capacity of both was similar (unpublished observations). This finding suggests that the low level of CD8+/Leu-8+ T cells in the lamina propria does not affect suppressor potential.

### 3. *Response of Lamina Propria T Cells to Antigens*

We evaluated the response of lamina propria T cells to specific antigens in studies of nonhuman primates immunized with *Chlamydia trachtomatis* (L2 serovar) per rectum (Zeitz *et al.*, 1988b). Surprisingly, T cells from peripheral blood, spleen, and mesenteric and draining lymph nodes proliferated vigorously when cultured with antigen, but T cells from the infection site in the rectal lamina propria and from distant uninfected lamina propria sites did not proliferate. We could not attribute this failure to proliferate to a lack of functional antigen presenting cells, to the presence of suppressor cells, nor to an idiosyncratic feature of *C. trachtomatis* infection. Despite this failure to proliferate, we found that lamina propria T cells at chlamydia infection sites contained antigen-reactive cells. Chlamydia antigen stimulated these T cells to assist in polyclonal Ig synthesis *in vitro.* Although their precise role in polyclonal Ig synthesis is unclear, it probably relates to their secretion of lymphokines that act on B cells in conjunction with antigen. This phenomenon probably plays a role in maintaining the relatively high level of terminal B cell differentiation seen in the lamina propria. In related assays, lamina propria T cells did not proliferate in response to BCG mycobacterial antigens, whereas they did proliferate in response to concanavalin A.

Thus, the state of activation of T cells in the lamina propria appears to affect their function. It may explain their generally low level of antigen-induced proliferation and their high helper activity. It may also explain why partially activated T cells are more refractory to antigen-initiated membrane events than resting cells (Otten *et al.*, 1986).

## IV. MUCOSAL IMMUNOREGULATORY FUNCTION AND THE PATHOGENESIS OF GASTROINTESTINAL DISEASE

Understanding the role of the normal mucosal immune system is important to understanding the pathogenesis of several gastrointestinal diseases, including food sensitivities of the gastrointestinal tract such as celiac disease (gluten-sensitive enteropathy), IgA immune-complex-mediated diseases, and inflammatory bowel disease.

### A. Gluten-Sensitive Enteropathy (GSE)

Gluten-sensitive enteropathy (GSE) or celiac disease is characterized by an exquisite sensitivity to the gliadin fraction of gluten, which leads to villus atrophy, malabsorption, and nutrient deficiencies. Mucosal lymphoid infiltrate from these patients consists of B and T cells in the lamina propria and T cells in intraepithelial areas (Strober, 1985). Because IgE antigliadin antibodies are not elevated in this disease, it is a sensitivity but not an allergy. The disease is controlled by eliminating gluten from the diet.

The high levels of circulating and mucosal antigliadin antibodies reported in many studies of patients with GSE were initially thought to be nonspecific effects of mucosal injury. However, current evidence suggests that these effects may be disease-specific because high titers of IgA antigliadin antibody are found only in GSE (Ribes-Koninckx *et al.*, 1984). This apparently unique response to gliadin is accompanied by a T cell-mediated response in which circulating cells produce lymphokines upon exposure to the offending antigen (Ashkinazi *et al.*, 1981). Mucosal tissue from GSE patients reacted to gliadin *in vitro*, but mucosal tissue from controls did not (Falchuk *et al.*, 1974). This immunological effector function is characteristic of GSE.

A major advance in understanding of GSE came with the demonstration of its strong association with the major histocompatibility markers HLA-B8, HLA-DR3, and HLA-DR7 (Strober, 1988). Many studies have concluded that GSE is brought about by two sets of MHC genes acting in concert as well as by one or more non-MHC genes. Because MHC genes are immune response genes, the HLA association encourages the view that GSE arises from in abnormality in an immune response gene that causes an abnormal response to gliadin.

It is reasonable to speculate that the normal mucosal immune mechanisms preventing response to gliadin may be subverted in GSE, thus leading to abnormal, pathological responses mediated by gliadin-specific effector cells in the lamina propria. Two pieces of indirect evidence support this view. First, GSE patients display excessive immune responses to gliadin. Second, in animals in which the normal mucosal unresponsiveness was subverted, oral administration of an antigen resulted in mucosal response to that antigen and gastrointestinal histopathology similar to that found in GSE (Mowat and Ferguson, 1981). Interestingly, the treatments used to subvert normal unresponsiveness also inhibited suppressor T cells.

It is also reasonable to suspect that the immune response genes postulated to cause GSE originally arose as host defenses against antigens associated with environmental pathogens. Because some of these antigens resemble gliadin, the genetically determined hypersensitivity they conferred may have become a disease factor when gliadin entered the diet. Support for this hypothesis comes from recent work demonstrating that gliadin crossreacts with a protein that is associated with an intestinal adenovirus (Kagnoff *et al.*, 1984).

## B. Other Food Hypersensitivities

Other food hypersensitivities, the most common of which is cow's milk hypersensitivity, cause villus atrophy and malabsorption (Savilahti and Verkasalo, 1984). Like GSE, these food hypersensitivities cannot be considered allergies because they are not associated with IgE-mediated immune abnormalities. Unlike GSE, which occurs in both adults and children, these other food hypersensitivities occur only in children. These transient sensitivities, which often follow infectious gastrointestinal illness, usually disappear as the child grows older.

Insight into the pathogenesis of food hypersensitivity comes from studies in which an enteropathy similar to GSE developed in weanling pigs that were not exposed to dietary antigens before weaning (Miller *et al.*, 1984). Exposure to dietary antigens before weaning did not lead to mucosal unresponsiveness because suppressor T cell potential is undeveloped at this age. Providing many new antigens together, however, may interfere with development of the normal mucosal unresponsiveness to at least some of them. These data suggest that exposure to a mucosal antigen at an inopportune time, such as early in life or after infection, may produce abnormal mucosal immune responses and immunologically induced villus atrophy. However, in the absence a genetic defect such as that found in GSE, normal mucosal unresponsiveness develops, and the enteropathy disappears.

## C. Mucosal Unresponsiveness and IgA Immune-Complex-Mediated Disease

Another defect in mucosal unresponsiveness may explain certain forms of immune-complex-mediated disease. This defect is most clearly seen in such diseases as Henoch-Schoenlein purpura or Berger's disease (IgA nephropathy), in which circulating or deposited IgA antibody-antigen complexes point to the mucosa as the locus of the abnormality (Miller *et al.*, 1984). IgA immune complexes are thought to arise when antibodies are formed in response to inciting antigens, which may be environmental antigens, crossreactive autologous antigens, or both. This theory, which is compatible with the fact that these diseases often follow oral infection, has received powerful support from recent animal models of IgA nephropathy (Emancipator *et al.*, 1987; Emancipator *et al.*, 1985). In these studies, mice fed low doses of antigens for many weeks produced high levels of IgA antibodies and progressively declining levels of IgM and IgG antibodies. This pattern may result from Ig class-specific regulation, mediated by T cells that enhance IgA responses and suppress IgG responses. Although IgA immune complex was deposited in the glomerular mesangium following antigen feeding, no renal injury occurred because IgA is a noninflammatory immunoglobulin. However, when antigen feeding was followed by parenteral administration of antigen, IgM and IgG antibody levels increased, immunoglobulin and complement were deposited in the kidney, and renal injury occurred. Thus, the key defect in IgA immune-complex disease may reside not in the lack of negative regulation of the IgA response per se but rather in the lack of regulation of the systemic IgM/IgG response.

## D. Mucosal Immunoregulation and Inflammatory Bowel Disease

The idiopathic inflammatory bowel diseases (IBD) ulcerative colitis and Crohn's disease may arise from disordered mucosal immunoregulation (Kirsner and Shorter, 1982). These diseases are characterized by gastrointestinal inflammation caused by an unidentified pathological agent. Ulcerative colitis, which is limited to the large bowel, causes superficial mucosal ulceration involving the rectum in mild disease and part or all of the colon in severe disease. Crohn's disease usually affects the terminal ileum and ascending colon, but lesions may occur anywhere in the gastrointestinal tract. Although this transmural disease is also associated with ulceration, it more frequently causes granulomas and obstruction consequent to bowel wall thickening. In both forms of IBD, the histological lesion consists of a chronic inflammatory infiltration, which, in acute disease, is associated with neutrophil accumulation and crypt abscesses.

Epidemiological studies show that IBD occurs primarily in industrialized, urbanized countries. Although these studies suggest the involvement of an environmental factor in its pathogenesis (Gilat and Rozen, 1979), the epidemiological pattern is not typical of infection. Moreover, no dietary component has been identified, and no single organism has been consistently isolated in patients. An atypical mycobacterial organism has been proposed as the cause of Crohn's disease (Chiodini *et al.*, 1984), but this is unlikely for two reasons: This organism has been isolated in both patients and controls without Crohn's disease, and no immune response to this agent has been found in patients (Graham *et al.*, 1987).

Because efforts to establish an infectious etiology for IBD have failed, many studies are now directed toward identifying an immunological abnormality (Strober and James, 1986). One line of investigation has led to the identification, especially in ulcerative colitis, of autoantibodies that have specificity for epithelial cell antigens or mucus substances associated with epithelial cells and that crossreact with bacterial antigens (Takahashi and Das, 1985). The occurrence of such antibodies may explain the presence of circulating and intestinal cytotoxic lymphocytes that are cytotoxic for colonic epithelial cells. These cytotoxic lymphocytes have been shown to be nonspecific killer cells that can be armed to kill epithelial cells by binding antibodies with antiepithelial-cell specificity (Shorter *et al.*, 1984). These findings are consistent with the hypothesis that IBD is an autoimmune disease in which epithelial cell damage is mediated by antiepithelial immune effector elements. However, certain features are inconsistent with this hypothesis: In Crohn's disease, epithelial cell damage is not a feature of the early pathologic lesions, and, in ulcerative colitis, the antiepithelial cell antibodies also occur in healthy relatives of patients.

The possibility that IBD results from an immunoregulatory defect has been explored in other studies. The earliest lesions of Crohn's disease appear as a collection of mononuclear cells that then become a follicular array of B and T cells surrounded by macrophages (Schmitz-Moorman and Becker, 1981). This pathologic picture suggests that the initial lesion of Crohn's disease is a normal response to mucosal immunogens, but one that occurs inappropriately in the diffuse mucosal area rather than in the Peyer's patches. This characteristic of Crohn's disease is consistent with the observation that responses to bacterial antigens and other immunogens are greater in Crohn's patients than in controls (Auer *et al.*, 1983).

In addition, Crohn's disease and ulcerative colitis have been shown to be associated with other immunoregulatory defects. One such defect is diminished mitogen-induced suppressor T cell function (Auer *et al.*, 1984). The T cell that mediates mitogen-induced suppression is the CD4+/Leu-8+ T cell, which, as previously discussed, is reduced in number in the lamina propria. Thus, even a minor alteration of the function of this cell could cause a pronounced change in the lamina propria. Suppressor T cell abnormalities correlate with advanced disease, which suggests that they are secondary to some other primary immunological abnormality. Regardless of the cause, diminished suppressor T cell function in the lamina propria coul lead to an excessive mucosal immune response.

Another immunoregulatory abnormality, identified in patients with mild Crohn's disease, is the presence of an excessive number of CD-8/Leu-7 suppressor T cells (Elson *et al.*, 1981), originally called "covert suppressor cells" because they were revealed only after cell purification. The CD-8/Leu-7 T cells also function as cytotoxic effector cells, and LFA-3 antigens on their cytotoxic targets may induce them to proliferate (unpublished observations). These data, along with the demonstration that CD-8/Leu-7 cells appear in several disorders involving chronic intracellular infection (Plaeger-Marshall *et al.*, 1987), suggest that the presence of these cells in IBD indicates that activation of cytolytic T cells by modified target cells is taking place. These phenomena may result from a primary immunoregulatory defect that leads to chronic cell activation.

The underlying immunological defect in IBD remains undefined. Yet it seems reasonable to view it as an antigen-nonspecific defect involving either a failure of the normally predominant downregulating T cell mechanism characteristic of the Peyer's patches or an imbalance in the normally upregulated T cell mechanism of the lamina propria. Either defect could cause ongoing, inappropriate immune response to one or more mucosal antigens, ultimately leading to acute cell inflammation and tissue injury.

## V. SUMMARY

Mucosal immune response in the GALT is oriented toward producing noninflammatory immunoglobulin with both host-defense and immune-exclusion functions. These activities prevent the entry of immunogens that could unnecessarily stimulate systemic immune responses and also suppress systemic immune responses to antigens that penetrate the mucosa. In contrast, mucosal immune response in the lamina propria is oriented toward producing helper T cells that rapidly and vigorously respond to antigens entering the mucosa. Because of this role, the lamina propria is especially vulnerable to abnormalities that might lead to excessive responses.

Knowledge of the immunoregulatory activities of the mucosal immune system forms a basis for understanding several gastrointestinal diseases. GSE and other food hypersensitivity diseases appear to be antigen-specific immunoregulatory defects centered primarily in the GALT. The same is true of diseases involving circulating IgA immune complexes, which appear to arise from inadequate downregulation of isotype-specific IgM/IgG responses. On the other hand, inflammatory bowel disease appears to be an antigen-nonspecific defect in mucosal immunoregulation that gives rise to an imbalance between helper and suppressor T cells in the lamina propria. Increased understanding of mucosal immunoregulation should lead to more effective therapeutic intervention in these gastrointestinal diseases.

## REFERENCES

Ashkinazi, A., Idar, D., Barzilai, N., Levin, S., Ayala, O. R., and Handzel, Z. T. (1981). Effect of gluten-free diet on an immunological assay for coeliac disease. *Lancet* **1**, 914–916.

Auer, I. O., Roder, A., Wesinck, F., van de Merwe, J. P., and Schmidt, H. (1983). Selected bacterial antibodies in Crohn's disease and ulcerative colitis. *Scand. J. Gastroenterol.* **18**, 217–223.

Auer, I. O., Roder, A., and Frolich, J. (1984). Immune status in Crohn's disease. VI. Immunoregulation evaluated by multiple, distinct T suppressor cell assays of lymphocyte proliferation, and by enumeration of immunoregulatory T lymphocyte subsets. *Gastroenterology* **86**, 1531–1543.

Bruce, M. G., and Ferguson, A. (1986). The influence of intestinal processing on the immunogenicity and molecular size of absorbed, circulating ovalbumin in mice. *Immunology* **59**, 295–300.

Challacombe, S. J., and Tomasi, T. B., Jr. (1980). Systemic tolerance and secretory immunity after oral immunization. *J. Exp. Med.* **152**, 1459–1472.

Chiodini, R. J., Van Kruiningen, H. J., Merkal, R. S., Thayer, W. R., Jr., and Coutu, J. A. (1984). Characteristics of an unclassified mycobacterium species isolated from patients with Crohn's disease. *J. Clin. Microbiol.* **20**, 966–971.

Elson, C. O., and Ealding, W. (1984). Cholera toxin feeding did not induce oral tolerance in mice and abrogated oral tolerance to an unrelated protein antigen. *J. Immunol.* **133**, 2892–2897.

Elson, C. O., Graeff, A. S., James, S. P., and Strober, W. (1981). Covert suppressor T cells in Crohn's disease. *Gastroenterology* **80**, 1513–1521.

Emancipator, S. N., Gallo, G. R., and Lamm, M. E. (1985). IgA nephropathy: Perspectives on pathogenesis and classification. *Clin. Nephrol.* **24**, 161–179.

Emancipator, S. N., Ovary, Z., and Lamm, M. E. (1987). The role of mesangial complement in the hematuria of experimental IgA nephropathy. *Lab. Invest.* **57**, 269–276.

Falchuk, Z. M., Gebhard, R. L., Sessoms, C., and Strober, W. (1974). An *in vitro* model of gluten-sensitive enteropathy. Effect of gliadin on intestinal epithelial cells of patients with gluten-sensitive enteropathy in organ culture. *J. Clin. Invest.* **53**, 487–500.

Gautam, S. C., and Battisto, J. R. (1985). Orally induced tolerance generates an efferently acting suppressor T cell and an acceptor T cell that together down-regulate contact sensitivity. *J. Immunol.* **135**, 2975–2983.

Gilat, T., and Rozen, P. (1979). Epidemiology of Crohn's disease and ulcerative colitis: Etiologic implications. *Isr. J. Med. Sci.* **15**, 305–308.

Graham, D. Y., Markesich, D. C., and Yoshimara, H. H. (1987). Mycobacteria and inflammatory bowel disease. Results of culture. *Gastroenterology* **92**, 436–442.

James, S. P., Fiocchi, C., Graeff, A. S., and Strober, W. (1986). Phenotypic analysis of lamina propria lymphocytes: Predominance of helper-inducer and cytolytic T cell phenotype and deficiency of suppressor-inducer phenotypes in Crohn's disease and control patients. *Gastroenterology* **91**, 1483–1489.

Jenkins, M. K., Pardoll, D. M., Mizuguchi, I., Quill, H., and Schwartz, R. H. (1987). T cell unresponsiveness *in vivo* and *in vitro*: Fine specificity of induction and molecular characterization of the unresponsive state. *Immunol. Rev.* **95**, 113–135.

Kagnoff, M. F., Austin, R. K., Hubsert, J. J., and Kasarda, D. D. (1984). Possible role of a human adenovirus in the pathogenesis of celiac disease. *J. Exp. Med.* **160**, 1544–1557.

Kansas, G. S., Wood, G. S., Fishwild, D. M., and Engleman, E. G. (1985). Functional characteristics of human T lymphocyte subsets distinguished by monoclonal anti-Leu-8. *J. Immunol.* **134**, 2995–3002.

Kanof, M. E., and James, S. P. (1987). Leu-8 antigen expression is modified by cell activation but does not correlate with effector function of activated T lymphocytes. *J. Immunol.* (In press.)

Kanof, M. E., Strober, W., and James, S. P. (1987a). Induction of CD4 suppressor T cells with anti-Leu-8 antibody. *J. Immunol.* **139**, 49–54.

Kirsner, M. B., and Shorter, R. G. (1982). Recent developments in "nonspecific" inflammatory bowel disease. *N. Engl. J. Med.* **306**, 775–837.

Kitamura, K., Kiyono, H., Fujihashi, K., Eldridge, J. H., Green, D. R., and McGhee, J. R. (1987). Contrasuppressor cells that break oral tolerance are antigen-specific T cells distinct from T helper (L3T4+), T suppressor (Lyt-2+), and B cells. *J. Immunol.* **139**, 3251–3259.

Kiyono, H., McGhee, J. R., Wannemueller, M. J., and Michalek, S. M. (1982). Lack of oral tolerance in C3H/HeJ mice. *J. Exp. Med.* **155**, 605–610.

Kotani, H., Mitsuya, H., Jarrett, R. F., Yenokida, G. G., James, S. P., and Strober, W. (1986). An autoreactive T cell clone which can be activated to provide both helper and suppressor function. *J. Immunol.* **136**, 1951–1959.

Mayer, L., and Shlein, R. (1987). Evidence for function of Ia molecules on gut epithelial cells in man. *J. Exp. Med.* **166**, 1471–1483.

Michalek, S. M., Kiyono, H., Wannemueller, M. J., Mosteller, L. M., and McGhee, J. R. (1982). Lipopolysaccharide (LPS) regulation of immune response: LPS influence and oral tolerance induction. *J. Immunol.* **128**, 1992–1998.

Miller, B. G., Newby, T. J., and Stokes, C. R. (1984). Influence of diet on postweaning malabsorption and diarrhea in the pig. *Res. Vet. Sci.* **36**, 187–193.

Mowat, A. McL., and Ferguson, A. (1981). Hypersensitivity in the small intestinal mucosa. V. Induction of cell-mediated immunity to a dietary antigen. *Clin. Exp. Immunol.* **43**, 574–582.

Mowat, M. I. A. (1987). The regulation of immune responses to dietary protein antigens. *Immunol. Today* **8**, 93–98.

Otten, G., Wilde, D. B., Prystowsky, M. B., Olshan, J. S., Rabin, H., Henderson, L. E., and Fitch, F. W. (1986). Cloned helper T lymphocytes exposed to interleukin 2 become unresponsive to antigen and concanavalin A but not to calcium ionophore and phrobal ester. *Eur. J. Immunol.* **16**, 217–225.

Plaeger-Marshall, S., Spina, C. A., Goigi, J. V., Mitsuyasu, R., Wolfe, P., Gottlieb, M., and Beall, G. (1987). Alterations in cytotoxic and phenotypic subsets of natural killer cells in acquired immunodeficiency syndrome (AIDS). *J. Clin. Immunol.* **7**, 16–23.

Reynolds, J. D. (1986). Evidence of extensive lymphocyte death in sheep Peyer's patches. *J. Immunol.* **136**, 2005–2010.

Ribes-Koninckx, C., Giliams, J. P., Polanco, I., and Pena, A. S. (1984). IgA antigliadin antibodies in celiac and inflammatory bowel disease. *J. Pediat. Gastroenterol. Nutr.* **3**, 676–682.

Richman, L. K. (1979). Immunological unresponsiveness after enteric administration of protein antigens. *In* "Immunology of Breast Milk" (P. L. Ogra and D. H. Dayton, eds.), p. 49. Raven Press, New York.

Richman, L. K., Chiller, J. M., Brown, W. R., Hanson, D. G., and Vaz, N. M. (1978). Enterically induced immunologic tolerance. I. Induction of suppressor T lymphocytes by intragastric administration of soluble proteins. *J. Immunol.* **121**, 2429–2434.

Richman, L. K., Graeff, A. S., Yarchoan, R., and Strober, W. (1981). Simultaneous induction of antigen-specific IgA helper T cells and IgG suppressor T cells in the murine Peyer's patches after protein feedings. *J. Immunol.* **126**, 2079–2083.

Savilahti, E., and Verkasalo, M. (1984). Intestinal cow's milk allergy: Pathogenesis and clinical presentation. *Clin. Rev. Allergy* **2**, 7–23.

Schmitz-Moorman, P., and Becker, H. (1981). Histologic studies on the formal pathogenesis of the epithelial cell granuloma in Crohn's disease. *In* "Recent Advances in Crohn's Disease" (A. S. Pena, I. T. Weterman, C. C. Booth, and W. Strober, eds.), p. 76. Martinus Nijhoff, The Hague.

Shorter, R. G., McGill, D. B., and Bahn, R. C. (1984). Cytotoxicity of mononuclear cells for autologous colonic epithelial cells in colonic diseases. *Gastroenterology* **86**, 13–22.

Strober, W. (1985). Gluten-sensitive enteropathy. An abnormal immunologic response of the gastrointestinal tract to a dietary protein. *In* "Gastrointestinal Immunity for the Clinician" (J. R. Kirsner and R. G. Shorter, eds.), p. 75. Grune & Stratton, Orlando.

Strober, W. (1988). The genetic basis of gluten-sensitive enteropathy. *In* "The Genetic Basis of Common Diseases" (R. A. King, J. I. Rotter, and A. Motulsky, eds.). Oxford Press, New York. (In press.)

Strober, W., and Brown, W. R. (1987). The mucosal immune system. *In* "Immunological Diseases" (M. Samter, ed.), 4th ed., pp. 79–139. W. B. Saunders, Philadelphia.

Strober, W., and James, S. P. (1986). The immunologic basis of inflammatory bowel disease. *J. Clin. Immunol.* **6**, 415–432.

Strober, W., Richman, L. K., and Elson, C. O. (1981). The regulation of gastrointestinal immune responses. *Immunol. Today* **2**, 156–161.

Takahashi, F., and Das, K. M. (1985). Isolation and characterization of a colonic autoantigen specifically recognized by colon tissue-bound immunoglobulin G from idiopathic ulcerative colitis. *J. Clin. Invest.* **76**, 311–318.

Zeitz, M., Green, W. C., Peffer, N. J., and James, S. P. (1988a). Lymphocytes isolated from the intestinal lamina propria in normal nonhuman primates have increased expression of genes associated with T cell activation. *Gastroenterology* **93**, 647–655.

Zeitz, M., Quinn, T. C., Graeff, A. S., and James, S. P. (1988b). Mucosal T cells provide helper function but do not proliferate when stimulated by specific antigen in hypergranuloma venereum proctitis in nonhuman primates. *Gastroenterology* **94**, 353–366.

# Index

## C

F



G

## R

## S